Compact Clinical Guide to

GERIATRIC PAIN MANAGEMENT

An Evidence-Based Approach for Nurses

Ann Quinlan-Colwell, PhD, RNC, AHNBC, DAAPM

Yvonne M. D'Arcy, MS, CRNP, CNS
Series Editor

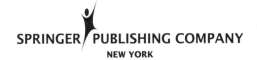

SPRINGER PUBLISHING COMPANY
NEW YORK

Springer Publishing Company, LLC
11 West 42nd Street
New York, NY 10036
www.springerpub.com

Acquisitions Editor: Margaret Zuccarini
Production Editor: Michael Lisk
Composition: S4Carlisle Publishing Serives

ISBN: 978-0-8261-0730-5
E-book ISBN: 978-0-8261-0731-2

11   12   13/   5   4   3   2   1

The author and the publisher of this Work have made every effort to use sources believed to be reliable to provide information that is accurate and compatible with the standards generally accepted at the time of publication. Because medical science is continually advancing, our knowledge base continues to expand. Therefore, as new information becomes available, changes in procedures become necessary. We recommend that the reader always consult current research and specific institutional policies before performing any clinical procedure. The author and publisher shall not be liable for any special, consequential, or exemplary damages resulting, in whole or in part, from the readers' use of, or reliance on, the information contained in this book. The publisher has no responsibility for the persistence or accuracy of URLs for external or third-party Internet Web sites referred to in this publication and does not guarantee that any content on such Web sites is, or will remain, accurate or appropriate.

Library of Congress Cataloging-in-Publication Data

Quinlan-Colwell, Ann.

Compact clinical guide to geriatric pain management : an evidence-based approach for nurses/ Ann Quinlan-Colwell.

p. ; cm. – (Compact clinical guide series)

Includes bibliographical references.
ISBN: 978-0-8261-0730-5
E-book ISBN: 978-0-8261-0731-2

I. Title. II. Series: Compact clinical guide series.

[DNLM: 1. Pain–therapy. 2. Aged. 3. Pain–nursing. 4. Pain Measurement. WL 704]

618.97'60472–dc23

2011036748

Printed in the United States of America by Bang Printing

This book is dedicated to

My father Bob Daly
and
My husband Clancy Colwell

Contents

Foreword   *ix*
Preface   *xi*
Acknowledgments   *xv*

SECTION I: AN OVERVIEW OF PAIN IN THE OLDER ADULT

1. Physiological Factors and Pain Processing
in the Older Adult   *1*

2. The Psychosocial Impact of Pain on the Older Adult Patient   *15*

SECTION II: ASSESSING PAIN IN THE OLDER ADULT

3. Pain Assessment in the Older Adult Patient   *31*

4. Assessing Pain in the Nonverbal, Cognitively
Impaired Older Adults   *47*

5. A Review of Pain Assessment Tools for
Use with the Older Adult Patient   *55*

SECTION III: MANAGING PAIN IN THE OLDER ADULT

6. Developing a Comprehensive Plan for Managing Pain in
Older Adults   *77*

7. Choosing the Right Medication for the Pain Complaint   *87*

8. Adjuvant Analgesic Medications   *119*

9. Managing Medication Side Effects and Specific
Recommendations for Using Medications with
Older Patients   *145*

SECTION IV: OTHER TREATMENT OPTIONS FOR PAIN RELIEF

10. Interventional Options Such as Vertebroplasty for Compression Fractures, Nerve Blocks, and Acupuncture   *167*

11. Complementary Interventions for Pain Management in Older Adults   *183*

12. The Role of Physical Therapy with Pain and Reconditioning   *211*

SECTION V: PAIN CONTROL FOR END OF LIFE CARE

13. Palliative Care: Techniques to Promote Comfort   *227*

14. When Is Hospice the Best Option?   *245*

SECTION VI: PAIN CONDITIONS COMMON IN OLDER ADULTS

15. Osteoarthritis and Gout   *257*

16. Chronic Back Pain and Osteoporosis   *283*

17. Neuropathic Pain Associated with Postherpetic Neuralgia and Diabetic Neuropathy   *299*

18. Central Poststroke Pain Syndrome   *317*

19. Facial Pain Associated with Temporal Arteritis and Trigeminal Neuralgia   *325*

20. Rheumatological Conditions   *335*

21. Fibromyalgia   *353*

SECTION VII: SPECIAL CONSIDERATIONS IN MANAGING PAIN IN OLDER ADULTS

22. Anxiety and Depression with Pain in Older Adults   *375*

23. Alcohol and Substance Use, Misuse, and Abuse   *403*

Index   *423*

Foreword

The care of older adults suffering with pain is a difficult task that calls for understanding as well as compassion. Dr. Quinlan-Colwell has written an excellent book that deals with every facet of the problems that are encountered by caregivers. Elderly people present challenges that call for recognition of the fact that pain affects sleep, appetite, social interactions, and many other facets of life that require attention. Dr. Quinlan-Colwell carries the reader into the lives of elderly people and provides the information necessary to bring psychological comfort as well as knowledge to help people control pains that destroy the quality of their lives. Needless pain is a tragedy that calls for a better understanding of the psychological, social, and medical dimensions of life. This book highlights all of these dimensions and provides the reader with valuable knowledge that will diminish suffering and enrich the lives of people confronting new, often frightening, problems.

The recognition that pain is a multidimensional experience determined by psychological as well as physical factors has broadened the scope of pain therapies. Patients with chronic pain need every possible therapy to battle the pain. Chronic pain is not a symptom but a syndrome in its own right and requires therapists from a wide range of disciplines.

Psychological therapies, which were once used as a last resort when drugs or neurosurgery failed to control pain, are now an integral part of pain management strategies. The recognition that pain is the result of multiple contributions gave rise to a variety of psychological approaches such as relaxation, hypnosis, and cognitive therapies. So too, transcutaneous electrical nerve stimulation and other physical therapy (PT) procedures emerged rapidly, bringing substantial pain relief to large numbers of people. Nursing is an integral part of all therapies and provides the binding unity essential for the elderly patient.

The field of pain continues to develop and there are reasons to be optimistic about its future. First, imaging techniques have confirmed pain-related activity in widely distributed, highly interconnected areas of the brain. An implication of the concept is that neural programs that evolved in the brain to generate acute pain as a result of injury or disease may sometimes go away and produce destructive chronic pain. Future imaging research may reveal the sites of abnormally prolonged activity in chronic pain patients. Second, the detailed knowledge and technical skills developed by scientists for research on the spinal cord can be used to explore brain mechanisms in humans and animals, especially in the brain stem reticular formation, which is known to play a major role on chronic pain. Third, our knowledge of the genetic basis of pain as well as the development of the brain is growing rapidly. Genetic factors are known to contribute to a large number of chronic pain syndromes, and future research will highlight their brain mechanisms. The inevitable convergence of these three approaches will hopefully lead to the relief of pain and suffering now endured by millions of people.

Ronald Melzack, PhD, FRSC
Professor Emeritus McGill University

Preface

As a nursing student, I most enjoyed caring for older adults. They were interesting in all ways—socially, emotionally, psychologically, and physically. Although my career path has taken me through a variety of settings, there have always been elders among the patients and family members with whom I worked.

During the last century, the prevalence of those individuals over 60 years of age who are being cared for in all areas of health care has dramatically grown. When I was given the opportunity to write this book about managing pain in older adults, it enabled me to blend my love of gerontology with my dedication to pain management, along with my extensive educational and professional experiences in these areas, to meet a vital need. As you will read, the percentage of older adults in society is consistently increasing. The chronic conditions with which they live often involve pain that requires particular expertise to manage it effectively.

Pain management among older people is a most important, but often neglected, area of health care. Not only are people living to increasingly advanced ages, they are living with more chronic illnesses. Those illnesses are often painful. Health care professionals (HCPs) want to help older adults to be comfortable and manage their pain; however, there are many barriers to accomplishing that goal. It is the intent of this book to provide information to guide HCPs to help older adults manage their pain as safely and effectively as possible.

To successfully address a challenging situation, it is important to understand what is involved in the challenge. This book begins with a general overview of pain among older adults. It includes physiological factors involved with aging that affect the process and occurrence of pain. As pain is a multi-dimensional experience, the psychosocial factors that impact the pain of older adults are also explored.

Good pain management begins with an effective assessment of pain. General concepts of assessing pain are provided. As barriers to assessing pain in older people often exist, the barriers that originate among older people and those that occur among HCPs are both presented. Awareness of these barriers is the first step in overcoming them. Techniques, tips, and tools for assessing pain in well elders and in those with cognitive impairment are presented.

Safe and effective pain management is best accomplished with a comprehensive plan, using a multimodal approach that involves pharmacological and nonpharmacological therapies and interventions. Several chapters focus on the various medications, including adjuvants, and the management of medication side effects. It is important for the reader to know that the intent of these chapters is to provide the most current information available in the most unbiased manner that is possible. With appropriate evaluation and monitoring, the majority of analgesic medications can be safely used with older adults. Although some medications, interventions, or therapies are not indicated, or are not preferred for older adults, information about them is provided for three reasons. It is important for the reader to know that there are contraindications for their use with older adults; there may be some instances when older adults have already been treated or are being treated with the medication or therapy; and there may be some instances when it is necessary for the medication, intervention, or therapy to be used with the older adult, even though it is not recommended. The information is provided so that the reader is aware of contraindications and side effects that must be considered and carefully monitored. All medications need to be evaluated in the context of the comorbidities and sensitivities of each individual older person.

Chapters, though not intended to be comprehensive, are devoted to interventional options, complementary therapies, and PT for reconditioning. These nonpharmacologic options offer good interventions to complement medications within the multimodal pain management plan.

Many illnesses and conditions that have pain associated with them are common among older adults. Overviews of pathophysiology and interventions available to manage arthritis, gout, chronic back pain, osteoporosis, neuropathic pain (postherpetic neuralgia and diabetic neuropathy), central poststroke syndrome, facial pains (temporal arteritis and trigeminal neuralgia), rheumatological conditions (rheumatoid arthritis and polymyalgia rheumatica) and fibromyalgia are provided.

Many of the chronic illnesses that occur among older people are appropriate for the symptom management that is characteristic of palliative care. This specialized area is discussed in comparison to the related specialized area of hospice care that can be most helpful for older adults as they near the end of life.

Anxiety and depression are common co-morbidities of chronic pain. Once identified, these disorders can be effectively managed in older adults. The prevalence of techniques and screening tools useful for identifying anxiety and depression among older adults are offered, as well as an overview of the pharmacological and nonpharmacological interventions.

As with other populations, when managing pain, older people may use, abuse, or misuse alcohol or substances. With age-related changes this can be of particular concern. Techniques for assessing, addressing, and intervening when alcohol or other substances are used, abused, or misused are presented.

It is intended that this book will provide a solid resource and strong base of information for nurses and other HCPs who care for older adults who experience pain in any setting. As the areas of pain management and gerontology are constantly evolving, future research may affect the information that is provided. The reader is encouraged to remain current with research in the areas of gerontology and pain management and to critically evaluate new information for evidence, validity and reliability. At the end of each chapter resources are listed through which new information may be accessed.

It was my intent to develop an easy-to-use resource for nurses and HCPs who care for older adults who experience pain. I sincerely hope that you find it as beneficial to use as I found it enjoyable to write.

Ann Quinlan-Colwell, PhD, RNC, AHNBC, FAAPM

Acknowledgments

Although many people contributed to me writing this book, I would like to acknowledge the following people who played particularly significant roles.

Most importantly, I am extremely grateful to my husband and soul mate Clancy. As always, he was the "wind beneath my wings." His support, love, patience, nurturing, technical support, and managing everything else in our lives made it possible for me to write.

I am eternally appreciative of my father who always taught me that I could accomplish anything that I desired and to believe in my abilities to do so. He also instilled in me a lifelong love of reading, learning, and writing.

Deep gratitude goes to Allison Matthews and Donna Flake at the SEAHEC Library for their wonderful and timely literature searches.

I appreciate the careful reviews of some of the chapters, with helpful suggestions by Leslie Kessler and Denise Phillips.

Although this was not a work-related project, I am very grateful for the support and encouragement of Sue Ballato and my co-workers at New Hanover Regional Medical Center.

I appreciate the editing suggestions and guidance of Yvonne D'Arcy as well as the support and guidance of Margaret Zuccarini at Springer Publishing, and careful editing and assistance of Nandini Loganathan.

Gratitude is extended to the International Association for the Study of Pain, Heela Kerr, Ronald Melzack, Daniel Segal, WHO, Chris Pasero, Ilan Lieberman, Center to Advance Palliative Care, the Rand Corporation, and Robert Bennett for developing their wonderful tools, figures and pictures, and for allowing me to use them.

Similar gratitude is extended to all of the researchers and authors who provided the evidence-based information used as reference materials in this book. Particular appreciation is extended to Dr. Ronald Melzack for reviewing and writing the forward to this book.

Finally, I am truly thankful to all the older adults, patients, family members, coworkers, and professors who have taught me how to care for older adults and help them in managing pain.

Physiological Factors and Pain Processing in the Older Adult

Pain is a subjective, multiphasic experience that is unique to each individual. This is true among older adults as well as among people in all other age groups. Rather than being resistant to the experience of pain, older adults can be particularly susceptible to the negative effects of pain that persists (Gibson & Farrell, 2004). Despite this, pain in older adults often is not recognized and is either poorly or inadequately treated (Gagliese, 2009; Gibson & Farrell, 2004; Herr & Decker, 2004; McCaffery & Pasero, 1999).

Pain is a complex subject. In addition to pain being subjectively experienced in multiple ways, there are various categorizations of pain. A brief description of each of these follows.

Nociception is the physiologic process through which pain is experienced. It begins with damage or irritation of peripheral nerve receptors and continues through a series of physiological processes to the perception of pain (Kingdon, Stanley, & Kizior, 1998).

Somatic pain is pain that is well localized and involves the skin, bones, joints, connective tissue, or blood vessels and is often described as aching (Kingdon et al., 1998; Polomano, 2002).

In comparison, *visceral pain* is characterized as more vague or diffuse, originating in smooth muscle or internal structures of the body. It is often described as cramping, dull, sharp, heavy, or splitting (Polomano, 2002).

Neuropathic pain was traditionally defined as pain that was "initiated or caused by a primary lesion or dysfunction of the nervous system" (Merskey & Bogduk, 1994). This definition was recently revised to be "pain arising as a direct consequence of a lesion or disease affecting the somatosensory system" (Haanpää et al., 2011).

The pain is frequently described as prickly, tingling, or like pins and needles (Bennett, 2001).

In addition, pain is generally categorized as being acute or chronic. *Acute pain* functions as a symptom that develops as a result of injury to the body and resolves as the body heals (American Pain Society, 2003). The cause of acute pain may be injury, surgery, or illness. Acute pain indicates that something in the body needs attention (Cox & Karpapas, 2002).

Chronic or persistent pain is pain that lasts for a period of time longer than expected for the course of an acute injury or illness, with the exact time frame ranging from 1 to 6 months longer than the expected time for acute pain. It may be nociceptive or neuropathic in nature (Cox & Karpapas, 2002).

The patient may experience a variety of pains in combination and in multiple areas of the body. Older adults experience pain while in their homes, hospitals, rehabilitation facilities, assisted living facilities, and long-term care facilities, or wherever they reside. Older adults experience pain as a result of acute illness and injuries, as well as chronic illness (Zyczkowska, Szczerbinska, Jantzi, & Hirdes, 2007).

Pearls	Pain is a subjective and multiphasic experience that is unique for each person.
	There are different types of pain with unique characteristics.

THE PROCESS OR PHYSIOLOGY OF NOCICEPTIVE PAIN

Nociceptive pain occurs through an involved process that begins with the affected tissue and progresses until a message to pay attention to the area is received, interpreted, and regulated. Acute pain may be considered the body's way of saying "pay attention." Nociception occurs in four distinct but interrelated steps. Although the process is complex, the following points are important to understand the process. Any part of this process can be altered by normal physiological changes of aging. These alterations are more significant if the older person has a chronic illness.

1. *Transduction* is the first step of the nociceptive process. It is a chemical process in which sensory messages are received through local

Table 1.1 ■ *Pain Nociceptors*

Nociceptor	Stimuli that Are Sensed	Tissue Type that Responds	Afferent Axon Fibers Involved
Mechanoreceptors	Cutting Twisting Pressure Trauma	Skin Joints Periosteum Viscera	A Beta (Aβ) C fiber
Thermoreceptors	Hot (burning) Cold	Skin	A Beta (Aβ)[a] C fiber[a]
Chemoreceptors	Inflammation Disease Ischemia Acid	Skin Muscle Joints Viscera	A Beta (Aβ) C fiber

[a]The thermal threshold of A Beta (Aβ) fibers is –53°C for Type I and –43°C for Type II and –43°C for C fibers.
Sources: From Clinical Coach for Effective Pain Management, by P. Arnstein, 2010, Philadelphia, PA: F. A. Davis Company; Pathophysiology of Pain (pp. 332–334), by J. Zhang, & M. L. Baccei, 2009, Philadelphia, PA: Saunders Elsevier.

nociceptors (see Table 1.1). The messages are initiated at the site of injury or potential harm and are transformed into electrical impulses that are then able to be transmitted by nerve tissue.

2. *Transmission* is the process through which the message is transferred by electrical impulses to the dorsal horn of the spinal cord. In response to these impulses, calcium channels open, releasing neurotransmitters (aspartate and glutamate) that initiate the message of pain being sent to higher brain regions, including the spinothalamic tract (STT) and subsequently the cerebral cortex.

3. *Perception* is how the older adult interprets the messages received in the higher brain. This interpretation involves a multitude of factors, including physical, emotional, psychological, and spiritual factors, past experiences with pain, and the meaning of the current pain.

4. *Modulation* is changing the amplitude of the pain message. Connections in the descending tract of the central nervous system can send messages that can alter the strength of the pain message to either increase or decrease it. The amplitude can be impacted by chemicals in the body. Although the release of substance P can increase the intensity of the message, the release of endorphins can decrease the strength of the message.

(Arnstein, 2010; Zhang & Baccei, 2009).

Pearl	Acute pain is the body's way of saying "pay attention" to an area that is injured or potentially injured.

SIGNIFICANCE OF PAIN IN OLDER ADULTS

It is estimated that on a regular basis nearly half of all community-dwelling elders experience pain and that between 70% and 80% of older adults who reside in nursing homes experience pain (Horgas, Nichols, Schapson, & Vietes, 2007).

These estimates are staggering. Older adults in the United States are an ever-increasing segment of the society. In 1900, there were 3.1 million older Americans, but in 1999 there were 34.6 million in that group. The estimate for 2050 is that there will be 82 million older Americans (U.S. Census Bureau, 2001). This growth is a significant increase in the proportion of the American population represented by older adults. In 1950, people of 65 years or older represented 8.3% of the US population, whereas in 2004 they represented 12.7%, and it is anticipated that in 2050 they will represent 20.6% of the total population (Centers for Disease Control and Prevention [CDC], 2005). This means that, in 2050, one in every five people in the United States will be 65 years or older.

The current and future aging populations are different from earlier groups of older adults. Current older adults are heterogeneous in characteristics and in health status. Although many elders have focused on being healthy, many others have not done so. Large numbers of older adults have physiologic changes related to aging that result in greater incidence of morbidities and iatrogenic illnesses as well as associated functional disabilities (CDC, 2005).

Although older adults are more likely to experience pain than younger adults, they are often less likely to report pain; thus the true prevalence of pain in older adults is most likely underestimated (Reyes-Gibby, Aday, & Cleeland, 2002). Accurate prevalence is difficult for agencies tracking this information to capture for several reasons:

■ Communication and terminology—older adults frequently use words other than pain (i.e., sore, tired, and achy) to describe instances that are considered painful.
■ Multiple categories—pain may be acute, chronic, or a combination of both.

■ Multiple locations/sites—pain may occur in more than one area of the body.
■ Older adults reside in a variety of settings—independently, with family, in assisted living facilities, nursing homes, and government facilities (psychiatric and corrections).

Pain has been referred to as a public health concern, with the prevalence of chronic or persistent pain among older adults having "reached epidemic proportions" (Fine, 2009). Reyes-Gibby et al., (2002) noted that among 5,807 community-dwelling older adults in the Asset and Health Dynamics Among the Oldest Old, 37% of women and 28% of men reported pain. In 2002, the American Geriatric Society Panel on Persistent Pain in Older Persons cited one survey in which 18% of older Americans reported taking analgesic medications on a regular basis (several times per week) and of them, 63% reported taking prescription analgesia for more than 6 months (Ferrell et al., 2002; Fine, 2009; Fox, Raina, & Jadad, 1999; Zyczkowska et al., 2007).

The prevalence of pain in older adults can differ by gender, culture, and socioeconomic factors. Although race and ethnicity are not necessarily correlated with pain, members of minority groups are often in a socioeconomic group that tends to suffer frequent pain. Socioeconomic factors that have been associated with more frequent or more severe pain are

■ less education
■ lower income
■ Medicaid recipient
■ psychological distress
■ female gender
■ chronic comorbid illnesses

(Portenoy, Ugarte, Fuller, & Haas, 2004; Reyes-Gibby et al., 2002; U.S. Department of Health and Human Services, 2010).

In 2004, the CDC reported that pain was diagnosed in 23% of nursing home residents (29% without dementia and 17% with dementia). In the same report it was noted that 24% of the nursing home patients with pain were whites and 17% were nonwhites. Of those with pain nearly half (44%) did not have appropriate care for that pain. Other sources have reported that nursing home residents do not receive appropriate pain management (CDC, 2005; Cook, Niven, & Downs, 1999).

Pearls	It is difficult to determine the exact number of older adults who experience or live with pain. Pain among older adults is a major health care problem. Pain experienced by many older adults is often not detected, diagnosed, or adequately managed.

The Experience of Pain in Older Adults

Research studies that investigate whether older adults experience more or less pain inhibition (the ability to modulate, repress, or quiet the pain experience) contradict each other. Riley, King, Wong, Fillingim, and Mauderli (2010) reported that when healthy older adults were compared with younger healthy adult controls, the older adults showed diminished endogenous pain inhibition—a process in which naturally produced substances in the body act to calm the pain experience (Arnstein, 2010). A number of studies have indicated that older adults may report low levels of pain (mild) as being lower than younger adults, and they may report higher (severe) levels of pain as being more intense than younger adults (Edwards, 2005). In a study that compared 788 of the oldest old (100 or older) with 192,370 older adults ranging in age from 65 to 100, the centurions experienced less pain even with adjustment for confounding variables (Zyczkowska et al., 2007).

Perception of pain in older adults, particularly those older than 79, may be different from young adults, with older adults being more sensitive to pain (Fine, 2009). In some instances, this altered perception of pain may be either caused or exacerbated by atrophy of the brain (Breuer, Pappagallo, & Tai, 2007; Fine, 2007).

In addition to an increased sensitivity to pain, a decreased ability to tolerate pain has been demonstrated in older adults. This was demonstrated through MRI studies in which there was reduced activity in processing of pain in the caudate and putamen (Cole, Farrell, Gibson, & Egan, 2010; Fine, 2007).

With aging, absorption and utilization of medications is affected by altered body functions, including the intestines, liver, and kidneys (Fine, 2007). Comorbidities such as diabetes, heart disease, renal failure, and obesity (Ray, Lipton, Katz, & Derby, 2011) need to be considered with medication management.

Pearls	There is conflicting research as to whether older adults experience pain the same as younger adults. Research studies have shown that although older adults may experience pain differently, they do experience pain and it is unique to each person. There is some evidence that many older adults experience intense pain as being more intense than younger adults experience it.

Pain and the Aging Body

It is important to remember that pain is very subjective and uniquely experienced by each older adult. Some factors that may affect how pain is experienced by older adults include the following:

- Individual differences regarding the perception of pain.
- Pain tolerance may decline with aging.
- Age-related changes of the nociceptive system.
- Some studies have found elevated heat and electrical pain thresholds among older adults.

Age-related changes in the deep tissues of the body may affect how pain is perceived and experienced. Geriatric syndromes such as frailty, falls, skin breakdown, and functional decline affect the perception of pain. It is conceivable that superficial pain perception may be altered related to fragile, aging skin with less subcutaneous tissue.

Three factors that are associated with the incidence of pain in older people have the potential for modification. These factors are

- depression
- smoking
- increased body mass

(Edwards, 2005; Gibson & Farrell, 2004; Inouye, Studenski, Tinetti, & Kuchel, 2007; Shi, Hooten, Roberts, & Warner, 2010).

Unique Challenges of Managing Pain in Older Adults

Advancing age causes successive physiological alterations that must be considered when assessing pain among older adults. Sensory impairments intensify with aging. During verbal questioning, it is important to speak clearly while facing the older adult. If the person uses hearing aids, ensure that they are functioning. Assessment tools should be produced in large font with clear colors to compensate for impaired vision. Often older adults fear what the pain may mean. Often there is an expectation that pain is a normal part of aging (Fine, 2009).

Comorbidities that can complicate assessment and management of pain include

- diabetes
- renal insufficiency/failure
- liver disease
- gastrointestinal (GI) disturbances
- cardiac disease
- skin alterations
- impaired nutrition
- obesity
- mental illness
- substance abuse including alcoholism

When prescribing analgesic medications, the absorption and excretion must be considered with regard to the possibility of

- GI disturbances
- liver disease
- renal insufficiency/failure
- medication side effects
- medication-medication interactions
- medication-food interactions

It is also important to consider the literacy level and any cognitive limitations. Instructions should be clear and appropriate for the educational level, health care literacy, and experience of the patient.

Pearl	Remember that general education and health care literacy are not necessarily related. Well-educated older adults may not be literate about health care issues and may need careful education about their condition, pain management, and medications.

Financial concerns are an important consideration. Many older adults live on fixed incomes. They have limited money to spend on health care and medications. Expensive medications may cause the patient to use money allocated for food for themselves or their pet animals. Alternatively, the person simply will not fill the prescription and will live with the pain or self-medicate the pain.

> *Pearls*
>
> Age-related changes cause the older adult to be at increased risk for experiencing pain on a regular basis.
>
> Age-related changes place the older adult at increased risk for complications related to pain.
>
> Age-related changes necessitate careful evaluation of pain management interventions.

Barriers to Appropriate Pain Management in Older Adults

A significant barrier to good pain management in older adults is the common belief by older adults that "pain is just part of getting older." Older adults must be reminded that pain is not a normal part of aging. Many older adults believe that health care providers (HCPs) will know best how to manage pain and that they do not need to report how severe the pain is for them. They may also believe that not much can be done to help the pain (Shea & McDonald, 2011).

Ageism by HCPs can also be a significant barrier to adequately managing pain among older adults. HCPs have a responsibility to assess their beliefs about older adults and educate themselves how to provide optimal care.

At times, professionals assume that people who live with significant pain, which often interferes with activities of daily living (ADLs), will complain in accordance with the degree of pain experienced. Shea and McDonald (2011) found that this was not the case among more than 300 older adults with arthritis pain. They caution that HCPs should not assume that pain will be reported or reported accurately. It is important that HCPs include assessment of pain as a standard of care (Reyes-Gibby et al., 2002).

> *Pearls*
>
> Many older adults are diagnosed with chronic illnesses that are known to be painful.
>
> Knowing that older adults may not offer complaints about pain, HCPs need to assess pain as a standard of care.

COMPLICATIONS OF UNRELIEVED PAIN IN OLDER ADULTS

Unrelieved pain impacts the daily life of the older adult with poor outcomes that include

- increased disability
- increased symptom burden
- depression
- anxiety
- alterations in sleep
- weight loss related to decreased appetite
- limitation or inability to perform usual ADLs
- increased utilization of health care services
- increased morbidity and mortality

(Gagliese, 2009; Schofield, O'Mahony, Collett, & Potter, 2008) Unrelieved or poorly managed pain is an obstacle when managing comorbidities that benefit from movement and exercise, such as cardiac and respiratory disorders. It is a barrier to rehabilitation efforts and collaborative care. Pain interferes with cognition and is a limiting factor when working with older adults who suffer from depression (Thielke, Fan, Sullivan, & Unutzer, 2007).

Pearls	Unrelieved pain negatively affects the health care and function of older adults. Comorbid illnesses can be negatively impacted by unrelieved pain.

GUIDELINES

American Geriatrics Society. (2009). Pharmacological management of persistent pain in older adults. *Journal of the American Geriatrics Society, 57,* 1331–1346.

An Interdisciplinary Expert Consensus Statement on Assessment of Pain in Older Persons. (2007). *Clinical Journal of Pain, 23,* S1–S43

Practice Guidelines for Assessing Pain in Older Persons with Dementia Residing in Long-Term Care Facilities. (2010). *Physiotherapy Canada, 62,* 104–113.

The American Geriatric Society Panel on Persistent Pain in Older Persons. (2002). *Journal of the American Geriatric Society, 50,* S205–S224.

Case Study

Mabel Jones is an 82-year-old African American woman who presents at clinic today. She has diagnoses of hypertension, obesity, diabetes, osteoarthritis of her knees and hips, and osteoporosis in her back. During assessment she tells you that she has not been sleeping well and feels "kind of nervous" lately and that her "knees are not what they used to be." When you ask her about her knees she says "they are just old." She tells you that the "burning" in the back of her legs is really bothering her. When you ask if she is taking the analgesic medicine prescribed, she tells you that the pharmacy in her neighborhood doesn't carry that, and she doesn't have the money to take a cab to one that does carry it. She says that she just uses some heat and some aspirin, but that bothers her stomach.

Questions

1. What barriers can you identify for assessing pain in Mrs. Jones?
2. What barriers can you identify to managing pain in Mrs. Jones?
3. What types of pain does Mrs. Jones describe?
4. How can her pain interfere with the other illnesses Mrs. Jones has?
5. What education do you need to provide to Mrs. Jones?

REFERENCES

American Pain Society. (2003). *Principles of analgesia use in the treatment of acute pain* (5th ed.). Glenview, IL: Author.

Arnstein, P. (2010). *Clinical coach for effective pain management.* Philadelphia, PA: F. A. Davis Company.

Bennett, M. (2001). The LANSS Pain Scale: The leeds assessment of neuropathic symptoms and sign. *Pain, 92,* 147–157.

Breuer, B., Pappagallo, M., & Tai, J. Y. (2007). U.S. board-certified pain physician practices: Uniformity and census data of their locations. *Journal of Pain, 8,* 244–250.

Centers for Disease Control. (2005). The proportion of older Americans is growing. *Health, United States, 2005*. Retrieved January 31, 2011, from http://www.cdc.gov/nchs/data/hus/hus05.[df database

Cole, L. J., Farrell, M. J., Gibson, S. J., & Egan, G. F. (2010). Age-related differences in pain sensitivity and regional brain activity evoked by noxious pressure. *Neurobiology of Aging, 31,* 494–503.

Cook, A. K., Niven, C. A., & Downs, M. G. (1999). Assessing the pain of people with cognitive impairment. *International Journal of Geriatric Psychiatry, 14,* 421–425.

Cox, D. S., & Karpapas, E. T. (2002). Taxonomy for pain management nursing. In B. St. Marie (Ed.), *Core curriculum for pain management nursing—American Society for Pain Management Nursing* (2nd ed., pp. 9–25). Dubuque, IA: Kendall Hunt.

Edwards, R. R. (2005). Age-associated differences in pain perception and pain processing. In S. J. Gibson & D. K. Weiner (Eds.), *Pain in older persons* (pp. 45–65). Seattle, WA: IASP Press.

Ferrell, B., Casarett, D., Epplin, J., Fine, P., Gloth, M., Herr, K., Weiner, D. (2002). The American Geriatric Society Panel on Persistent Pain in Older Persons. *Journal of the American Geriatric Society, 50,* S205–S224.

Fine, P. G. (2009). Chronic pain management in older adults: Special considerations. *Journal of Pain and Symptom Management, 38,* S4–S14.

Fox, P. L., Raina, P., & Jadad, A. R. (1999). Prevalence and treatment of pain in older adults in nursing homes and other long-term care institutions: A systematic review. *Canadian Medical Association Journal, 160,* 329–333.

Gagliese, L. (2009). Pain and aging: The emergence of a new subfield of pain research. *The Journal of Pain, 10,* 343–353.

Gibson, S. J., & Farrell, M. (2004). A review of age differences in the neurophysiology of nociception and the perceptual experience of pain. *Clinical Journal of Pain, 20,* 227–239.

Haanpää, M., Attal, N., Backonja, M., Baron, R., Bennett, M., Bouhassira, D., Treede, R. D. (2011). NeuPSIG guidelines on neuropathic pain assessment. *Pain, 152,* 14–27.

Herr, K., & Decker, S. (2004). Older adults with severe cognitive impairment: Assessment of pain. *Annals of Long-Term Care: Clinical Care and Aging, 12,* 46–52.

Horgas, A. L., Nichols, A. L., Schapson, C. A., & Vietes, K. (2007). Assessing pain in persons with dementia: Relationships among the non-communicative patient's pain assessment instrument, self-report and behavioral observations. *Pain Management Nursing, 8*(2), 77–85.

Inouye, S. K., Studenski, S., Tinetti, M. E., & Kuchel, G. A. (2007). Geriatric syndromes: Clinical, research, and policy implication of a core geriatric concept. *Journal of the American Geriatric Society, 55,* 780–791.

Kingdon, R. T., Stanley, K. J., & Kizior, R. J. (1998). *Handbook for pain management*. Philadelphia, PA: W. B. Saunders Company.

McCaffery, M., & Pasero, C. (1999). *The clinical manual of pain* (2nd ed.). St. Louis, MO: Mosby.

Merskey, H., & Bogduk, N. (1994). *Classification of chronic pain*. Seattle, WA: IASP Press.

Polomano, R. C. (2002). Neurophysiology of pain—Part one: Anatomy and physiology of pain. In B. St. Marie (Ed.), *Core curriculum for pain management nursing—American Society for Pain Management Nursing* (2nd ed., pp. 63–90). Dubuque, IA: Kendall Hunt.

Portenoy, R. K., Ugarte, C., Fuller, I., & Haas, G. (2004). Population-based survey of pain in the United States: Differences among White, African American and Hispanic subjects. *The Journal of Pain, 5,* 317–328.

Ray, L., Lipton, R. B., Katz, M. J., & Derby, C. A. (2011). Mechanisms of association between obesity and chronic pain in the elderly. *Pain, 152,* 53–59.

Reyes-Gibby, C. C., Aday, L., & Cleeland, C. (2002). Impact of pain on self-rated health in the community-dwelling older adults. *Pain, 95,* 75–82.

Riley, J. L., King, C. D., Wong, F., Fillingim, R., & Mauderli, A. P. (2010). Lack of endogenous modulation and reduced decay of prolonged heat pain in older adults. *Pain, 150,* 153–160.

Schofield, P., O'Mahony, S., Collett, B., & Potter, J. (2008). Guidance for the assessment of pain in older adults: A literature review. *British Journal of Nursing, 17,* 914–919.

Shea, M., & McDonald, D. D. (2011). Factors associated with increased pain communication in older adults. *Western Journal of Nursing Research, 32,* 196–206.

Shi, Y., Hooten, M., Roberts, R. O., & Warner, D. O. (2010). Modifiable risk factors for incidence of pain in older adults. *Pain, 151,* 366–371.

Thielke, S. M., Fan, M. Y., Sullivan, M., & Unutzer, J. (2007). Pain limits the effectiveness of collaborative care for depression. *American Journal of Geriatric Psychiatry, 15,* 699–707.

U.S. Census Bureau. (March 13, 2001). Press Release: The number of older Americans is growing. *U.S. Census Bureau.* Retrieved February 02, 2011, from http://www.census.gov/database

U.S. Department of Health and Human Services. (2010). *Summary health statistics for U.S. adults: National Health Interview Survey* [Brochure]. Hyattsville, MD: Author.

Zhang, J., & Baccei, M. L. (2009). Pathophysiology of pain. In H. S. Smith (Ed.), *Current therapy in pain* (pp. 332–334). Philadelphia, PA: Saunders Elsevier.

Zyczkowska, J., Szczerbinska, K., Jantzi, M. R., & Hirdes, J. P. (2007). Pain among the oldest old in community and institutional settings. *Pain, 129,* 167–176.

2

The Psychosocial Impact of Pain on the Older Adult Patient

Pain is a multiphasic experience that generally involves all aspects of the life of the older person. In addition to physiologic manifestations, it both affects cognition, emotions, function, activities, finances, education, socialization, and interpersonal relationships and is affected by each of them. Since each of these areas is also affected by the natural aging process, pain experienced by older adults can be very complicated (Eliopoulos, 2001; Parmelee, 2005).

There is generally a circular or bidirectional path that develops between pain and the psychosocial impact it has on older adults (Gibson, 2005). Pain can be the source of

- anxiety
- fear
- depression
- poor self-image
- impaired cognition
- impaired function
- financial challenges
- limited socialization
- damaged relationships

At the same time, each of those can affect the patient's perception of pain. How pain is experienced is affected by

- the culture of the person
- the social context
- health beliefs
- personality characteristics
- attitudes (Gibson, 2005)
- previous experiences with pain
- life challenges

The literature about the psychosocial manifestations of pain can seem conflicting or challenging to interpret for the health care provider (HCP). In one study by Green and Hart-Johnson (2010) it was noted that caffeine and alcohol use, which are frequently part of social interactions, were associated with better outcomes among white men with chronic pain. Although such a finding may sound strange, the interpretation was that the socialization experience, rather than the use of caffeine or alcohol, contributed to the improved outcomes. This underscores the importance of socialization in the management of pain. In older adults, social interactions become curtailed as a result of impaired function (limited mobility, vision, eyesight), fatigue, incontinence, and impaired self-concept (Eliopoulos, 2001), in addition to pain. Although many of these factors may not be modifiable in the older adult, pain and its resultant affect on function and fatigue can be managed.

Adding to the challenge of unraveling this complexity of information is that many of the psychosocial factors related to the experience of pain (i.e., depression, function, self-concept) are also known to change with aging (Eliopoulos, 2001; Gibson, 2005; Parmelee, 2005). In addition, older adults are a heterogeneous group who experience various degrees of pain with associated negative impacts in different ways (British Pain Society and British Geriatric Society, 2007).

Pearl	For the older patient, psychological and social influences, such as depression, the death of a spouse, or financial concerns, both affect how pain is experienced and are affected by the pain experience.

COGNITION

Much has been written about the effect of cognition on pain. Recent research has investigated the effect of pain on cognition with strong indications that impaired concentration and cognitive impairment can develop when pain is not relieved (Cook, Niven, & Downs, 1999).

Weiner, Rudy, Morrow, Slaboda, and Lieber (2006) reported that older adults living with chronic low back pain (CLBP) did not perform as well as their pain-free counterparts on neuropsychological tests. In a large sample of 3,107 middle-aged and older participants in the European Male Ageing Study, cognitive testing revealed slower psychomotor speed among the men with chronic widespread pain compared with the men who were pain free (Lee et al., 2010). When pain-free older adults were compared with older adults suffering with CLBP, those with pain showed impaired neuropsychological functioning on memory, language, and mental flexibility scales (Weiner, Rudy, Morrow, Slaboda, & Lieber, 2006).

PAIN LOCUS OF CONTROL

What patients believe about their health and pain is critical to their experience of pain. People may believe that their pain is under their own control (internal locus of control); under the control of others, including HCPs (external locus of control); or that it is randomly influenced (external locus of control). A variety of research has indicated that older adults more frequently have an external locus of control, believing that pain is under the control of strong others or chance. The strongest predictor of depression (Table 2.1) in patients with pain was having a low internal locus of control (Gibson & Helme, 2000).

For the HCP it is important to know how the older patients perceive their pain. If the patient thinks that the HCP is in control, the

Table 2.1 ■ *Pain Locus of Control Characteristics*

Perceived Internal Locus of Control	*Perceived External Locus of Control*
Less intense pain	More intense pain
Less perceived interference from pain	More perceived interference from pain
Less depression	Greater depression
Less catastrophizing	More catastrophizing
Better compliance with treatments	Poorer compliance with treatments
More behavioral activities	More praying and hoping
Self-rated ability to control pain	Less ability to decrease or control pain
More behavioral activities	More depression
Perception of ability to self-control or decrease pain	

Source: "Cognitive Factors and the Experience of Pain and Suffering in Older Persons," by S. J. Gibson, & R. D. Helme, 2000, *Pain, 85*, pp. 375–383.

patient may not assume active steps to alleviate pain independently. If the older person feels he or she is in control of the pain, he or she will want to work actively with the HCP in developing a plan of care.

DEPRESSION

Depression is a mood disorder involving a disturbance of cognition that is characterized by negative thoughts, self-criticism, and pessimism (Wenzlaff & Wegner, 2000). It is estimated that 8%–20% of community-dwelling older adults, with up to 37% in primary care settings, experience symptoms of depression. Although treatment is generally successful in older adults (60%–80% response rate), it generally requires more time to achieve success than is required with younger people (U.S. Public Health Service, 1999a, 1999b).

Depression can preexist pain; there may be predisposition to depression or depression may be a sequel of pain (Chou, 2007; Miller & Cano, 2009; Mossey & Gallagher, 2004; Vaccarino, Sills, Evans, & Kalali, 2009). In general, reports of comorbidity widely range from 4% to 66% (Miller & Cano, 2009).

At every routine assessment, clinic visit, or hospitalization the older adult should be screened and assessed for symptoms of depression. A simple and easy-to-use depression screening using a tool such as the Geriatric Depression Index or the five-item Geriatric Depression Scale (see Chapter 5) can help determine if the patient is clinically depressed (Herr, Bjorg, Steffensmeier, & Rakel, 2006).

The reader is referred to Chapter 22 for a detailed discussion of the relationship between pain and depression in older adults.

Pearl	It is important to assess patients with pain for comorbid depression and intervene using a geriatric depression assessment tool.

SUICIDE

Depression is a significant risk factor among people who complete suicide, and chronic pain has been correlated with suicide ideation (SI), suicide attempts (SA), and suicide completions (SC)—with SI and SA two or three times more common among persons with chronic pain than their peers without pain. In addition to depression, it has been suggested that patients living with chronic pain are at risk for suicide for the following reasons:

- Low levels of tolerance for pain when treatment is not effective
- Stress related to physical disability
- Seeking escape from suffering
- Feelings of demoralization
- Insomnia related to chronic pain
- Feelings of hopelessness related to pain

(Edwards, Smith, Kudel, & Haythornwaite, 2006; Ilgen, Zivan, Mc-Cammon, & Valenstein, 2008; Ratcliffe, Enns, Belik, & Sareen, 2008; Ploghaus, et al, 2001; Smith, Edwards, Robinson, & Dworkin, 2004)

Research in this area is relatively new; however, several studies have reported important insights. In a study of 1512 patients, Edwards et al. (2006) found that, regardless of severity of pain, SI was significantly associated with older age, depressive symptoms, and pain interfering with function, but not with pain severity. They also found that SI was associated with using pain catastrophizing and prayer as coping mechanisms. However, the relationships need further research. Ratcliffe et al. (2008) reported a positive correlation between one or more chronic pain conditions, with migraine headaches having the greatest association. This was consistent with the work of Ilgen et al. (2008) who found a strong correlation between head pain and SI and SA. They also found an association of patients with chronic nonarthritic pain with SAs. In a study by Smith et al. (2004), abdominal pain was highly associated with SI but again not correlated with pain severity. The reader is referred to Chapter 22 for additional information on suicide.

> *Pearls*   Chronic pain is associated with increased risk of suicide, regardless of whether depression is evident.
> Patients with chronic pain should be considered at risk for suicide and assessed for SI.
> SI among patients with chronic pain is not necessarily related to the severity of pain.

ANGER

When pain interferes with continuing usual and pleasurable activities, the person may become apathetic, depressed, irritable, or angry (Baumann, 2009). A 2007 study of 79 community-dwelling married individuals found correlations between pain and anger/hostility and sadness (Johansen & Cano, 2007). Anger related to pain may be the cause of elderly patients physically striking caregivers, which is often seen among patients who have a working diagnosis of dementia but who are still physically active.

ANXIETY

Anxiety, which is the emotion that involves the sense and apprehension of an impending threat or harm (Tang & Gibson, 2005), has been associated with chronic pain (Meredith, Strong & Feeney, 2006; Smith & Zautra, 2008; Tang & Gibson, 2005). As with depression, a more detailed discussion of anxiety is found in Chapter 22. Among a national sample of individuals with arthritis pain, anxiety was more closely correlated with pain than was depression (McWilliams, Cox, & Enns, 2003). This was consistent with other studies showing similar relationships (Blyth et al., 2011). Subsequently, the correlations of both arthritis and chronic back pain with panic attacks and general anxiety disorders were statistically similar (McWilliams, Goodwin, & Cox, 2004). Migraines have also been positively correlated with anxiety disorders (Swartz, Pratt, Armenian, Lee, & Eaton, 2000).

OBESITY

Obesity has recently been studied as a correlate with chronic pain (Hitt, McMillen, Thornton-Neaves, Koch, & Cosby, 2007). In a recent study of 840 New York City residents ranging from 70 to 101 years of age, 52% reported chronic pain. In another study, the odds ratio was 2.1 that older adults who were obese would have chronic pain, and for those who were extremely obese the odds ratio was 4 to 4.5 times more likely that they would have chronic pain (McCarthy, Bigal, Katz, Derby & Lipton, 2009).

BMI as well as abdominal girth were positively associated with chronic pain. Almost twice the probability of developing chronic pain was noted among obese older adults, and this remained true when investigators controlled for confounding variables. In fact, the relationship with BMI was so strong that "the relative odds of chronic pain increased with each unit of BMI" (Ray, Lipton, Zimmerman, Katz, & Derby, 2011, p. 56). In many instances, surgery that could be helpful for the chronic pain situation is precluded because of the risks related to obesity (Arnoff, 2009). As with other psychosocial factors, there is a circular path. Pain can lead to limited activity that can lead to further weight gain that can increase the risk or intensity of pain (McCarthy et al. 2009).

INTERFERENCE WITH ACTIVITIES

A number of functions and activities of daily living can be negatively impacted by pain.

Sleep disturbances, including restless sleep (Bergh et al., 2003), are common among older adults with inadequately managed pain (Eliopoulos, 2001; Nicholson & Verma, 2004). Arthritic pain is noted as one of the conditions that limits sleep, which leads to untoward outcomes (Vaz Fragoso & Gill, 2007). Oncology patients (*n* = 182) with an average age of 58 years reported markedly impaired sleep related to pain, and this held true when controlled for age (Buffum et al., 2011).

Chronic pain has been associated with fatigue. Fatigue and lack of sleep negatively affect cognitive function, interpersonal relationships, safety, and quality of life. Fatigue related to lack of sleep is predictive of mortality in older adults, especially when associated with activities of daily living and among those who are members of minority groups (CDC, 2011a, 2011b; Hardy & Studenski, 2008; Schultz-Laresen & Avlund, 2007).

At each visit, HCPs should ask their older patients about the quality and duration of sleep. For patients with pain that negatively affects sleep, interventions should be used to decrease the pain so sleep and sleep hygiene can be improved. Good sleep hygiene involves

- managing pain to promote relaxation
- limiting caffeine
- increasing daytime activity
- participating in relaxing activities prior to bed time

MOBILITY

Mobility is often limited as a result of pain because older people tend to remain in a position that is most comfortable and movement often is painful. Disability is noted to result from muscle weakness and pain. Limited activity is associated with arthritic pain. Loss of skeletal muscle mass and strength (sarcopenia), which occurs with aging leading to decreased physical activity, can result in increased falls, fractures, morbidity, and mortality (Leveille et al., 2011; Patel et al., 2010; Whitson et al., 2009). The sites of pain commonly associated with limited activities are the lower back, knees, and legs, which are also common sites of arthritis-related pain in older adults (Duong, Kerns, Towle, & Reid, 2005; Leveille, Bean, Ngo, McMullen, & Guralnik, 2007; Vaz Fragoso & Gill, 2007).

Again there is a circular relationship between disability related to musculoskeletal pain and depression. Chronic pain has also been implicated as a factor of falling among older adults living in the community. The relationship may be due to joint disease, neuromuscular disorders, or pain interfering with cognition as well as impaired balance or weakness (Leveille, et al., 2011; Reid, Williams, & Gill, 2003).

Referrals for interventions to improve strength, balance, and mobility include
- physical therapy
- occupational therapy
- yoga
- tai chi
- exercise physiology

(Adler, Good, Roberts, & Snyder, 2000; Buettner, 2001; Cheung, Wyman, & Halcon, 2007; Hinman, Heywood, & Day, 2007)

Pearls	Quality of life is impaired by sleep disturbances and impaired mobility related to chronic pain. Patients with chronic pain may be at increased risk for falling. Older adults should be assessed for sleep disturbances and risk of falling.

INTERPERSONAL RELATIONSHIPS

Interactions with others, particularly with one's spouse, are often affected by chronic pain. The degree of congruence to which a person living with chronic pain and the spouse perceive the pain is an important factor. One study reported that spouses considered the person in pain to have less physical disability and interference with activities than the person in pain perceived (Cano, Johansen, & Franz, 2005). They also noted that the greater degree of incongruence, the greater the degree of distress experienced.

SOCIAL WITHDRAWAL

The relationship between social connections and pain can also be considered circular. Social interactions can be helpful in managing pain and limiting disability, but pain can interfere or prevent those interactions, thus reducing or eliminating a beneficial feature of pain management. Peat, Thomas, Handy, and Croft (2004) reported that there is a protective effect of social networks in the development and progression of disability and that fewer social ties are associated with greater pain interference. This protective quality of social contacts is true regardless of age. Social support also tends to be protective of depression (which also negatively impacts chronic pain). With increasing age, this is a particular concern since the social network often becomes smaller as family and friends die (Gibson, 2005; Keefe, et al., 2002).

Chronic pain also interferes with

- shopping
- work
- recreation
- leisure time activities
- attendance at religious services

In some instances the way these activities are carried out must be modified, whereas in other instances the activities and associated socialization are abandoned (Duong et al., 2005).

Pearl	Older adults with chronic pain are at risk for social isolation. Explore social networks and encourage participation.

SOCIAL ENVIRONMENT

Jordan, Thomas, Peat, Wilkie, and Croft (2008) suggested that regardless of their own health status, individuals who live in socioeconomically deprived areas may be at greater risk for developing chronic pain. The risk could be related to social factors, such as environment, health care services, access to health care, and opportunities for managing chronic pain.

African American women may be more negatively impacted by pain (Green, Baker, & Ndao-Brumblay, 2004). Although more research is needed, a recent study of 1,600 men noted that African American men (6%) who live with chronic pain often have greater incidence of depression, disability, and distress than their Caucasian counterparts (96%) (Green & Hart-Johnson, 2010). Possible factors that may contribute to this difference include

■ poorer general health of the African American men
■ lower marriage rates
■ lower income
■ less education
■ litigation processes related to the origin of the pain
■ difficulty obtaining analgesic medications in their neighborhoods (related to transportation or availability)

(Green et al. 2004; Green & Hart-Johnson, 2010)

It is very important to be sensitive to the culture of the older adult persons and how their culture impacts the pain experience. Some important cultural considerations that can affect pain management are as follows:

■ Language, including the connotation of words
■ The meaning of the pain from a cultural perspective
■ What folk medicines (i.e., herbs) or treatments (i.e., "coining") is the person using to manage pain
■ Who in the family is the gate keeper for information about the person in pain
■ Who in the family does the person in pain trust or rely on, and to whom does he or she defer for important decisions
■ Understand that not all cultures in a country or nationality are the same (e.g., there are significant differences in the cultures of the various South American and Central American countries)

Whenever possible use a professional medical translator or translation telephone service and approved translations of assessment and education materials. This is important to ensure that the HCP is accurately hearing what the patient is saying as well as to ensure that the patient is accurately hearing what the HCP is saying. Translators who are not professionals in medical translation may not fully understand what is being said or how to accurately communicate it.

Not only is this true for family members, but also family members may screen what is being translated in an effort to protect the patient.

Pearls	As individuals age, the scope of their social interactions shrinks. Pain often interferes with the interpersonal relationships of the older person in pain. Pain is experienced in a cultural setting and cultural factors are important to consider when assessing and planning care. Sometimes the greatest challenge is to see the diversity in the person who seems the most like us.

RESOURCES AND GUIDELINES

Acute pain management in older adults. (2006). Herr, K., Bjoro, K., Steffensmeier, J., Rakel, B. Iowa City, IA: University of Iowa. Gerontological Nursing Interventions Research Center, Research Translation and Dissemination Core. http://www.guideline.gov/content.aspx?id=10198&search=persistent+pain+and+iowa

American Pain Society. www.ampainsoc.org

American Psychiatric Association. www.psych.org

American Psychological Association. www.apa.org

Institute of Medicine. www.iom.edu

International Association for the Study of Pain. www.iasp-pain.org/terms-p.html

Mental Health – A Report of the Surgeon General. http://www.surgeongeneral.gov/library/mentalhealth/home.html

National Alliance of Hispanic Health. ftp://ftp.hrsa.gov/hrsa/Quality HealthServicesforHispanics.pdf

National Institute on Aging. http://www.nia.nih.gov/

National Institute of Health Senior Health. http://nihseniorhealth.gov/index.html

University of Michigan Multicultural health program: Cultural competency. www.med.umich.edu/multicultural/ccp/background.htm

Case Study

Mr. Evans is an 83-year-old African American. Since his wife died about 3 months ago, he lives alone. He comes to clinic today for a routine diabetes follow-up visit. You notice that he is moving

(continued)

slower than usual and isn't as interactive as on past visits. When you ask him how he is feeling, he tells you "I'm doing." When you assess his pain, he reports 6/10 pain in his lower back and 7/10 pain in his lower legs that he tells you is "burning something wicked" and keeps him awake most nights. When asked how he copes with his pain, he tells you that he just prays about it.

Questions

1. Does Mr. Evans have risk factors for suicide?
2. What activities has Mr. Evans modified or curtailed?
3. What psychological factors will you assess in Mr. Evans?
4. What referrals will you make to other HCPs?
5. What community resources may be of help to Mr. Evans?

REFERENCES

Adler, Good, Roberts, & Snyder. (2000). Musculoskeletal conditions in the United States. *American Academy of Orthopaedic Surgeons Bulletin, 47,* 34–36.

Arnoff, G. (2009). Chronic pain, smoking, and obesity: A pain physician's perspective on patient selection. *Pain Medicine, 10,* 962–965.

Baumann, S. (2009). A nursing approach to pain in older adults. *MEDSURG Nursing, 18,* 77–82.

Bergh, I., Steen, G., Waern, M., Johansson, B., Oden, A., Sjostrom, B., & Steen, B. (2003). Pain and its relation to cognitive function and depressive symptoms: A Swedish population study of 70-year-old men and women. *Journal of Pain and Symptom Management, 2003,* 903–912.

Blyth, F. M., Cumming, R. G., Nicholas, M. K., Creasey, H., Handelsman, D. J., Le Couteur, D. G., Waite, L. M. (2011). Intrusive pain and worry about health in older men: The CHAMP study. *Pain, 152,* 447–452.

British Pain Society and British Geriatric Society. (2007). *Guidance on the assessment of pain in older adults* (2007 ed.) [Brochure]. London: Author.

Buettner, L. L. (2001). Therapeutic recreation in the nursing home: Reinventing a good thing. *Journal of Gerontological Nursing, 27,* 8–13.

Buffum, D., Koetters, T., Cho, M., Macera, L., Paul, S. M., West, C., Miaskowski, C. (2011). The effects of pain, gender, and age on sleep/wake and circadian rhythm parameters in oncology patients at the initiation of radiation therapy. *The Journal of Pain, 12,* 390–400.

Cano, A., Johansen, A. B., & Franz, A. (2005). Multilevel analysis of couple congruence on pain, interference, and disability. *Pain, 118,* 369–379.

CDC (Centers for Disease Control and Prevention). (2011a). Effect of short sleep on daily activities – United States, 2005–2008. *Morbidity and Mortality Weekly Report (MMWR), 60*(08), 239–242.

CDC (Centers for Disease Control and Prevention). (2011b). Unhealthy sleep-related behaviors – 12 states, 2009. *Morbidity and Mortality Weekly Report (MMWR), 60*(08), 233–238.

Cheung, C. K., Wyman, J. F., & Halcon, L. L. (2007). Use of complementary and alternative therapies in community-dwelling older adults. *The Journal of Alternative and Complementary Medicine, 3,* 997–1006.

Chou, K-L. (2007). Reciprocal relationship between pain and depression in older adults: Evidence from the English Longitudinal Study of Ageing. *Journal of Affective Disorders, 102,* 115–122.

Cook, A. K., Niven, C. A., & Downs, M. G. (1999). Assessing the pain of people with cognitive impairment. *International Journal of Geriatric Psychiatry, 14,* 421–425.

Duong, B. D., Kerns, R. D., Towle, V., & Reid, M. C. (2005). Identifying the activities affected by chronic nonmalignant pain in older veterans receiving primary care. *Journal of the American Geriatrics Society, 53,* 687–694.

Edwards, R. R., Smith, M. T., Kudel, I., & Haythornwaite, J. (2006). Pain-related catastrophizing as a risk factor for suicidal ideation in chronic pain. *Pain, 126,* 272–279.

Eliopoulos, C. (2001). *Gerontological nursing* (5th ed.). Philadelphia, PA: Lippincott.

Gibson, S. J. (2005). Age differences in psychosocial aspects of pain. In S. J. Gibson & D. K. Weiner (Eds.), *Pain in older persons* (pp. 87–107). Seattle, WA: IASP Press.

Gibson, S. J., & Helme, R. D. (2000). Cognitive factors and the experience of pain and suffering in older persons. *Pain, 85,* 375–383.

Green, C. R., Baker, T. A., & Ndao-Brumblay, S. (2004). Patient attitudes regarding healthcare utilization and referral: A descriptive comparison in African- and Caucasian Americans with chronic pain. *Journal of the National Medical Association, 96,* 31–42.

Green, C. R., & Hart-Johnson, T. (2010). The impact of chronic pain on the health of black and white men. *Journal of the National Medical Association, 102,* 321–331.

Hardy, S. E., & Studenski, S. A. (2008). Fatigue predicts mortality in older adults. *Journal of the American Geriatrics Society, 56,* 1900–1914.

Herr, K., Bjorg, L., Steffensmeier, J., & Rakel, B. (2006). Acute pain management in older adults. *Gerontological Nursing Interventions Research Center, Research Translation and Dissemination Core.* Retrieved March 13, 2011, from http://www.guideline.gov/content.aspx?id=10198&search=persistent+pain+and+iowa

Hinman, R. S., Heywood, S. E., & Day, A. R. (2007). Aquatic physical therapy for hip and knee osteoarthritis: Results of a single-blind randomized controlled trial. *Physical Therapy, 87,* 32–43.

Hitt, H. C., McMillen, R. C., Thornton-Neaves, T., Koch, K., & Cosby, A. G. (2007). Comorbidity of obesity and pain in a general population: Results from the Southern Pain Prevalence Study. *Journal of Pain, 8,* 430–436.

Ilgen, M. A., Zivan, K., McCammon, R. J., & Valenstein, M. (2008). Pain and suicidal thoughts, plans and attempts in the United States. *General Hospital Psychiatry, 30,* 521–527.

Johansen, A. B., & Cano, A. M. (2007). A preliminary investigation of affective interaction in chronic pain couples. *Pain, 132,* S86–S95.

Jordan, K. P., Thomas, E., Peat, G., Wilkie, R., & Croft, P. (2008). Social risks for disabling pain in older people: A prospective study of individual and area characteristics. *Pain, 137,* 652–661.

Keefe, F. J., Smith, S. J., Buffington, A. L. H., Gibson, J., Studts, J. L., & Caldwell, D. (2002). Recent advances and future directions in the biopsychosocial assessment and treatment of arthritis. *Journal of Consulting and Clinical Psychology, 70,* 640–655.

Lee, D. M., Pendleton, N., Tajar, A., O'Niell, T. W., O'Connor, D. B., Bartfai, G., McBeth, J. (2010). Chronic widespread pain is associated with slower cognitive processing speed in middle-aged and older European men. *Pain, 151,* 30–36.

Leveille, S. G., Bean, J., Ngo, L., McMullen, W., & Guralnik, J. M. (2007). The pathway from musculoskeletal pain to mobility difficulty in older disabled women. *Pain, 128,* 69–77.

Leveille, S. G., Jones, R. N., Kiely, D. K., Hausdorff, J. M., Shmerling, R. H., Guarlnik, J. M., Bean, J. F. (2011). Chronic musculoskeletal pain and the occurrence of falls in an older population. *Journal of the American Medical Association, 302,* 2214–2221.

McCarthy, L. H., Bigal, M. E., Katz, M., Derby, C., & Lipton, R. B. (2009). Chronic pain and obesity in elderly people: Results from the Einstein Aging Study. *Journal of the American Geriatric Society, 57,* 115–119.

McWilliams, L. A., Cox, B. J., & Enns, M. W. (2003). Mood and anxiety disorders associated with chronic pain: An examination in a nationally representative sample. *Pain, 106,* 127–133.

McWilliams, L. A., Goodwin, R. D., & Cox, B. J. (2004). Depression and anxiety associated with three pain conditions: Results from a nationally representative sample. *Pain, 111,* 77–83.

Meredith, P., Strong, J., & Feeney, J. A. (2006). Adult attachment, anxiety, and pain self-efficacy as predictors of pain intensity and disability. *Pain, 123,* 146–154.

Miller, L. R. & Cano, A. (2009). Comorbid chronic pain and depression: who is at risk? *The Journal of Pain, 10,* 619-627.

Mossey, J. M., & Gallagher, R. M. (2004). The longitudinal occurrence and impact of comorbid chronic pain and chronic depression over two years in continuing care retirement community residents. *Pain Medicine, 5,* 335–347.

Nicholson, B., & Verma, S. (2004). Comorbidities in chronic neuropathic pain. *Pain Medicine, 5,* S9–S27.

Parmelee, P. A. (2005). Measuring mood and psychosocial function associated in pain in late life. In S. J. Gibson & D. K. Weiner (Eds.), *Pain in older persons* (pp. 87–107). Seattle, WA: IASP Press.

Patel, H. P., Syddall, H. E., Martin, H. J., Steward, C. E., Cooper, C., & Sayer, A. A. (2010). Hartfordshire sarcopenia study: Design and methods. *BMC Geriatrics, 10*(43), 1–25.

Peat, G., Thomas, E., Handy, J., & Croft, P. (2004). Social networks and pain interference with daily activities in middle and old age. *Pain, 112,* 397–405.

Ploghaus, A., Narian, C., Beckmann, C.F., Clare, S., Bantick, S., Wise, R., Tracey, I. (2001). Exacerbation of pain by anxiety is associated with activity in a hippocampal network. *The Journal of Neuroscience, 21,* 9896–9903.

Ratcliffe, G. E., Enns, M. W., Belik, S. L., & Sareen, J. (2008). Chronic pain conditions and suicidal ideation and suicide attempts: An epidemiologic perspective. *Clinical Journal of Pain, 24,* 204–210.

Ray, L., Lipton, R. B., Zimmerman, M. E., Katz, M. J., & Derby, C. A. (2011). Mechanisms of association between obesity and chronic pain in the elderly. *Pain, 152,* 53–59.

Reid, M. C., Williams, C. S., & Gill, T. M. (2003). The relationship between psychological factors and disabling musculoskeletal pain in community-dwelling older persons. *Journal of the American Geriatric Society, 51,* 1092–1098.

Schultz-Laresen, K., & Avlund, K. (2007). Tiredness in daily activities: A subjective measure for the identification of frailty among non-disabled community-dwelling older adults. *Archives of Gerontology and Geriatrics, 44,* 83–93.

Smith, B.W., & Zautra, A. J. (2008). The effects of anxiety and depression on weekly pain in women with arthritis. *Pain, 138,* 354–361.

Smith, M. T., Edwards, R. R., Robinson, R. C., & Dworkin, R. H. (2004). Suicidal ideation, plans, and attempts in chronic pain patients: Factors associated with increased risk. *Pain, 2004,* 201–208.

Swartz, K. L., Pratt, L. A., Armenian, H. K., Lee, L. C., & Eaton, W. W. (2000). Mental disorders and the incidence of migraine headaches in a community sample: Results from the Baltimore epidemiologic catchment area follow-up study. *Archives of General Psychiatry, 57,* 945–603.

Tang, J., & Gibson, S. J. (2005). A psychophysical evaluation of the relationship between trait anxiety, pain perception, and induced state anxiety. *The Journal of Pain, 6,* 612–619.

U.S. Public Health Service. (1999a). *Mental health: A report of the surgeon general – Depression in older adults*. Retrieved March 08, 2011, from http://www.surgeongeneral.gov/library/mentalhealth/chapter5/sec3.html

U.S. Public Health Service. (1999b). *Mental health: A report of the surgeon general – Other mental health disorders in older adults*. Retrieved March 08, 2011, from http://www.surgeongeneral.gov/library/mentalhealth/chapter5/sec5.html#anxiety

Vaz Fragoso, C. A., & Gill, T. M. (2007). Sleep complaints in community-living older persons: A multifactorial geriatric syndrome. *Journal of the American Geriatric Society, 55,* 1853–1866.

Vaccarino, A. L., Sills, T. L., Evans, K. R., & Kalali, A. H. (2009). Multiple pain complaints in patients with major depressive disorder. *Psychosomatic Medicine, 71,* 159–162.

Wenzlaff, R. M. & Wegner, D. M. (2000). Thought suppression. *Annual Review of Psychology, 51,* 59-91.

Whitson, H. E., Sanders, L. L., Pieper, C. F., Morey, M. C., Oddone, E. Z., & Gold, D. T. (2009). Correlation between symptoms and function in older adults. *Journal of the American Geriatrics Society, 57,* 676–682.

Weiner, D. K., Rudy, T. E., Morrow, L., Slaboda, J., & Lieber, S. (2006). The relationship between pain, neuropsychological performance, and physical function in community-dwelling older adults with chronic low back pain. *Pain Medicine, 7*(1), 60–70.

3

Pain Assessment in the Older Adult Patient

To provide adequate pain management for a patient of any age, a good pain assessment is essential. However, for the older patient special considerations related to assessment are necessary to make it a more complete and consistent process. The plan for managing pain in older patients will depend upon various components of the pain assessment.

The objectives of assessing pain in older adults are to:
1. determine whether pain exists,
2. accurately identify the characteristics of pain,
3. obtain information to guide in appropriate management of pain,
4. identify potential barriers to good pain management,
5. understand the beliefs of the older adult about pain,
6. identify comorbid diagnosis,
7. identify opportunities for intervention to relieve pain and minimize disability (Yonan & Wegener, 2003).

GENERAL ASSESSMENT

Before asking about pain, it is essential to determine whether the older adult is a good historian and able to adequately participate in the assessment of pain. Ensure that the person is comfortable both physically and emotionally. It is difficult to concentrate and remain attentive when in pain or uncomfortable. Similarly, information will be guarded if the person feels that he or she is being judged or negatively perceived. Assess the cognitive function of the older adult. Determine orientation to person, place, and time as well as short-term memory ability. (See Chapter 4 for discussion of the older adult with cognitive limitations.)

Once it is determined that the older adult is cognitively intact and able to participate adequately in the pain assessment, begin by asking the person if he or she is experiencing pain at this time. Self-report of pain by the patient is "the single most reliable indicator of the existence and intensity of pain" (American Pain Society [APS], 2008; National Guideline Clearing House, 2009, p. 4). Using a simple tool such as the numeric rating scale (NRS) to rate pain will enhance the patient's ability to provide an accurate report of pain.

To provide adequate pain management, a good pain assessment is essential. The plan for managing pain will depend upon what is discovered in the various components of the pain assessment.

| *Pearls* | Adequate pain management depends upon a good pain assessment. |
| | Ensure that the older adult is comfortable and feels safe during the pain assessment. |

Barriers to Pain Assessment

There are a variety of barriers that can interfere with good pain assessment in older adults. These can originate with the patient, with the health care provider (HCP), or with the health care system.

Patient barriers

Beliefs

Many older adults believe that pain is a normal part of aging and that it must be accepted as such. Many also believe that the HCP will know that they are in pain without being told.

Misconceptions

The older person and/or family members may believe that "the pain is all in my/her/his head" because the pain does not seem to be an issue when the person is playing cards, knitting, carving, or participating in other activities that require concentration. It is important to explain to the older person and the family that these activities can have considerable analgesic effects, that the pain is "real", and older persons may be using these activities as a technique to distract themselves from their pain.

Fears
Older adults may fear that the pain means that they have a serious illness that may impair their ability to function or live in their homes. They may fear that they will need to have tests or be hospitalized; that they will need to take more medications; that they will get addicted to those medications; or that the medications will negatively affect their cognition. Some also fear that talking about pain will take time or attention of the HCP away from more serious health care concerns (Forrest, 1995; Herr, 2005).

Desire
Many older adults want to be considered a "good patient" and they do not want to be considered a "bother" or "burden." Older adults may want to be considered independent and vibrant, which they may not consider to be consistent with having pain. They may not want to be considered "complaining" or "whining." They may believe that the fewer medications they take the healthier they are, so they do not want to take additional medications. This may lead them to stop taking pain medications that have been ordered.

Cultural factors
There are many cultural influences on the beliefs about and experience of pain. These include unique beliefs and language differences. Language differences include different connotations of the same word. Older adults may use the word pain only for excruciating experiences. More commonly they use "ache," "sore," "tingling," or "hurt." They may use other words not necessarily associated with pain such as "bothersome" or "aching." One woman with severe pathology, always described the sensation we considered painful as "tight." Some cultures expect people in pain to be stoic and accepting of the pain, whereas others feel a more emotional expression is appropriate.

Sensory impairments
Assessment of pain requires communication. Hearing loss and decreased visual acuity may be significant obstacles. Encourage use of hearing aids and eye glasses during the assessment. When the HCP eliminates extraneous noise, faces the person, speaks slowly, and carefully enunciates words, communication often improves. Remember also that pain can be very distracting and make it difficult to concentrate (Ardery, Herr, Titler, Sorofman, & Schmitt, 2003).

Finances

Many older adults have limited financial resources. At the same time, they may have pride in being self-sufficient and do not want anyone to know that they struggle financially. Medicare may cover HCP costs but either not cover or not fully cover the cost of medications that are prescribed. Many older adults must choose between buying food and pain medicine or buying food for their pet and pain medicine. In either situation, they most often do not buy the pain medicine. These are facts not commonly shared with HCPs. As a part of the pain assessment when medication choices are being made, a discussion of ability to purchase the medications that may be prescribed is essential to the success of the therapy.

HCP barriers

Cultural factors

As with older adults, HCPs have unique cultural backgrounds. Among people born within the same community in the United States, there are often different cultural beliefs and practices that have been passed down through generations. It is important to be aware of these and how they may affect assessment and care of patients.

Beliefs

HCPs may also have particular beliefs about pain, namely that pain is a normal part of aging, that older adults do not "feel" pain the way younger people do, that older adults have a greater threshold for tolerating pain, or more general ageism beliefs. It is important to dispel unsupported myths and replace them with evidence-based information. HCPs may also erroneously believe that all older adults have adequate insurance to cover all health care costs, including medications.

Education

Despite the amount of literature available on the subject, assessment and management of pain are often not part of the education of health care professionals. Myths and misconceptions about pain and pain management persist among health care professionals.

Some common misconceptions include the beliefs that
- prescribing opioids will cause addiction,
- older adults do not experience as much pain as younger adults,

- patients overrate their pain, and
- medications should be prescribed based on actual body weight.

Communication skills

Because of generational differences between HCPs and older adult patients, there may be different connotations of words and phrases. One study noted that when HCPs interrupted older adults, more than half of the assessment information was not reported (McDonald & Fedo, 2009).

System barriers

These generally include limitations of time for the HCP to assess and financial restrictions. Other system barriers may include availability of evidence-based health care information, absent or inadequate practice standards, and pain not being an organizational priority. In the American Pain Society Monograph "Pain: Current Understanding of Assessment, Management and Treatments" it is noted that "the greatest systems barrier to appropriate pain management is a lack of accountability for pain management practices" (200, p. 21).

Pearls	There are many patient and HCP barriers to assessing pain in older adults. These barriers can be removed once they are identified.

Pain Screening

In addition to being aware of the potential barriers, assessment of pain in the cognitively intact older adult requires being patient, persistent, and attentive to detail. After an initial introduction, begin with screening questions such as "How are you doing today? Are you comfortable? Are you having any discomfort today?" The topic of discomfort can then be explored through a thorough assessment that starts with a careful review of history and physical assessment (National Guideline Clearing House, 2004).

Assess the History

Review of the history of the patient can provide clues to pain that may be experienced. Identify the following:

- Any parameters that have changed since the last visit or during the past year
- New co morbidities or medicines
- Previous experiences of pain and how the person responded to pain in those instances
- Medications and other interventions that were successful
- Any side effects experienced
- Any allergic responses to analgesic medications
- Medications or other interventions that did not work

If a medication did not work previously, no matter how appropriate it is for the current pain, it probably will not be effective. Once a medication has been negatively experienced, the chances of it being effective are very low. In some cases, it may be just that the dose provided was too low to provide adequate pain relief. Ascertain what dose was prescribed and what dose the patient was taking when last prescribed. Explain that the dose may have been too low and therefore not effective, but be prepared to accept that this medication may not be effective for the person.

Physical Examination

A logical starting point is to identify the location or locations of pain. Begin assessment in the general area where pain is described and then assess closer and closer to the area of pain, rather than beginning at the site of pain. Particular attention should be given to the musculoskeletal and neurological systems because many pains experienced by older adults originate in these systems. During physical examination, be attentive to grimacing, flinching, guarding, or other behavioral signs that may indicate areas of tenderness or pain.

Pain Assessment Interview

Identify the *onset* of each pain. With older adults, the onset may be recent or it may have started many years prior. Pain may also be acute and related to an exacerbation of a chronic disorder, or it may be acute in addition to a chronic pain state.

Identify the *location* of the pain. This should include assessing
- where it feels most intense,
- where the pain begins,

■ where it moves or radiates to other parts of the body,
■ where else in the body there is pain, and
■ how many different parts of the body are affected by different pains.

Each pain must be assessed separately. One patient may experience somatic pain related to osteoarthritis (OA) of the knees and visceral pain related to chronic pancreatitis, as well as neuropathic pain (NP) subsequent to herpes zoster (HZ) and an acute pain in the hip as a result of a fall the day before. Although the hip pain may be the presenting complaint, each site of pain needs to be assessed individually because each may require different intervention.

Identify the *duration* of the pain. Determine whether the pain is acute, occurring for less than 3 months, or whether it is chronic, with a long duration. It is important to differentiate acute from chronic pain. Acute pain is a symptom of a change or injury, and the underlying pathology must be assessed and treated. While the origin of the pain is being investigated, the pain must be treated. Current evidence (Thomas & Silen, 2003; Thomas et al., 2003; Vermeulen et al., 1999) informs that treating pain does not mask symptoms or confuse diagnosis. Chronic pain is no longer a symptom, but rather a syndrome that requires treatment.

Determine the *character* of the pain. Ask the patient to describe the pain in his or her own words. Words such as burning, aching, shooting, tingling, throbbing, and stabbing can give insight into the type of pain and the type of medication that will be most appropriate to manage it.

Asking what *aggravates* the pain or makes it worse can lead to important assessment information regarding the etiology of the pain. This also provides insight into the functional limitations that result from the pain.

Asking what *relieves* the pain or makes it feel better can also provide insight into the etiology of the pain, as well as the interventions that have worked. Interventions that have been effective need to be incorporated into the treatment plan unless they are contraindicated by a comorbidity or are known to cause harm.

It is important to know the timing aspects of the pain. Identify during a 24-hour period when the pain generally occurs and how long it generally lasts. This information will provide diagnostic insight (pain related to OA typically is worse upon rising and improves with activity), as well as insight into the types of medications that may be most appropriate in helping to manage the pain.

The *severity* of pain is best assessed using a consistent pain assessment tool. Although these will be discussed in detail in Chapter 5, the most commonly used tools are the numeric analog/rating scale (NAS/NRS), the FACES scale, and the word descriptor scale (none, mild, moderate, severe, and worst possible).

Assess the Meaning of Pain Being Experienced

It is important to identify what experiencing this pain means to the person and what activities have been altered by the pain. The person may believe that the pain is

- a "normal" part of the aging process,
- punishment for something done in the past, or
- an indicator of terminal illness.

Assess Pain-Related Goals

Determine what goal the person has for pain management and whether the goal is reasonable. If the goal is too low, it could compromise the patient's safety considering the etiology of pain, comorbidities, and medication limitations. If the goal is too high, it could interfere with effective functioning and quality of life. Creating realistic expectations for pain relief can significantly contribute to the success of the care plan.

Assess Medication Use

Determine what medications, over the counter (OTC) as well as prescription, the person takes to manage the pain. Ask if the medication is being taken correctly, what doses are used, and how frequently they are taken. Ask if the medication that is being taken is adequately managing the pain.

It is essential to discuss this in a nonjudgmental manner to identify how the person is really taking the medication. Very often people take medications differently than the way they are prescribed or recommended. If this is not honestly reported, there is a risk of either under or over prescription of medicine. Lab tests to determine the level of medication can be helpful. Determine whether there is someone other than the older adult who is taking some or all of the analgesia prescribed. This should be investigated whenever an older adult does not have the expected response to opioids. Using a simple urine screen can determine whether the medications are being taken at all.

As older patients may have some type of liver or renal dysfunction, it is important to monitor the amount of acetaminophen being taken. It is important to identify how much acetaminophen is taken from all sources. If the person is taking a combination analgesic that contains an opioid and acetaminophen for pain while taking an OTC acetaminophen product as well, there is a risk of excessive acetaminophen use leading to liver damage.

Assess Finances

It is important to understand the financial ability of older adults to obtain medications that have been prescribed and participate in other interventions, such as physical therapy (PT) and nonpharmacological techniques. The most appropriate medication or treatment cannot be effective if the person cannot afford to purchase it. It may be most appropriate to refer the older adult to a case manager or social worker who can assist with financial issues. Some pharmaceutical companies have coupons or programs to financially assist patients who cannot afford medications.

Assess Alcohol and Other Substance Use

Ask whether the older adult is drinking alcohol and, if so, the frequency and usual amount. It is imperative that alcohol use be assessed in a nonjudgmental manner. Asking patients how much wine, beer, or mixed drinks they have daily in a matter-of-fact manner is best. Determine whether alcohol use is social/cultural or self-medicating for pain. It is important to educate about contraindications of alcohol with certain medications, such as those containing acetaminophen, or the potential for complications with opioids resulting from synergistic effects.

Ask the patient if he or she is using any other substances. Some older people use marijuana, cocaine, amphetamines, heroin, or other illegal substances. This is another area where it is important to provide a nonjudgmental and safe environment in which the person can be honest about use. Screening laboratory tests can also be helpful in identifying use. Lab reports for patients in their eighties have been positive for marijuana, cocaine, and other substances. The reader is referred to Chapter 23 for a more detailed discussion of substance misuse and abuse.

Assess Nonpharmacological Interventions

Ask what culturally based methods of managing pain the person is using. Determine whether these have any potential for harm or whether they have a problematic interaction with any medications that are taken. Educate the person accordingly.

Ask if he or she uses exercise to manage pain. Determine if the form of exercise is appropriate for the type of pain experienced and if there is a possibility that the exercise may cause more damage rather than benefit.

Ask about use of meditation, progressive muscle relaxation, breathing, or other relaxation techniques to manage pain and if spirituality is an important coping mechanism. Ask about the use of distraction with hobbies, music, art, and other activities that can be enjoyable as well as distracting.

Assess Function

There are many tools that can assess the physical, psychosocial, and cognitive function, as well as activities of daily living (ADLs) of older adults. The following assessment points are highlights. Positive findings indicate a need for more detailed assessment.

Activities of Daily Living

Determine the effect of pain on ADL. Identify what activities he or she had been doing successfully and that are now challenging because of pain. Ask if the person now needs assistance to:

■ rise from a chair (painful knees and hips can make rising from a chair difficult),
■ walk (musculoskeletal or neurologic pain can impair gait),

- bathe (moving in and out of a tub requires joint agility),
- dress (arthritic fingers may limit the ability to button),
- manage medications (pain in fingers and hands can interfere with or prohibit fine motor tasks),
- cooking (lifting pots, stirring foods, or even turning can be difficult with musculoskeletal or neurologic pain),
- do laundry (reaching into washing machines and dryers may be difficult with back or upper extremity pain),
- clean the home (lifting a pail of water, sweeping, and pushing a vacuum can be limited by painful joints),
- drive a car (turning the neck and pressing the brake pedal can limit the ability to drive),
- shop for groceries and other items, and
- usual leisure activities (walking, jogging, biking, golfing, swimming, dancing, reading, knitting, sewing, quilting, scrap booking, painting, playing tennis, or playing a musical instrument may all be negatively impacted and limited by pain).

Assess Function in the Physical Domain

Pain can limit usual function and activities. Assess balance, posture, range of motion, dexterity, and proprioception (Rudy & Lieber, 2005). Assess patients when they stand in the waiting room. They may need to use their arms to get up, have a unsteady gait, or limp when walking.

Ask if pain interferes with or negatively affects sleep (delayed or interrupted), sexual activity, appetite, ingestion, or digestion. Pain may contribute to incontinence if it causes delays in getting to the toilet.

Assess Function in the Psychosocial Domain

Determine whether pain negatively affected the person's self-confidence in social activities. Chronic pain can lead to depression. A general question is to ask if he or she feels sad often or most of the time. Ask if he or she

- avoids usual social activities because they may be painful,
- feels irritable,
- avoids other people, and
- is worried about the meaning of the pain.

Assess Function in the Cognitive Domain

Pain can interfere with concentration and the ability to read, write, and communicate well. Determine whether there has been a change in the cognitive ability of the person since the onset or worsening of pain. Family members may be a good source for this information.

Assess the Strengths and Assets of the Older Person

Determine whether the older adult is cognitively able to participate in a plan for managing pain.

Is he or she able to:

- follow an education plan?
- physically participate in an exercise plan, PT, or strengthening exercises?
- afford medications, therapies, and interventions recommended?

Does he or she have an effective coping strategy and family/community support system?

Assessment of Pain Types

Acute Pain

Acute pain is pain that has a recent onset. It is a symptom that indicates something has changed or is injured. Acute pain may be calling attention to an emerging myocardial infarction, appendicitis, small bowel obstruction, thrombosis, or joint damage. With acute pain, treatment of the cause is most important.

Chronic Pain

Chronic pain is pain that last longer than the expected time of healing, generally 3 to 6 months (APS, 2008). Chronic pain may occur in any part of the body, and there may no longer be an etiology for the pain (D'Arcy, 2010).

Neuropathic Pain

One type of chronic pain is NP. As a result of physiological aging changes, older adults are at greater risk for developing NP, which "results from a lesion or a malfunction within the nervous system" (Arnstein, 2010). Assessment tools specific to NP are discussed in Chapter 5.

NP may be a sequel to HZ, chronic low back pain (sciatic nerve involvement), diabetes, coronary artery disease, and amputations to name a few. NP is characterized by word descriptors that include numb, tingling, shock-like, and burning. Physical examination may be positive for *allodynia*, which is pain that occurs from light touch or other stimulation that normally does not cause pain (Pasero & McCaffery, 2010).

Assessment Guides

There are a variety of methods that can be used to guide the assessment of pain in older adults. One of these is an algorithm to guide assessment and management. It is available from the Royal College of Physicians, British Geriatrics Society and British Pain Society (2007).

The mnemonic OLD CARTS can be helpful in remembering the essential components of a pain assessment (Goldberg, 2009). The components are as follows:

Onset
Location
Duration
Character
Aggravating factors
Relieving factors
Timing
Severity

Communication

Communication is a critical element of successful assessment. Being specific in what is communicated and paraphrasing what has been said are helpful. Communicating with older adults requires patience, especially when the patient repeats information.

Health care professionals often ask "what number is your pain?" rather than asking open-ended questions that do not convey prejudice or bias (McDonald, Shea, Rose, & Fedo, 2009). Open-ended questions such as "Can you tell me how your pain affects you?" or "Can you tell me the differences in your pain when you are resting and moving?" encourage older adults to contribute important assessment information (McDonald, 2009) that may be lost by closed questioning.

Patience and time are needed to allow patients to think of the answers and the right words for their responses (Hanks-Bell, Halvey, & Paice, 2004). Several years ago, while trying to assess cognition, a patient was asked who was president. The patient named the counties of the state out loud. The HCP was ready to document the patient as confused when the patient said "Clinton," who was then president. His way of remembering the name was to work his way through the counties until he reached the county named Clinton. He was not confused, he merely needed time to remember things in his own way.

Follow-up and Ongoing Assessment

Ongoing assessment must include the following:
- effectiveness of analgesia
- current pain in relation to realistic pain goal
- patient satisfaction with analgesia
- side effects or untoward symptoms of analgesia

Side effects such as urinary retention, gastric irritation, confusion, and constipation may be as bothersome as pain and require a change of analgesia.

ASSESSMENT GUIDELINE RESOURCES

Acute pain management in older adults. (2009). http://www.guideline .gov/summary/summary.aspx?ss=15&doc_id=10198&nbr=5382

British Pain Society and British Geriatric Society Recommendations for Pain Assessment http://www.britishpainsociety.org/pub_professional. htm#assessmentpop

Best Practices in Nursing Care of Older Adults. The Hartford Institute for Geriatric Nursing. www.hartfordign.org and www.ConsultGeriRN.org

Pain Management. In: Evidence-based geriatric nursing protocols for best practice. (2004). http://www.guideline.gov/summary/summary. aspx?ss=15&doc_id=12268&nbr=6352

Pain Management. In: Evidence-based geriatric nursing protocols for best practice. (2004). http://www.guideline.gov/summary/summary.aspx?ss=15& doc_id=12268&nbr=6352

Registered Nurses' Association of Ontario Nursing Best Practice Guidelines Program. *Assessment and management of pain supplement.* www.rnao.org

Case Study

Mr. Jones is an 83-year-old man who presents for a routine annual physical. He tells you that he is fine but has slowed down a lot during the past year and is no longer playing golf, which he loved. You noticed that when he walked from the waiting room, his gait was slower and stiffer than you remembered. Upon questioning he tells you that he stopped playing golf about a month ago, after he fell in the bathroom. Ever since then he has "not been as spry as I used to be." He denies pain but admits to having an ache in his back and a tingling sensation in his right leg. He tells you that he expects to have some aches and pains at his age. On further questioning he tells you that he is not sleeping well and has not been able to enjoy sexual activities with his wife. X-rays and an MRI confirm a herniation in the lumbar spine.

Questions

1. What indications of pain did Mr. Jones report?
2. What types of pain is Mr. Jones describing?
3. What additional information needs to be assessed before an appropriate pain management plan can be developed?

REFERENCES

American Pain Society. (2008). *Principles of analgesic use in the treatment of acute pain and cancer pain* (6th ed.). Glenview, IL: Author.

Ardery, G., Herr, K. A., Titler, M. G., Sorofman, B. A., & Schmitt, M. B. (2003). Assessing and managing acute pain in older adults: A research base to guide practice. *MEDSURG Nursing, 12,* 7–18.

Arnstein, P. (2010). Assessment of nociceptive versus neuropathic pain in older adults. *Try this, SP1,*. Retrieved December 30, 2010, from www.hartfordign .org database

D'Arcy, Y. (2010). *Compact clinical guide to chronic pain management.* New York, NY: Springer.

Forrest, J. (1995). Assessment of acute and chronic pain in older adults. *Journal of Gerontological Nursing, 21,* 15–20.

Goldberg, C. (2009). A comprehensive physical examination and clinical education site for medical students and other health care professionals. *A practical guide to clinical medicine.* Retrieved January 15, 2010, from http://meded .ucsd.edu/clinicalmed/history.htm database

Hanks-Bell, M., Halvey, K., & Paice, J. A. (2004). Pain assessment and management in aging. *Online Journal of Issues in Nursing, 9*(3).

Herr, K. (2005). Pain assessment in the older adult with verbal communication skills. In S. J. Gibson & D. K. Weiner (Eds.), *Pain in older persons* (pp. 111–133). Seattle, WA: IASP Press.

McDonald, D. (2009). Older adults' pain descriptions. *Pain Management Nursing, 10,* 142–148.

McDonald, D. D., & Fedo, J. (2009). Older adults' pain communication: The effect of interruption. *Pain Management Nursing, 10,* 149–153.

McDonald, D., Shea, M., Rose, L., & Fedo, J. (2009). The effect of pain question phrasing on older adult pain information. *Journal of Pain and Symptom Management, 37,* 1050–1060.

National Guideline Clearing House. (2004). *Pain Management In: Evidence-based geriatric nursing protocols for best practice.* Retrieved February 16, 2010, from http://www.guideline.gov/summary/summary.aspx?ss=15&doc_id=12268&nbr=6352 database

National Guideline Clearing House. (2009). *Acute pain management in older adults.* Retrieved February 16, 2010, from http://www.guideline.gov/summary/summary.aspx?ss=15&doc_id=10198&nbr=5382 database

Pasero, C., & McCaffery, M. (2010). *Pain assessment and pharmacologic management* (3rd ed.). St. Louis, MO: Mosby Elsevier.

Royal College of Physicians, British Geriatrics Society and British Pain Society (2007). *The assessment of pain in older people. National guidelines. Concise guidance to good practice series* (Number 8). London, UK: RCP.

Rudy, T. E., & Lieber, S. J. (2005). Functional assessment of older adults with chronic pain. In S. J. Gibson & D. K. Weiner (Eds.), *Pain in older persons: Progress in pain research and management* (Vol. 35, pp. 153–174). Seattle, WA: IASP Press.

Thomas, S. H., & Silen, W. (2003). Effect on diagnostic efficiency of analgesia for undifferentiated abdominal pain. *British Journal of Surgery, 90,* 5–9.

Thomas, S. H., Silen, W., Cheema, F., Reisner, A., Aman, S., Goldstein, J. N., Stair, T. O. (2003). Effects of morphine analgesia on diagnostic accuracy in emergency department patients with abdominal pain: A prospective randomized trial. *Journal of the American College of Surgeons, 196,* 18–31.

Vermeulen, B., Morabia, A., Unger, P. F., Goehring, C., Skljarov, I., & Terrier, F. (1999). Acute appendicitis: Influence of early pain relief on the accuracy of clinical and US findings in the decision to operate–A randomized trial. *Radiology, 1999,* 639–643.

Yonan, C. A., & Wegener, S. T. (2003). Assessment and management of pain in the older adult. *Rehabilitation Psychology, 48,* 4–13.

4

Assessing Pain in the Nonverbal, Cognitively Impaired Older Adult

In this chapter, the assessment needs of older adults who are nonverbal and/or cognitively impaired will be discussed. "Age is the highest risk factor for both dementia and pain" (Scherder et al., 2009, p. 276). It is estimated that approximately 5% of all those between 65 and 75 years of age have Alzheimer's disease (AD) – that is, the dementia for which most statistics are available. Among those over 85 years of age, up to 50% may have AD (Centers for Disease Control and Prevention, 2010). In 2010, the Alzheimer's Association estimated that 5.1 million Americans over 65 years of age were diagnosed with AD. Communication about what is being experienced (i.e., pain) can be very difficult when there is cognitive impairment.

Assessment of pain is always challenging because pain is a subjective experience, and no one other than the experiencing person can totally understand it. This challenge is dramatically increased when the pain assessment is with an older adult who is nonverbal or who has cognitive impairments. As with any individual, appropriate treatment is dependent upon the results of a thorough assessment. When traditional assessment techniques are used with individuals suffering from cognitive impairment, pain may go unrecognized, which may lead to delays in diagnosis and result in unrelieved pain (Defrin, Lotan, & Pick, 2006).

Traditional assessment may be limited or not possible when older adults have significant cognitive impairments. Language, comprehension, interpretation, and/or abstract reasoning may be impaired. This impairment can occur when the older adult receives a message such as an assessment question, or attempts to send a message as in responding to the question, or both.

It is important to understand that individuals with mild or moderate cognitive impairment are able to report pain and participate in assessment. Older adults with mild or moderate cognitive impairment can reliably use the verbal descriptor scale and numeric rating scale when instructions are clear and explanations are patiently repeated (Chibnall & Tait, 2001; Closs, Barr, Briggs, Cash, & Seers, 2004; Gagliese, 2009). In contrast, some older adults with more severe cognitive impairment can feel pain sensation but do not necessarily identify it as pain (Ferrell, Ferrell, & Rivera, 1995). Cognitive impairments may be long standing as with developmental disability and brain trauma, or they may be more recent as with dementia, AD, or trauma. The etiology and degree of impairment will influence how pain is assessed. The ability to accurately assess pain is affected by the source of the impairment and the part of the brain affected. For example, older adults who have had a cerebral vascular accident that affected speech may be able to point at pain levels on a written pain scale, whereas those with an injury or disease in another area of the brain may no longer have that ability.

A common cognitive impairment in older adults is dementia, which is a "progressive and debilitating disease characterized by severe cognitive deficits, loss of language, and the ability to carry out ADLs" (Herr, Bjoro, & Decker, 2006, p. 170). As dementia is progressive, the limitations associated with it change and become more intense over time. Rather than using words to describe pain, the person with progressive dementia may express pain through behavior, such as increased confusion, withdrawal, gait changes, aggressive behavior, or other behaviors that may not usually be associated with pain (Gordon, 1999; Herr et al., 2006; Kaasalainen, 2007).

In addition to the barriers to assessing pain in general among older adults (Chapter 3), there are barriers specific to assessing pain in older adults with cognitive impairment. Older adults with dementia may not complain of pain and limitations, or inability to communicate about pain may be a constraint experienced by them (Defrin et al., 2006; Horgas, Nichols, Schapson, & Vietes, 2007). Often people living with dementia do not have the ability to understand changes over time regarding pain and are not able to report the character or quality of pain (Kelley, Siegler, & Reid, 2008). Some common misconceptions include the following:

- Older patients do not experience or perceive pain.
- Appropriate and thorough assessment of older adults with cognitive impairment is more time consuming than normal (that may or may not be true).
- A flat emotional affect indicates an absence of pain.

It is known that pain in older adults with cognitive impairment is both underestimated and undertreated (Kaasalainen, 2007; Shega et al., 2007).

Pearl	Many patients diagnosed with cognitive impairment *are* able to self-report pain.

Using simple assessment tools, pain can be successfully assessed in older adults who have cognitive impairment (Feldt, 2000). Generally, individuals who have a score of 18 or higher on the mini mental status exam are able to reliably self-report pain (Hadjistavropoulos, 2005). It is important to remember that even when older adults with dementia may not be able to report pain, it is believed that they experience pain in a normal way (Benedetti et al., 2004; Shega et al., 2007).

Even those patients who cannot self-report pain in the traditional way can participate in the assessment of pain through their behavior. Some behaviors that indicate pain include guarding, moaning, calling out, or restlessness. Clinicians must be attentive to the behaviors that these patients exhibit.

Family members or caregivers of individuals with long-standing cognitive limitations will be able to share communication methods that are effective with the patient. When the patient has been nonverbal or lived with cognitive impairment for an extended time, the family and caregivers most likely know what cues and behaviors indicate pain or discomfort. Even family members or caregivers of older adults with more recent onset of cognitive impairment may be able to share communication techniques, cues, or behaviors that indicate pain. Often, behaviors such as withdrawal, agitation, increased confusion, sleep alterations, decreased appetite, or change in activity indicate pain in older adults with cognitive impairment (Shega et al., 2007).

Pearl	Pain management in older adults who have comorbid dementia is complicated, and the assessment must be individualized with awareness that behaviors, including those not usually associated with pain, may indicate pain.

In recent years, many tools were developed to assess pain in older adults with cognitive impairment. They vary in reliability and validity and will be discussed in detail in Chapter 5. A commonality among tools is assessment of behaviors. As pain at rest may be different and less severe than pain with activity, the behaviors should be observed both at rest and with activity (Herr et al., 2006).

The American Geriatric Society listed six categories of behavior that indicate pain. These categories are as follows:

- *Facial expressions,* including grimacing, frowning, closed eyes, and rapid blinking.
- *Vocalizations* such as moaning, groaning, chanting, noisy breathing, and calling for help.
- *Body movements,* including muscle tension, pacing, fidgeting, rocking, and rubbing a body area.
- *Interpersonal interactions* that may include aggression, disruptive behavior, resistance, and withdrawal.
- *Changes in activity patterns* of eating, sleeping, or usual activities.
- *Changes in mental status* that may include increased confusion, sadness, crying, or irritability.

In a study comparing pain-related behaviors in 53 cognitively intact and 35 cognitively impaired older adults, no significant differences were noted. Pain behaviors were noted as vocalizations, grimaces, bracing, rubbing, restlessness, as well as verbal complaints of pain (Feldt, 2000).

Common painful conditions that occur in older adults with cognitive impairment include the following:

- Musculoskeletal injuries, pathologies, or fractures
- Urinary tract infections or urinary retention
- Pressure ulcers
- Poststroke syndrome
- Postherpetic neuralgia
- Cancer
- Peripheral vascular disease
- Diabetic neuropathy
- Polymyalgia
- Body position and contractures
- Dental problems
- Ear impaction or infection
- Eye infections
- Constipation

(Kerr, Cunningham, & Wilkinson, 2006; Shega et al., 2007)

Assessment of pain in the older adult with cognitive impairment may include self-report, use of assessment tools, physical examination, assessment of behavior, and information reported by family or caregivers. Once these various components are considered, the next step is an analgesic trial with medications appropriate to manage the pain indicated, with consideration of medications currently prescribed for other comorbidities (Pasero & McCaffery, 2010).

Pearl	It is important to consider self-report from the patient, as well as unusual behaviors, changes in usual behavior, assessment tool findings, information from caregivers, physical exam findings, and analgesic trial results in pain assessment of the cognitively impaired older adult.

GUIDELINES

American Geriatric Society. (2002). AGS panel on persistent pain in older persons. *JAGS, 50,* S205–S224.

American Pain Society. (2005). Current understanding of assessment, management, and treatments.

ASPMN Position Statement. (2006). Pain assessment in the nonverbal patient: Position statement with clinical practice recommendations. *Pain Management Nursing, 7(2),* 44–52.

Interdisciplinary Expert Consensus Statement on Assessment of Pain in Older Adults. (2007). *Clinical Journal of Pain, 23,* S1–S43.

Practice Guidelines for Assessing Pain in Older Persons with Dementia Residing in Long-Term Care Facilities. (2010). *Physiotherapy Canada, 62,* 104–113.

Case Study

Today, Mrs. Jackson was driven to her appointment by her daughter. Although Mrs. Jackson was diagnosed with early dementia 19 months ago, she has actively participated in her physical assessments every 3 months. Today her affect is flat and she is not responding to many questions. When asked about pain, she nods but does not speak. Her daughter reports that Mrs. Jackson fell after slipping on a scatter rug 3 weeks ago and has been quieter ever since. During physical assessment, it is noted that her breathing is shallow and breath sounds are diminished on the right side. When her right ribs are touched, Mrs. Jackson guards the area,

(continued)

flinches, and makes a slight moaning sound. When asked if the rib area is painful, she nods but does not respond to questions about a number for the pain or the character of the pain.

Questions

1. What is your assessment of pain in Mrs. Jackson?
2. Do you think that her flat affect is related to the pain?
3. Do you have enough information to start Mrs. Jackson on a trial of analgesic medication?
4. What education do you provide to Mrs. Jackson and her daughter?
5. What additional tests are indicated?

REFERENCES

Alzheimer's Association. (2010). Alzheimer's disease facts and figures, Alzheimer's & Dementia. *Alzheimer's disease facts and figures, 2010, 6.* Retrieved February 27, 2011, from http://www.alz.org/documents_custom/report_alzfactsfigures2010.pdf database

Benedetti, F., Arduino, C., Vighetti, S., Asteggiano, G., Tarenzi, L, & Rainero, I. (2004). Pain reactivity in Alzheimer patients with different degrees of cognitive impairment and brain electrical activity deterioration. *Pain, 111,* 22–29.

Centers for Disease Control. (2010). Alzheimer's disease. *Healthy aging.* Retrieved February 27, 2011, from http://www.cdc.gov/aging/aginginfo/alzheimers.htm database

Chibnall, J. T., & Tait, R. C. (2001). Pain assessment in cognitively impaired and unimpaired older adults: A comparison of four scales. *Pain, 92,* 173–186.

Closs, S. J., Barr, B., Briggs, M., Cash, K., & Seers, K. (2004). A comparison of five pain assessment scales for nursing home residents with varying degrees of cognitive impairment. *Journal of Pain and Symptom Management, 27,* 196–205.

Defrin, R., Lotan, M., & Pick, C. G. (2006). The evaluation of acute pain in individuals with cognitive impairment: A differential effect of the level of impairment. *Pain, 124,* 312–320.

Feldt, K. (2000). The checklist of nonverbal pain indicators (CNPI). *Pain Management Nursing, 1,* 13–21.

Ferrell, B. A., Ferrell, B. R., & Rivera, L. (1995). Pain in cognitively impaired nursing home patients. *Journal of Pain and Symptom Management, 8,* 591–598.

Gagliese, L. (2009). Pain and aging: The emergence of a new subfield of pain research. *The Journal of Pain, 10,* 343–353.

Gordon, D. (1999). Pain management in the elderly. *Journal of Perianesthesia Nursing, 14,* 367–372.

Hadjistavropoulos, T. (2005). Assessing pain in older adults with severe limitations in ability to communicate. In S. J. Gibson & D. K. Weiner (Eds.), *Pain in older adults: Progress in pain research and management* (Vol. 35, pp. 135–151). Seattle, WA: IASP Press.

Herr, K., Bjoro, K., & Decker, S. (2006). Tools for assessment of pain in nonverbal older adults with dementia: A state-of-the-science review. *Journal of Pain and Symptom Management, 31,* 170–192.

Herr, K., Coyne, P., Key, T., Manworren, R., McCaffery, M., Merkel, S., Wild, L. (2006). Pain assessment in the nonverbal patient: Position statement with clinical practice recommendations. *Pain Management Nursing, 7,* 44–52.

Horgas, A. L., Nichols, A. L., Schapson, C. A., & Vietes, K. (2007). Assessing pain in persons with dementia: Relationships among non-communicative patient's pain assessment instrument, self-report, and behavioral observations. *Pain Management Nursing, 8,* 77–85.

Kaasalainen, S. (2007). Pain assessment in older adults with dementia. *Journal of Gerontological Nursing, 33*(6), 6–10.

Kelley, A. S., Siegler, E. L., & Reid, M. C. (2008). Pitfalls and recommendations regarding the management of acute pain among hospitalized patients with dementia. *Pain Medicine, 9,* 581–586.

Kerr, D., Cunningham, C., & Wilkinson, H. (2006) *Responding to the pain experiences of people with a learning difficulty and dementia. Joseph Rowntree Foundation.* Retrieved February 01, 2011, from www.jrf.org.uk/bookshop

McCaffery, M., & Pasero, C. (2010). *Pain: Clinical Manual (2nd Ed.).* St. Louis, MO: Mosby Elsevier.

Scherder, E., Herr, K., Pickering, G., Gibson, S., Benedetti, F. & Lautenbacher, S. (2009). Pain in dementia. *Pain, 145,* 276-278.

Shega, J., Emanuel, L., Vargish, L., Levine, S. K., Bursch, H., Herr, K., Weiner, D. K. (2007). Pain in persons with dementia: Complex, common, and challenging. *The Journal of Pain, 8,* 373–378.

5

A Review of Pain Assessment Tools for Use with the Older Adult Patient

Appropriate pain management is dependent upon thorough pain assessment. One aspect of pain that can be assessed using objective tools is pain intensity. Using the same tool consistently, it is possible to monitor over time the effectiveness of pain management interventions with the individual patient.

SELECTING THE CORRECT TOOL

There are numerous tools available for assessing pain. No one assessment tool has been found to be particularly effective in assessing pain in older adults (Gordon, 1999). It is important that older adults are able to respond to and to use a tool that will provide the most accurate assessment of pain possible. Cognitive, psychological, social, and communication issues may affect the ability to use a particular tool.

Each pain assessment tool has strengths and limitations. Two factors need to be considered when selecting the most appropriate tool for the individual patient:

■ Ensure that the tool meets the sensory and cognitive needs of the patient.
■ Ensure that the tool you selected is reliable and valid.

It is important that all members of the health care team are willing to use the same tool to ensure consistency of assessment.

Once the most appropriate tool has been selected, ensure that the sensory needs of the patient are met. Regardless of the tool selected, use clear copies with large fonts and obvious contrasting colors or shading if it is in black and white. Verbal instructions or verbal versions of the scales should be clearly spoken, providing adequate time and opportunity for questions.

One-Dimensional or Unidimensional Pain Scales

They assess a single dimension of the pain experience, which is generally a measure of pain intensity. The most common one-dimensional pain scales used with older adults are the visual analog scale (VAS), the numeric rating scale (NRS), and the verbal descriptor scale (VDS) or verbal rating scale (VRS). In several studies, significant association was seen among these three scales (Deconno et al., 1994). They are discussed in greater detail below.

Visual Analog Scale

It is a simple tool that consists of a 100 mm line that is free of words and numbers. It must be explained to the person that no pain at all (zero) is on the left and the most possible pain to experience is on the right. The patient is then instructed to put a single mark on the line that is consistent with the pain being experienced. The health care provider (HCP) then measures where on the line the person made the mark. That measurement is the pain score. If the person marked the line at 77 mm the score is 77/100 mm, which would be comparable to 7.7 on the NRS of 0 to 10. The VAS is often used in research because it is considered the most sensitive to statistical analysis (Huskisson, 1982).

Limitations

- Use of the VAS requires abstract thought (conveying the pain being experienced to a single place on a line). That may be difficult for some older adults, especially those with cognitive impairment.
- Some older adults have difficulty putting a single mark on the line where they believe their pain ranks.
- Accuracy of measurement is dependent upon the instructions given to the patient. With any individual, the accuracy of clinically significant changes in subsequent VAS scores may be related to the degree of pain first rated on the initial VAS.
- Recording the report of pain requires the HCP to accurately measure along the 100 mm line (Price, Bush, Long, & Harkins, 1994). This can be tedious and time consuming.

(Bird & Dickson, 2001; D'Arcy, 2011; Herr & Mobily, 1993; Price et al., 1994).

Strengths

- The VAS is considered a very sensitive gauge of pain intensity.
- Because no language is used after the initial instructions, there is less bias or influence through the connotation of words or numbers.

- The possible rating of pain is limitless since there are no numeric or word limitations.
- When used to measure pain, the VAS is reported as reliable and generalizable, with good internal consistency when used clinically and in research studies.
- It is highly correlated with other pain assessment tools, including the NRS and pain thermometer.

(Hadjistavropoulos et al., 2007; Herr & Mobily, 1993; Huskisson, 1982; Price et al., 1994).

Numeric Rating Scale

There are many varieties of this scale, but the basic scale consists of the person rating pain using a number between 0 and 10. The number indicates the intensity of the pain being experienced.

The paper copy of the scale has a line with 11 numbers ranging from 0 to 10. Sometimes there are word descriptors used along with the scale (Figure 5.1), and sometimes there are colors used ranging from blue at 0 and 1 fading to green, yellow, orange, and red at 9 and 10.

Whether a paper copy of the scale is used or not, the verbal instructions to the person are the same. The instructions are "on a scale of 0 to 10 with 0 being no pain at all and 10 being the worst pain you can imagine, what number describes your pain now?"

Often patients ask what the numbers mean. It may be helpful to explain that the numbers are individual for the patient. There is no right or wrong number, and they are not compared with numbers other people use to identify their pain. It can also be helpful to give some examples of assigning a number to pain. No pain is the easiest because it is 0. Many people rate mild pain as 3 when they are able to read, play cards, watch television, visit, or fall asleep. Moderate pain is often rated as 5 and may be the pain that occurs with moving after surgery or an injury. It is pain that may be bearable for a brief time but not for longer. Pain that is in varying degrees of greater severity

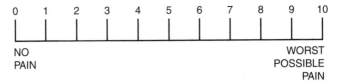

Figure 5.1 ■ Numeric rating scale.

tends to be 6 or greater. Pain that is 10 on the NRS is the worst pain that can be imagined, not the worst pain that has been experienced.

Interestingly in their study with older adults, Herr and Mobily (1993) reported that 36.4% of the subjects with a high-school education or less preferred the NRS, whereas none of the participants with more than a high-school education preferred it.

Limitations

- Use of this scale requires abstract thought that may not be possible for some older adults, particularly those with cognitive impairment.
- Many patients become frustrated with using numbers to rate their pain.
- Test–retest reliability is diminished in older adults with cognitive impairment.
- When compared with previous scores, the NRS provides information on whether pain has increased or decreased, but it is not possible to calculate a true percentage of change, which may be less important clinically.

(Hadjistavropoulos et al., 2007; Price et al., 1994).

Strengths

- This is the preferred tool by some older adults.
- It is sensitive to changes in pain and can be used with multiple pain sites.
- Internal consistency is high.
- Test–retest reliability is generally adequate.
- Strong positive correlations have been reported with other pain scales.
- It has been used effectively by older adults with cognitive impairment.
- It is a very common pain assessment tool that is widely used in many health care organizations.

(Hadjistavropoulos et al., 2007; Ware, Epps, Herr, & Packard, 2006).

VDS or VRS

There is a variety of VDS tools, with choices ranging from four to seven words that can describe the pain being experienced. The simplest uses four choices of "no pain," "a little pain," "medium pain," or "a lot of pain." An example of a VDS with seven descriptors is in Figure 5.2 (Hadjistavropoulos et al., 2007; Herr, 2005).

Limitations

- This scale can be difficult for some older adults because it requires abstract thought to quantify in words the degree of pain being experienced.

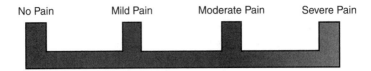

| No Pain | Mild Pain | Moderate Pain | Severe Pain |

Figure 5.2 ■ Verbal descriptors.

■ For many people, it is difficult to categorize pain using the limited number of word choices (Hadjistavropoulos et al., 2007).

Strengths

■ It is often preferred by older adults.

■ It has been used effectively by older adults with cognitive impairment.

■ In their study with older adults, Herr and Mobily (1993) reported that most participants found the VDS was the easiest to use of the five scales tested.

■ It has strong positive correlations with other pain assessment scales. (Gordon, 1999; Hadjistavropoulos et al., 2007; Ware et al., 2006).

Faces Pain Scale—Revised

Bieri, Reeve, Champion, Addicoat, and Ziegler (1990) developed the original faces pain scale (FPS) in 1990 as an adaptation of the Wong-Baker FACES pain scale. The FPS was later adapted (Figure 5.3) by Hicks to be consistent with the 0 to 10 of the NRS.

The FPS-R consists of six faces illustrated with expressions ranging from smiling to distress.

There is no cost to reproduce the FPS-R for clinical use. To ensure clarity, it is recommended to download the FPS-R directly from the official FPS-R website www.usask.ca/childpain/fpsr, where it is available with instructions in 47 different languages.

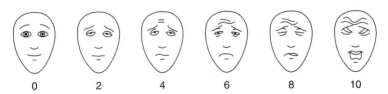

| 0 | 2 | 4 | 6 | 8 | 10 |

Figure 5.3 ■ Faces pain scale—revised
©2001 International Association for the Study of Pain.

Limitations

- Some reports are that correlation with other scales is weaker.
- Whether it is assessing only the intensity of pain is not clear; it may also be assessing affective aspects of pain.

(Hadjistavropoulos et al., 2007).

Strengths

- The cartoon faces do not appear childlike.
- The absence of tears avoids any connotations or associations with crying and pain.
- Validity and reliability have been demonstrated in various groups of older adults.
- Test–retest reliability and reproducibility of the FPS and FPS-R over time have been good.
- Preferred by many older adults, especially those with African American, Spanish, and Chinese backgrounds.
- The FPS was used effectively with older adults with cognitive impairment.
- Since it does not require language, it is helpful when language is a barrier.

A preliminary study indicated that a vertical version of the FPS was valid and reliable in patients who had experienced a left hemispheric stroke.

(Benaim et al., 2007; Hadjistavropoulos et al., 2007; Herr, Mobily, Kohout, & Wagenaar, 1998; Herr, 2010; Li, Liu, & Herr, 2007; Stuppy, 1998; Taylor & Herr, 2003; Ware et al., 2006).

Iowa Pain Thermometer

This tool combines a picture of a thermometer (Figure 5.4) with word descriptors indicating that the pain intensifies as the temperature rises on the thermometer (Herr, 2007). The patient is shown the picture and asked to think of pain rising in the same manner as the temperature rises on the thermometer.

Limitations

- It is not commonly used by clinicians.

Strengths

- The thermometer provides a concrete focus for what is otherwise abstract thinking of pain.
- In their study with older adults, Herr and Mobily (1993) found that the pain thermometer was the second most popular pain assessment tool among the participants.

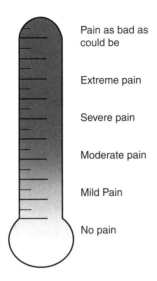

Figure 5.4 ■ Iowa pain thermometer scale.

Source: Used with permission from Keela Herr, PhD, RN, FAAN, AGSF, The University of Iowa, College of Nursing.

■ It is used effectively by older adults with cognitive impairment.
■ Its use is consistent with national guideline recommendations. It is reliable and valid.

(Hadjistavropoulos et al., 2007; Herr, 2007; Taylor & Herr, 2003; Ware et al., 2006).

Assessment of Neuropathic Pain—The Leeds Assessment of Neuropathic Symptoms and Signs

The Leeds Assessment of Neuropathic Symptoms and Signs (LANSS) is a two-part screening tool that was designed to identify pain that is predominantly of neuropathic origin. The first part consists of five self-report questions, each of which has two response options. The second part of the tool is completed by the HCP assessing allodynia and pin prick threshold. The score indicates that it either is or is not likely that neuropathic mechanisms contribute to the pain that is being experienced. A short version is the S-LANSS that includes the self-assessment questions but not the physical examination portion (Bennett, 2001; Bennett et al., 2007; Bouhassira & Attal, 2011; CSL Biotherapies, n.d.).

Limitations

■ It is a screening, not a diagnostic, tool.

- It was not designed to be a measurement tool.
- If more than one body area needs to be assessed, the LANNS needs to be administered for each body part. This is true of all currently available neuropathic assessment tools.

(Bennett et al., 2007; Bouhassira & Attal, 2011).

   Strengths
- LANNS is simple and easy to use.
- It is effective in identifying patients with pain that is primarily of a neuropathic origin.
- Although not designed as a measurement tool, sensitivity to the effects of treatment has been reported.
- It is validated in several settings with good sensitivity and specificity.
- The short version has also been validated. It is comparable to clinical, positive predictive value in diagnosis of NP.
- LANNS has been studied in patients with radiculopathies and complex regional syndrome type 1 as well as NP.

(Bennett, Smith, Torrance, & Lee, 2006; Bennett et al., 2007; Bouhassira & Attal, 2011).

Multidimensional Pain Scales

Although pain is most commonly assessed using a unidimensional scale to measure severity, pain is a multidimensional experience that includes affective, sensory, and functional components. Multidimensional pain scales can be used to measure those components.

The Short-form McGill Pain Questionnaire

The short-form McGill pain questionnaire (SF-MPQ) (Figure 5.5) derived from the McGill pain questionnaire is short and easy to use in the clinical setting, with 11 sensory and 4 affective descriptors that are also rated on a 4-point scale ranging from none (0) to severe (3). Total scores can range from 0 to 40, with 0 being no pain and 40 being maximum pain. The questionnaire allows for three summary pain scores to be obtained. In addition to the total score, the current pain intensity as perceived by the subject is measured using the VAS. It usually takes between 2 and 5 minutes to complete. This tool assesses both intensity and quality of pain (Dudgeon, Raubertas, & Rosenthal, 1993; Katz & Melzack, 1999; McDonald & Weiskopf, 2001; Melzack, 1975; Melzack, 1987).

Selecting the Correct Tool **63**

Appendix IV (i)

SHORT-FORM McGILL PAIN QUESTIONNAIRE AND PAIN DIAGRAM

(Repoduced with permission of author © Dr. Ron Melzack, for publication and distribution)

Date: _____

Name: _____

Check the column to indicate the level of your pain for each word, or leave blank if it does not apply to you.

	Mild	Moderate	Severe
1 Throbbing	_____	_____	_____
2 Shooting	_____	_____	_____
3 Stabbing	_____	_____	_____
4 Sharp	_____	_____	_____
5 Cramping	_____	_____	_____
6 Gnawing	_____	_____	_____
7 Hot-Burning	_____	_____	_____
8 Aching	_____	_____	_____
9 Heavy	_____	_____	_____
10 Tender	_____	_____	_____
11 Splitting	_____	_____	_____
12 Tiring-Exhausting	_____	_____	_____
13 Sickening	_____	_____	_____
14 Fearful	_____	_____	_____
15 Cruel-Punishing	_____	_____	_____

Mark or comment on the above figure where you have your pain or problems.

Indicate on this line how bad your pain is—at the left end of line means no pain at all, at right end means worst pain possible.

No Pain	_____	Worst Possible Pain

S	/33	A	/ 12	VAS	/ 10

Figure 5.5 ■ Short-form McGill pain questionnaire. Used with permission of Dr. R. Melzack.

Limitations
- It requires language and reading ability.
- Although the term gnawing is considered a sensory descriptor in the SF-MPQ, it has also been shown to be characterized as an affective descriptor.

(Wright, Asmundson, & McCreary, 2001).

Strengths
- SF-MPQ is short and easy to use.
- Validity and reliability for the SF-MPQ among patients with various conditions in a variety of settings have been strong.
- It has proven reliability and validity when used specifically with older adults.

(Dudgeon et al., 1993; Grafton, Foster, & Wright, 2005; Herr, 2005; McDonald & Weiskopf, 2001; Melzack, 2005; Wright et al., 2001).

Short-form McGill Pain Questionnaire revised (SF-MPQ-2)

Recently the SF-MPQ was revised to include descriptions that reflected symptoms of NP. Initial testing was done with 882 subjects, of whom 226 lived with painful diabetic neuropathy (PDN).

Limitations
- At this point, it is intended to be used for epidemiological and clinical research.
- Additional research is needed.

Strengths
- The reliability and validity were reported as excellent.
- A single instrument measures nociceptive and NP.

(Dworkin et al., 2009).

Brief Pain Inventory (BPI)

It is a 16-item tool that can be used to assess pain severity, as well as the effect of pain on function during a 24-hour period. Pain severity is assessed on a 0 to 10 scale at its worst, at its least, on the average, and right now. The person is asked to shade the areas of full-body diagrams with both front and back views and to mark the area where the greatest pain is felt. Two analgesia questions ask what medications are taken for pain and what percentage of relief those medications have provided during the last 24 hours.

From a functional perspective, on a 0 to 10 scale, it asks how pain interferes with
- general activity
- mood
- walking ability
- normal work (both work outside the home and housework)
- relations with other people
- sleep
- enjoyment of life

(Cleeland & Syrjala, 1992; Mendoza et al., 2004)

Limitations
- Brief pain inventory requires an ability to read and think abstractly.
- It requires short-term memory ability.

Strengths
- It provides greater insight into the pain experience over time.
- It assesses pain intensity as well as social and functional limitations.
- It is valid with older adults following surgery.

(Mendoza et al., 2004).

Combined Thermometer Scale

It is a modification of the Iowa Pain Thermometer that includes words that describe pain distress and pain intensity. It also includes numbers ranging from 0 to 10. Both the words and the numbers reflect an increase in the intensity of the pain experience. It often is colored, ranging from blue at the bottom of the thermometer to bright red at the top of the thermometer, indicating agonizing or the worst pain possible. It combines the VDS and the NRS, which are one-dimensional scales measuring pain intensity (D'Arcy, 2011). As it also includes word descriptors that measure distress, it is listed in the multidimensional pain scales category.

Limitations
- Some older adults may be confused by words, numbers, and colors all in one tool.
- There is no documented reliability or validity for the combined tool.
- It is difficult to determine whether pain intensity or pain distress is being measured.

Strengths
- Some considered it to be a simple and easy to use format.
- It is expected that pain ratings can be duplicated for reassessment.

(D'Arcy, 2011).

Behavioral Pain Scales—The Pain Behavior Checklist

As noted by Kerns et al. (1991), it is important to include pain behavior measures when the goal of care is to better understand the etiology of pain. The pain behavior checklist (PBC) is used to measure thoughts, feelings, and behaviors that the patient associates with living with pain. The PBC, which contains 17 items that are rated on a 7-point scale, was developed as a self-report tool.

Limitations
- It is an additional tool for the patient to complete.

Strengths
- It does not take much time (generally 5 to 10 minutes) to complete.
- It gives additional insight into the pain experience of the individual patient.
- Reliability and validity tests were strong.

(Kerns et al., 1991).

Pain Behavior Tools to Evaluate Pain in Older Adults with Cognitive Impairment

In recent years, a number of tools have been developed with the intent of assessing pain in older adults who have cognitive impairments. Although assessment of pain in this population is important, it is essential to note that these tools continue to be tested psychometrically and need additional testing in larger samples of cognitively impaired older adults (Herr, Bjoro, & Decker, 2006; Kaasalainen, 2007; Zwakhalen, Hamers, Abu-Saad, & Berger, 2006). As pain is a subjective experience, it must be remembered that self-report is the most reliable method of assessment and that agreement of pain scores and observed behavior is not established (Jordan, Hughes, Pakresi, Hepburn, & O'Brien, 2011).

All pain tools that assess pain other than self-report rely on information that is construed as indicating pain.

The Checklist for Nonverbal Pain Indicators

The checklist for nonverbal pain indicators (CNPI) is one of the early tools designed to specifically assess pain in cognitively impaired older adults (Feldt, 2000). This tool is used by observing three aspects of behavior (verbalization, facial expressions, and body movements) in older adults. The observer rates the behavior as either being 0 if not present or 1 if present and are then added. The sum for activity is one score and the sum for at rest is a separate score. The specific indicators that are assessed with movement and at rest are

- vocal complaints (including "moans, groans, grunts, cries, gasps, sighs")
- facial grimaces (including "furrowed brow, narrowed eyes, tightened lips, dropped jaw, clenched teeth, distorted expression")
- bracing (including clutching or holding onto furniture, person, or body area)
- restlessness (including "constant or intermittent shifting position, rocking, intermittent hand motions, inability to keep still")
- rubbing (or massaging the affected area)
- Vocal complaints (verbal expressions of pain using words, e.g., 'ouch' or 'that hurts', cursing during movement or exclamation of protest, e.g., 'stop' or 'that's enough')

(Feldt, 2000; Nygaard & Jarland, 2006).

Limitations

- Additional testing is needed to establish validity.
- The indicators are not unique to pain. In one study it was noted that of 46 patients, 6 who reported pain did not exhibit the behaviors, whereas 6 who denied pain did exhibit some of the behaviors.
- Behaviors were seen less frequently at rest, leading the developer to conclude that the CNPI is more useful during activities.
- The CNPI includes only three—facial expression, vocalization, and body movements—of the six behavior categories listed in the American Geriatric Society guidelines for assessing persistent pain."
- Additional study is needed to strengthen the validity and reliability of the CNPI.
- The tool does not account for changes in mental status, interpersonal interactions, or activity patterns.
- Research and data are needed to determine how effective this tool is when used by staff nurses; however, interrater reliability among Norwegian nursing home staff was adequate (Nygaard & Jarland, 2006).
- As pain is a subjective experience, it is difficult to determine what the scoring means (Kaasalainen, 2007).
- Additional psychometric testing is needed in larger samples.
- Breathing and consolability are not known to be significant to pain in the older adults.

(Feldt, 2000; Herr, Bjoro et al., 2006; Herr, Coyne, et al., 2006; Kaasalainen, 2007; Nygaard & Jarland, 2006; Stolee et al., 2005; Zwakhalen et al., 2006).

Strengths

■ Instructions for use are clear and easy to follow.
■ Scoring is simple and does not require interpretation.
■ It is easy to use at the bedside (Nygaard & Jarland, 2006); however, in one study observations took 5 minutes before scoring.
■ It is considered to be a useful instrument for measuring pain during activities in patients after surgery.
■ Reliability was considered adequate (Stolee et al., 2005).
■ Interrater reliability was very high in one small study.

(Dewaters, Popovich, & Faut-Callahan, 2003; Herr, Coyne, et al., 2006; Zwakhalen et al., 2006).

Pain Assessment in Advanced Dementia

The pain assessment in advanced dementia (PAINAD) is a tool (Figure 5.6) that measures pain in people with severe dementia using five indicators:

■ Breathing
■ Negative vocalizations
■ Facial expression
■ Body language
■ Consolability

It is used by observing the person with regard to each of the five categories. A score is given in each of the categories of 0, 1, or 2, depending upon what is observed (see Figure 5.6). A total score can range from 0 to 10. The PAINAD guideline for use includes definitions of the various descriptor terms in each category (Warden, Hurley, & Volicer, 2003).

Limitations

■ Additional research is needed to establish stability, internal consistency, and validity (Herr, Coyne, et al., 2006).
■ The behavior indicators are not unique to pain.
■ One study reported a high false-positive rate (33%), with psychosocial factors accounting for the observed behaviors rather than pain.
■ The PAINAD includes only three (facial expression, vocalization, and body movements) of the six behavior categories listed in the American Geriatric Society guidelines for assessing persistent pain.

Instructions: Observe patient for 5 minutes before scoring behaviors. Score behaviors according to the following chart. The patient can be observed under different conditions (e.g., at rest, during a pleasant activity, during caregiving, after administration of pain medication).

Behavior	0	1	2	Score
Breathing Independent of vocalization	• Normal	• Occasional labored breathing • Short period of hyperventilation	• Noisy labored breathing • Long period of hyperventilation • Cheyne-Stokes respirations	
Negative vocalization	• None	• Occasional moan or groan • Low-level speech with a negative or disapproving quality	• Repeated troubled calling out • Loud moaning or groaning • Crying	
Facial expression	• Smiling or inexpressive	• Sad • Frightened • Frown	• Facial grimacing	
Body language	• Relaxed	• Tense • Distressed pacing • Fidgeting	• Rigid • Fists clenched • Knees pulled up • Pulling or pushing away • Striking out	
Consolability	• No need to console	• Distracted or reassured by voice or touch	• Unable to console, distract, or reassure	
			TOTAL SCORE	

Scoring: Total score ranges from 0–10 points. Possible interpretations: 1–3 = mild pain; 4–6 = moderate pain; 7–10 = severe pain. Ranges are based on a standard 0–10 pain scale, but have not been substantiated in the literature for this tool. *Source:* Development and Psychometric Evaluation of the Pain Assessment in Advanced Dementia (PAINAD) Scale, by V. Warden, A. C. Hurley, and L. Volicer, 2003, *Journal of the American Medical Directors Association, 4,* pp. 9–15.

Figure 5.6 ■ Pain assessment in advanced dementia tool.

The tool does not account for changes in mental status, interpersonal interactions, or activity patterns.
- Many studies using the PAINAD did not solely involve subjects with severe dementia.
- The 0 to 10 scores can be confused with the NRS of 0 to 10 that reflects a self-report pain score. The score from the PAINAD does not equal the self-report of the NRS.
- It is not possible to interpret the summed score means.

(Herr, Coyne, et al., 2006; Jordan et al., 2011; Zwakhalen et al., 2006).

Strengths
- It has good interrater reliability (Herr, Coyne, et al. 2006).
- It is relatively easy to use.
- Sensitivity and assessing behavior as pain when pain is present have been reported as high with older adults with dementia.

(Jordan et al., 2011).

Assuming Pain Is Present

"Assuming pain is present" is not an assessment scale, but rather an assessment process that includes consideration of the following:
- Pain and medication history (including all preexisting painful conditions).
- Current pathology or trauma and the degree of pain associated with the diagnosis.
- Behaviors that may indicate pain (may need to utilize a pain behavior tool or reference).
- Consider information from family or others who know the patient well regarding behaviors indicative of pain.

Once this information is considered it should be used to start an analgesic trial with adjustments based upon reassessments of behavior and condition.

Limitations
- This is not a specific tool and there is no score.

Strengths
- The unique pain history, analgesia history, condition, and behaviors of the patient are considered.
- This process is consistent with nursing and medical critical thinking processes and professional patient care.

(Pasero, 2009; Pasero & McCaffery, 2005).

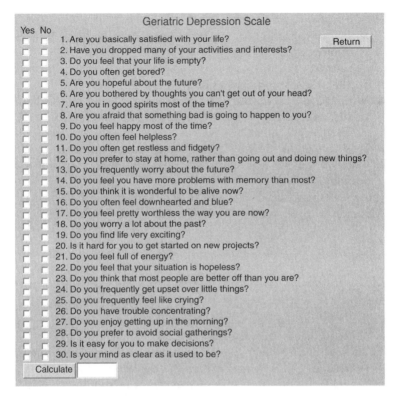

Figure 5.7 ■ Geriatric Depression Scale.

Geriatric Depression Scale

Because depression is common among older patients with chronic or persistent pain, using a tool to assess depression is helpful as a part of the assessment process. The Geriatric Depression Scale (GDS) (Figure 5.7) is a 30-item instrument that is considered to be the most effective tool to screen for depression in older adults. A unique aspect of the self-report GDS is that it is effective in distinguishing between depression and dementia in older adults (Brown & Schinka, 2005). The person responds yes or no to the questions regarding the past week. When compared with the longer version, the 15-item GDS proved to be comparable in effectiveness (Brown & Schinka, 2005; Kurlowicz, 2001).

Limitations

■ Specificity of the 15-item tool was lower than seen on the 30-item instrument.

Strengths

■ Scoring is simple and requires little time.

■ When the 15-item GDS was compared with the longer version, both validity and reliability were reported as good and consistent with the earlier version.

■ Sensitivity of the 15-item tool was higher than on the 30-item tool.

■ Criterion validity was equal to or higher than other geriatric screening tools.

(Brown & Schinka, 2005; Sheikh & Yesavage, 1986; Wancata, Alexandrowicz, Marquart, Weiss, & Friedrich, 2006).

GUIDELINES

AGS Panel on Persistent Pain in Older Persons. The management of persistent pain in older persons. *Journal of the American Geriatric Society (2002)50,* Supplement 205–224.

An Interdisciplinary expert consensus statement on assessment of pain in older adults. *Clinical Journal of Pain, 23,* Supplement 1-S43.

Faces Pain Scale—Revised (2010) www.usask.ca/childpain/fpsr

International Association for the Study of Pain (IASP) http://www .iasp-pain.org

PainKnowledge.org available at http://www.painknowledge.org

> *Case Study*

> Ronald Hawke is a 72-year-old man who is admitted to the hospital after falling from a ladder and landing on his right hip. He cannot remember the accident or why he was on the ladder. He reports that he has a 10-year history of diabetes and chronic low back pain. Now he is complaining about "really bad" pain in his right leg and tells you that this is the last straw. He does not want to have to deal with recuperating from this fall.

Questions

1. What information do you need to assess the pain in Mr. Hawke?
2. What tool or tools are most appropriate for assessing him?
3. Why have you selected the tools you did?
4. Could other tools provide additional information that could be important?

REFERENCES

Benaim, C., Froger, J., Cazottes, C., Gueben, D., Porte, M., Desneulle, C., & Pelissier, J. Y. (2007). Use of the faces pain scale by left and right hemispheric stroke patients. *Pain, 128,* 52–58.

Bennett, M. I. (2001). The LANSS pain scale: The leeds assessment of neuropathic symptoms and signs. *Pain, 92,* 147–157.

Bennett, M. I., Attal, N., Backonja, M. M., Baron, R., Bouhassira, D., Freynhagen, R., & Jensen, T. S. (2007). Using screening tools to identify neuropathic pain. *Pain, 127,* 199–203.

Bennett, M. I., Smith, B. H., Torrance, N., & Lee, A. J. (2006). Can pain be more or less neuropathic? Comparison of symptom assessment tools with ratings of certainty by clinicians. *Pain, 122,* 289–294.

Bieri, D., Reeve, R., Champion, G., Addicoat, L., & Ziegler, J. B. (1990). The faces pain scale for the self-assessment of the severity of pain experienced by children: Development, initial validation, and preliminary investigation for ratio scale properties. *Pain, 41,* 139–150.

Bird, S. B., & Dickson, E. W. (2001). Clinically significant changes in pain along the Visual Analog Scale. *Annals of Emergency Medicine, 38,* 639–643.

Bouhassira, D., & Attal, N. (2011). Diagnosis and assessment of neuropathic pain: The saga of clinical tools. *Pain, 152,* S74–S83.

Brown, L. M., & Schinka, J. A. (2005). Development and initial validation of a 15-item informant version of the Geriatric Depression Scale. *International Journal of Geriatric Psychiatry, 20,* 911–918.

Cleeland, C. S., & Syrjala, K. L. (1992). How to assess cancer pain. In D. C. Turk & R. Melzack (Eds.), *Handbook of pain assessment* (pp. 362–387). New York, NY: The Guilford Press.

CSL Biotherapies. (n.d.). Appendix 4 LANSS. *PAINXCHANGE Tailoring pain education on line.* Retrieved February 24, 2011, from http://www.painxchange.com.au/AssessmentTools/Appendices/PDF/Apx4_LANSS.pdf database

D'Arcy, Y. (2011). *Compact clinical guide to chronic pain management: An evidence-based approach for nurses.* New York, NY: Springer

Deconno, F., Caraceni, A., Gamba, A., Mariani, L., Abbattista, A., Brunelli, C., Ventafridda, V. (1994). Pain measurement in cancer patients: A comparison of six methods. *Pain, 57,* 161–166.

Dewaters, T., Popovich, J., & Faut-Callahan, M. (2003). An evaluation of clinical tools to measure pain in older people with cognitive impairment. *British Journal of Community Nursing, 8,* 226–234.

Dudgeon, D., Raubertas, R. F., & Rosenthal, S. N. (1993). The short-form McGill pain questionnaire in chronic cancer pain. *Journal of Pain and Symptom Management, 8,* 191–195.

Dworkin, R. F., Turk, D. C., Revicki, D. A., Harding, G., Coyne, K. S., Peirece-Sandner, S., Melzack, R. (2009). Development and initial validation of an expanded and revised version of the short-form McGill pain questionnaire (SF-MPQ-2). *Pain, 144,* 35–42.

Feldt, K. (2000). The Checklist of Nonverbal Pain Indicators (CNPI). *Pain Management Nursing, 1,* 13–21.

Gordon, D. (1999). Pain management in the elderly. *Journal of Perianesthesia Nursing, 14,* 367–372.

Grafton, K. V., Foster, N. E., & Wright, C. C. (2005). Test-retest reliability of the short-form McGill pain questionnaire: Assessment of intraclass correlation coefficients and limits of agreement in patients with osteoarthritis. *The Clinical Journal of Pain, 21,* 73–82.

Hadjistavropoulos, T., Herr, K., Turk, D. C., Fine, P. G., Dworkin, R. H., Helme, R., Williams, J. (2007). An interdisciplinary expert consensus statement on assessment of pain in older adults. *Clinical Journal of Pain, 23,* S1–S43.

Herr, K. (2007). Pain Thermometer Scale Overview. *PainKnowledge.org.* Retrieved February 21, 2011, from http://www.painknowledge.org/physician-tools/Pain_Thermometer/Pain%20Thermometer%20Scale%20Overview.pd database

Herr, K. (2010). Pain in the older adult: An imperative across all health care settings. *Pain Management Nursing, 11,* S1–S10.

Herr, K. A. (2005). Pain assessment in the older adult with verbal communication skills. In S. J. Gibson & D. K. Weiner (Eds.), *Pain in older adults* (pp. 111–133). Seattle, WA: IASP Press.

Herr, K., Bjoro, K., & Decker, S. (2006). Tools for assessment of pain in nonverbal older adults. *Journal of Pain and Symptom Management, 31,* 170–192.

Herr, K., Coyne, P. J., Manworren, R., McCaffery, M., Merkel, S., Pelosi-Kelly, J., & Wild, L. (2006). Pain assessment in the nonverbal patient: Position statement with clinical practice recommendations. *Pain Management Nursing, 7*(2), 44–52.

Herr, K., & Mobily, P. R. (1993). Comparison of selected pain assessment tools for use with the elderly. *Applied Nursing Research, 6,* 39–46.

Herr, K. A., Mobily, P. R., Kohout, F. J., & Wagenaar, D. (1998). Evaluation of the Faces Pain Scale for use with the elderly. *The Clinical Journal of Pain, 14,* 29–38.

Huskisson, E. C. (1982). Measurement of pain. *Journal of Rheumatology, 9,* 768–769.

Jordan, A., Hughes, J., Pakresi, M., Hepburn, S., & O'Brien, J. T. (2011). The utility of PAINAD in assessing pain in a UK population with severe dementia. *International Journal of Geriatric Psychiatry, 26,* 118–126.

Kaasalainen, S. (2007). Pain assessment in older adults with dementia. *Journal of Gerontological Nursing, 33*(6), 6–10.

Katz, J., & Melzack, R. (1999). Measurement of pain. *Surgical Clinics of North America, 79,* 231–252.

Kerns, R. D., Haythornthwaite, J., Rosenberg, R., Southwick, S., Giller, E. L., & Jacob, J. C. (1991). The Pain Behavior Check List (PBC): Factor structure and psychometric properties. *Journal of Behavioral Medicine, 14,* 155–167.

Kurlowicz, L. H. (2001). Benefits of psychiatric consultation-liaison nurse interventions for older hospitalized patients and their nurses. *Archives of Psychiatric Nursing, 15,* 53–61.

Li, L., Liu, X., & Herr, K. (2007). Postoperative pain intensity assessment: A comparison of four scales in Chinese adults. *Pain Medicine, 8,* 223–234.

McDonald, D. D., & Weiskopf, C. S. (2001). Adult patients' postoperative pain descriptions and response to the short-form McGill pain questionnaire. *Clinical Nursing Research, 10,* 442–452.

Melzack, R. (1975). The McGill Pain Questionnaire: Major properties and scoring methods. *Pain, 1,* 277–299.

Melzack, R. (1987). The short-form McGill pain questionnaire. *Pain, 1987,* 191–197.

Melzack, R. (2005). The McGill Pain Questionnaire: from description to measurement. *Anesthesiology, 103,* 199-202.

Mendoza, T. R., Chen, C., Brugger, A., Mendoza, T. R., Chen, C., Hubbard, R., Snabes, M., Palmer, S. N., Cleeland, C. C. (2004). The utility and validity of the Modified Brief Pain Inventory in a multiple-dose post-operative analgesic trial. *Clinical Journal of Pain, 20,* 357–362.

Nygaard, H. A., & Jarland, M. (2006). The Checklist of Nonverbal Pain Indicators (CNPI): Testing of reliability and validity in Norwegian nursing homes. *Age and Aging, 35*(1), 79–81.

Pasero, C. (2009). Challenges in pain assessment. *Journal of Perianesthesia Nursing, 24,* 550–554.

Pasero, C., & McCaffery, M. (2005). No self-report means no pain-intensity rating. *American Journal of Nursing, 105,* 50–53.

Price, D. D., Bush, F. M., Long, S., & Harkins, S. W. (1994). A comparison of pain measurement characteristics of mechanical visual analogue and simple numerical rating scales. *Pain, 56,* 217–226.

Sheikh, J. I., & Yesavage, J. A. (1986). Geriatric Depression Scale: Recent evidence and development of a shorter version. *Clinical Gerontology, 1986,* 165–172.

Stolee, P., Hillier, L. M., Esbaugh, J., Bol, N., McKellar, L., & Gauthier, N. (2005). Instruments for the assessment of pain in older persons with cognitive impairment. *Journal of the American Geriatric Society, 53,* 319–326.

Stuppy, D. J. (1998). The Faces Pain Scale: Reliability and validity with mature adults. *Applied Nursing Research, 11,* 84–89.

Taylor, L. J., & Herr, K. (2003). Pain intensity assessment: A comparison of selected pain intensity scales for use in cognitively intact and cognitively impaired African American older adults. *Pain Management Nursing, 4,* 87–95.

Wancata, J., Alexandrowicz, R., Marquart, B., Weiss, M., & Friedrich, F. (2006). The criterion validity of the Geriatric Depression Scale: A systematic review. *Acta Psychiatrica Scandinavica, 114,* 398–410.

Warden, V., Hurley, A. C., & Volicer, L. (2003). Development and psychometric evaluation of the Pain Assessment in Advanced Dementia (PAINAD) scale. *Journal of the American Medical Directors Association, 4,* 9–15.

Ware, L. J., Epps, C. D., Herr, K., & Packard, A. (2006). Evaluation of the revised Faces Pain Scale, Verbal Descriptor Scale, Numeric Rating Scale, and Iowa Pain Thermometer in older minority adults. *Pain Management Nursing, 7,* 117–125.

Wright, K. D., Asmundson, G. J., & McCreary, D. R. (2001). Factorial validity of the short-form McGill pain questionnaire (SF-MPQ). *European Journal of Pain, 5,* 279–284.

Zwakhalen, S. M., Hamers, J. P., Abu-Saad, H. H., & Berger, M. P. (2006). Pain in elderly people with severe dementia: A systematic review of behavioral pain assessment tools. *BMC Geriatrics, 6,* 3.

6

Developing a Comprehensive Plan for Managing Pain in Older Adults

A comprehensive plan for managing pain in older adults must be evidence based and personalized for the individual (Herr, 2010; Lawson, Revelino, & Owen, 2006). Although each plan needs to be individualized, there are certain elements that should be included in all comprehensive plans for pain management:

- Assessment
- Diagnosis
- Identification of goals and anticipated outcomes
- Identification of multidisciplinary team members
- Developing a specific plan for accomplishing the goals and outcomes
- Reviewing the plan with the patient and family
- Implementation of the plan
- Reassessment and evaluation of the plan
- Revising the plan as needed

Before developing the actual plan for pain management, it is important to consider certain factors. These include the following:

- Assessment
- Diagnosis
- Outcomes and goals desired
- Resources available in the community
- Universal precautions of pain management

ASSESSMENT

Any comprehensive plan for managing pain begins with a thorough assessment. This is essential to obtain the information needed to guide the plan. The specific aspects of pain assessment are described in Chapters 1, 2, and 3.

When developing a comprehensive plan, pain assessment should minimally include the following:

- Current pain description, including location, duration, quality, and intensity
- The effect of pain on various aspects of the person's life
- Activities or factors that increase the pain
- Interventions that alleviate the pain
- History of pain medication use, including what has been effective and what has been ineffective
- The nonpharmacological interventions being used and what is the effectiveness of them
- A screening of the risk of substance misuse or abuse

(Gourlay, Heit, & Almahrezi, 2005)

DIAGNOSIS

When working with patients in pain, a challenge is to remember that acute pain is a symptom that is calling attention to something that is not normal in the body (Brand & Yancey, 1997). Patients who live with chronic pain may have acute pain in addition to the chronic pain or they may have a change in the chronic pain. Either of these can indicate that something is different in the body and needs further assessment. A process of differential diagnosis will determine the etiology of the pain. This along with the assessment information will guide treatment.

In addition to assessment, medical diagnosis may involve physical examination, radiographic testing, laboratory testing, or even specialist consultation (Dubois, Gallagher, Lippe, & Anello, 2009). Nursing diagnosis focuses on identifying what the patient needs to best manage the pain and how to accomplish that. It is important to consider the following:

- Being knowledgeable about the role of pain in the medical diagnosis
- Understanding the meaning of this pain to the patient
- Being aware of the patient's history of pain and interventions to manage pain
- Identifying psychosocial and spiritual factors that contribute to the pain experience

> *Pearl*
>
> Assessment and diagnosis of pain must be individualized to address the unique physical, psychological, emotional, social, and spiritual needs of each older adult.

OUTCOMES AND GOALS

Identification of outcomes and goals for managing pain provides focus for the plan that will be developed. It is similar to determining the destination for a road trip. Once the person has been assessed and diagnosed, work with the person to develop a goal for pain management. Some points to consider when developing a goal for pain management are as follows:

- Recognize the importance of balancing comfort with safety.
- Identify the level of function and activity that are important and reasonable for the person.
- The goal must be realistic and reasonable.
- Pain goals are not limited to an intensity score.
- The level of function and activity important to the person must be included (Herr, 2010).
- Identify which outcomes are expected or desired.

IDENTIFY MULTIDISCIPLINARY TEAM MEMBERS

Since pain is a multifaceted and multidimensional experience, it is often necessary to include a variety of health care members in the comprehensive pain management plan (Dubois et al., 2009). In addition to primary care providers, the following practitioners may significantly contribute to the comprehensive plan of care:

- Physical therapists (PTs)
- Psychologists
- Occupational therapists
- Energy work practitioners (i.e., therapeutic touch, reflexology, and craniosacral)
- Recreational therapists
- Movement therapists
- Nutritionists
- Massage therapists
- Music and art therapists
- Yoga and Tai Chi instructors

(Adler, Good, Roberts, & Snyder, 2000; Ardery, Herr, Titler, So-
rofman, & Schmitt, 2003; Buettner, 2001; Cheung, Wyman, &
Halcon, 2007; Clair & Memmott, 2008; Kuczmarski et al., 2010;
Gloth, 2001; Gregory & Verdouw, 2005; Hinman, Heywood, &
Day, 2007; Messier et al., 2000; Rakel, 2003; Sherman, Cherkin,
Erro, Miglioretti, & Deyo, 2005)

An essential caveat to remember when referring older adults to other
practitioners is that older adults may experience pain and interventions differently than younger people. It is therefore important to
ensure that the practitioner is knowledgeable and experienced in
working safely with older adults (Rakel, 2003).

Pearls   Pain is a multidimensional and multiphasic experience.
Various practitioners are helpful in the comprehensive
plan of care.
It is imperative that practitioners are experienced in working with the special needs of older adults.

DEVELOP A SPECIFIC PLAN

After identifying the goal for pain intensity and for function with
the older adult, review the options for achieving those goals. The
plan is the roadmap to achieving the goals of pain management. Just
as some travelers prefer the scenic route, whereas others prefer the
by-pass roads and still others prefer a combination of the two, patients have preferences on how to reach their goals for pain control.

Although some older adults will prefer to manage pain by taking medication only, others will not want to take medication at all
because they fear addiction or side effects (Herr, 2005). Still others
will want to manage pain with a combination of pharmacological
and nonpharmacological methods.

If the older adult is not able to participate in developing the plan
for pain management, it is important to obtain information from
family members or others close to the person. The more consistent the
plan is with the individual preferences of the person, the more successful it is likely to be. Including the older adults in the development
of the plan will increase the sense of autonomy (Lawson et al., 2006).

Goal setting provides an opportunity to educate the person
about misconceptions, as well as the various options currently

available. Education may be a two-step process with older adults who have acquired a life time of information. Some of the information may be erroneous or outdated. Listening to questions and asking for clarification of grimaces, shrugs, or other nonverbal behavior that indicate negative responses will help to gain insight into what misconceptions need to be corrected.

When setting goals with older adults, it is important to consider accessibility. In many communities, certain medications or treatments are not readily available (Green et al., 2003). The most effective analgesia or intervention will not be helpful if it is not covered by insurance or the person cannot afford the cost of the medication, treatment, or transportation (Gottlieb, 2011).

Once the most appropriate interventions that are agreeable to the patient are identified, education and referral to other providers can be started.

Pearls	The anticipated outcomes can be achieved only if the plan is appropriate, meaningful, and feasible for the older adult. Whenever possible, the older adult needs to be part of developing the plan.

PATIENT EDUCATION

Eliopoulos (2001) suggests the following generalized guidelines when providing education to older adults:

■ Assess readiness to learn.

When assessing the readiness to learn in older adults with pain, the pain or associated anxiety or depression may be a barrier. It may be necessary to provide minimal education and schedule an education session when it is anticipated the patient will be more comfortable and/or ready to learn.

■ Assess learning capacities and limitations.

Identify the health care literacy, language barriers, education level, cultural factors, preconceptions, previous experiences, and cognitive status.

■ Outline the content of the information.

Develop an outline of what needs to be taught, understanding that not everything can be taught. Consider the needs and limitations of the patient and family. Know that there will be information that will need to be reinforced at later times.

■ Alter the teaching plan in view of capacities and limitations.

The patient may or may not be interested in the physiology that is causing the pain or why it is expected that certain modalities will be helpful. Focus education on what is meaningful to the person and what the person needs to know. Time constraints may also be a limiting factor. It is important to identify and teach the most important information first and be prepared to alter the plan to meet the needs of the patient.

■ Prepare the patient for the teaching–learning session.

Explain the importance of the patient understanding the information that will be taught. Ascertain if family members or caregivers need to be present. It may be necessary to identify a subsequent time for teaching.

■ Provide environment conducive to learning.

The physical environment is particularly important for the older adult experiencing pain. Physical discomfort is a significant barrier to comprehension and learning. The environment should also be relaxed, with minimal distractions, and safe.

■ Use the most effective individualized educational material.

The material that is most effective for the person will depend upon several factors. Educational level and literacy must be considered when choosing language. Visual and hearing limitations can be barriers to understanding. Handouts should be in large font with vivid color contrast. Copies should be clear. Speech and audio tools should be clear, with adequate volume and pace of words.

■ Use several approaches to the same body of knowledge.

Using a variety of methods of communicating the same information can enhance learning. Verbal teaching can be reinforced with written or audiovisual materials.

■ Leave material with the patient for later review.

Although the information is familiar to health care providers (HCPs), it may contain completely new concepts for the older adult in pain. Providing information that can be taken home and reviewed later will enable patients to review it in their own time. It also enables patients to share it with significant others and professional caregivers.

■ Reinforce key points.

Key concepts need to be reviewed frequently and consistently. Providing opportunity to ask questions and clarify points enables reiteration of important information.

■ Obtain feedback and evaluate understanding.

Education is a two-way street. It is important to determine to what degree the information taught was understood. Discussion, questions and answers, and return demonstrations are techniques that can be used to determine the level of comprehension.

■ Reevaluate periodically.

Although the information may be comprehended at the time of teaching, it may be forgotten or confused. Periodic reevaluation of what older adults and their families have retained is important and provides the opportunity to reinforce important points.

■ Document.

After the education session, it is imperative to record the following:

■ What was taught
■ To whom it was taught
■ What methods were used in teaching
■ Handouts that were given to the patient and family
■ The response of the patient and family
■ Plans for reevaluation and future education

REVIEW THE PLAN

As noted with education, an important aspect of developing a comprehensive plan is to review it with the older adults, family members, and/or caregivers. All those involved need to have the same information and understand the importance of consistency. If the patient receives care through a nursing home, assisted living facility, or home health agency, it is important to share the plan and education with those nurses (Eliopoulos, 2001).

IMPLEMENTATION OF THE PLAN

Once the necessary assessment, planning, and education have been accomplished, the plan can be implemented. This will involve medication prescription, referral to other providers, and educational materials.

| *Pearl* | Regardless of the intervention, a good axiom when working with older adults is to "Start low and go slow." |

REASSESSMENT AND EVALUATION
OF PROGRESS TOWARD GOALS

It is easiest to assess progress when goals are clear and specific. Consistent use of assessment tools enables progress to be clearly identified.

Reassessment should also include appraisal of the "Four A's" plus one:

■ **A**nalgesia—the use and effectiveness of medicines prescribed to control pain.
■ **A**ctivities—the degree to which the person is able to participate in their activities of daily living.
■ **A**dverse effects—side effects (also see Chapter 9).
■ **A**berrant behaviors—any behaviors that indicate misuse or abuse of prescribed medications (also see Chapter 23).
■ **A**ffect—the mood and disposition (depression, anxiety, and anger) are important considerations. (Gourlay et al., 2005) (also see Chapter 22).

Progress may be slow. If it is consistent over time, slight adjustments may be needed. If no progress or too little progress is seen, the plan needs to be revised.

In most situations, the pain experienced by older adults can be managed by their primary HCP; however, in complex situations or when the pain is not responding to treatments as expected, referral to a pain specialist or pain clinic is recommended. Ideally, referrals should be made prior to the development of maladaptive coping, considerable disability, or decline in function (Pujol, Katz, & Zacharoff, 2007).

RESOURCES AND GUIDELINES

Dietary Guidelines for Americans, 2005 (6th ed.). (2005). Washington, DC: US Government Printing Office.

Eliopoulos, C. (2001). *Gerontological nursing* (5th ed.). Philadelphia, PA: Lippincott.

Gourlay, D. L., Heit, H. A., & Almahrezi, A. (2005). Universal precautions in pain medicine: A rational approach to the treatment of chronic pain. *Pain Medicine, 6,* 107–112.

PainEDU.org

The American Academy of Pain Medicine. Pain Medicine Position Paper (2009). *Pain Medicine, 10,* 972–1000.

Case Study

Ms. Perez is an 87-year-old retired professor of Hispanic Studies. She lives with her significant other of many years who is 89 years old. Ms. Perez presents with complaints of polyuria and bilateral knee pain that has intensified over the last few months. The pain is interfering with her playing golf and bowling. She is reluctant to take medication because she does not want to "get hooked on them."

Questions

1. Who needs to be included in developing the plan of care for Ms. Perez?
2. What issues need to be considered when identifying treatment options?
3. What outcome measures can be used to assess progress toward goal attainment?
4. What psychosocial and cultural factors should be considered when developing the plan of care?
5. What multidisciplinary team members should be included in the plan for pain management?

REFERENCES

Adler, P., Good, M., Roberts, B., & Snyder, S. (2000). The effects of Tai Chi on older adults with chronic arthritis pain. *Journal of Nursing Scholarship, 32,* 377.

Ardery, G., Herr, K. A., Titler, M. G., Sorofman, B. A., & Schmitt, M. B. (2003). Assessing and managing acute pain in older adults: A research base to guide practice. *MEDSURG Nursing, 12*(1), 7–18.

Brand, P. & Yancey, P. (1997). *The gift of pain: Why we hurt and what we can do about it.* Grand Rapids, MI: Zondervan Publishing House.

Buettner, L. L. (2001). Therapeutic recreation in the nursing home: Reinventing a good thing. *Journal of Gerontological Nursing, 27,* 8–13.

Cheung, C. K., Wyman, J. F., & Halcon, L. L. (2007). Use of complementary and alternative therapies in community-dwelling older adults. *The Journal of Alternative and Complementary Medicine, 3,* 997–1006.

Clair, A. A., & Memmott, J. (2008). *Therapeutic uses of music with older adults* (2nd ed.). Silver Spring, MD: American Music Therapy Association.

Dubois, M. Y., Gallagher, R. M., Lippe, P. M., & Anello, M. (2009). Pain medicine position paper. *Pain Medicine, 10,* 972–1000.

Eliopoulos, C. (2001). *Gerontological nursing* (5th ed.). Philadelphia, PA: Lippincott.

Gloth, F. M. (2001). Pain management in older adults: Prevention and treatment. *Journal of the American Geriatrics Society, 49,* 188–199.

Gottlieb, S. (2011, March 10). Medicaid is worse than no coverage at all. *The Wall Street Journal,* Opinion.

Gourlay, D. L., Heit, H. A., & Almahrezi, A. (2005). Universal precautions in pain medicine: A rational approach to the treatment of chronic pain. *Pain Medicine, 6,* 107–112.

Green, C. R., Anderson, K. O., Baker, T. A., Campbell, L. C., Decker, S., Fillingim, R. B., . . . Vallerand, A. H. (2003). The unequal burden of pain: Confronting racial and ethnic disparities in pain. *Pain Medicine, 4,* 277–294.

Gregory, S., & Verdouw, J. (2005). Therapeutic touch: Its application for residents in aged care. *Australian Nursing Journal, 12,* 23–25.

Herr, K (2005). Pain assessment in the older adult with verbal communication skills. In S. J. Gibson, Herr, K., & Weiner, D. K. (Eds.), *Pain in older persons* (pp. 111–133). Seattle, WA: IASP Press.

Herr, K. (2010). Pain in the older adult: An interpretive across all health care settings. *Pain Management Nursing, 11,* S1–S10.

Hinman, R. S., Heywood, S. E., & Day, A. R. (2007). Aquatic physical therapy for hip and knee osteoarthritis: Results of a single-blind randomized controlled trial. *Physical Therapy, 87,* 32–43.

Kuczmarski, M. F., Sees, A. C., Hotchkiss, L., Cotugna, N., Evans, M. K., & Zonderman, A. B. (2010). Higher healthy eating index-2005 scores associated with reduced symptoms of depression in an urban population: Findings from the Healthy Aging in Neighborhoods of Diversity across the Life Span (HANDLS) Study. *Journal of the American Dietetic Association, 110,* 383–389.

Lawson, D., Revelino, K., & Owen, D. (2006). Clinical pathways to improve patient outcomes. *Physical Therapy Reviews, 2006,* 269–272.

Messier, S. P., Loesser, R. F., Mitchell, M. N., Valle, G., Morgan, T. P., Rejeski, W. J., & Ettinger, W. H. (2000). Exercise and weight loss in obese older adults with knee osteoarthritis: A preliminary study. *Journal of the American Geriatrics Society, 48,* 1062–1072.

Pujol, L. M., Katz, N. P., & Zacharoff, K. L. (2007). *PainEDU.org manual: A pocket guide to pain management* (3rd ed., Rev.). Newton, MA: Inflexxion.

Rakel, B. (2003). Physical modalities in chronic pain management. *Nursing Clinics of North America, 38,* 477–494.

Sherman, K. J., Cherkin, D. C., Erro, J., Miglioretti, D. L., & Deyo, R. A. (2005). Comparing yoga, exercise, and a self-care book for chronic low back pain: A randomized, controlled trial. *Annals of Internal Medicine, 143,* 849–856.

7

Choosing the Right Medication for the Pain Complaint

It is important for the reader to understand that the intent of this chapter is to provide the most recent information regarding safe use of analgesic medications for older adults. In no instance is any one medication recommended. It is critical that prior to prescribing or administering any analgesic medication to an older adult, all relevant patient and medication factors be considered. It is intended that the information in this chapter will assist the reader with this effort.

Older adults are at particular risk for inadequate pain management (Kumar, 2007). Choosing the most appropriate and safest medication to control pain experienced by older adults requires careful consideration of the following:

■ Each older person as a unique individual with various physical, emotional, cultural, spiritual, and social needs
■ The pain etiology (somatic, visceral, and neuropathic)
■ Severity of the pain
■ Patient beliefs about
  ■ the pain being experienced (cause and meaning)
  ■ what medications have and have not been effective previously (if the older person believes a particular medication did not work previously, it probably will not work now)
■ Safety issues, including
  ■ usual activities and function of the elder
  ■ possible side effects of medications
  ■ cognitive impairment that may affect how to best schedule medications (remembering to take them)
■ Route of administration limitations, including
  ■ impaired swallowing can limit oral analgesia
  ■ poor skin integrity or scarce suicide completion (SC) fat will limit transdermal administration

- changes in the liver (reduced mass)
- fewer glomeruli in the kidneys
- less total-body water
- religious beliefs that limit rectal administration
- Comorbid illnesses, including
  - renal or hepatic disease that affects excretion
  - gastrointestinal (GI) disorders
  - cardiac disorders
  - after effects of trauma
- Physiologic changes of aging, including
  - decreased creatinine clearance
  - limited cardiac output
  - decreased GI absorption
  - reduced vital capacity of lungs
  - decrease in muscle and lean body mass
  - less total water volume
- Potential interactions with current medications
  - polypharmacy is a particular concern in older adults
  - ascertain current use of medications, including over-the-counter (OTC) preparations
- Health literacy
  - well-educated elders may not be knowledgeable of health care issues
  - elders with limited education may be quite knowledgeable about health care issues
  - illiteracy is not necessarily acknowledged
- Cultural influences and beliefs, including
  - stoicism
  - traditional interventions
  - folk remedies
  - complementary modalities, including herbs
  - religious beliefs
  - fear of addiction
  - prohibition of IV medications
- Limited finances can prohibit purchase of some medications (financial assistance of some pharmaceutical companies may be available)
- Availability of the medication where the patient lives
- Safety of the older adult to use medications within the family or neighborhood (ascertain any fear of abuse or robbery for medication).

(Eliopoulos, 2001; Freedman, 2002; Gagliese & Melzack, 2003; Green, Ndao-Brumblay, Nagrant, Baker, & Rothman, 2004; Kingdon,

> | |
> |---|
> | *Pearls* | Pain management in older adults must be individualized. Pain management must consider the unique physical, emotional, cognitive, psychosocial, educational, and financial factors. Pain control must be balanced with safety for the older adult. |

Stanley, & Kizior, 1998; Kumar, 2007; Reuben et al., 2005; Zacharoff, Zeis, Frayjo, Chiauzzi, & Reznikova, 2009)

ANALGESIC SELECTION PROCESS

Older adults are at increased risk for polypharmacy and adverse effects of medications, but this should not be a barrier to good pain management when the class of analgesic medication most appropriate to manage pain is used (American Geriatrics Society [AGS], 2009). In general, analgesic medications are not appreciably altered with normal aging (Kingdon et al., 1998); however, it is imperative to judiciously administer and monitor their use.

With each older adult it is important to consider how the medication is absorbed, distributed, metabolized, and eliminated because each of these processes is affected with normal aging (Eliopoulos, 2001; Reuben et al., 2005). Some general age-related changes to consider are as follows.

Absorption is not appreciably altered with aging, however:
- Concomitantly administered medications may affect absorption.
- Food interactions may affect absorption.
- Comorbid pathologies resulting in decreased cardiac output, slower metabolism, elevated gastric pH, reduced intracellular fluid, sluggish gastric motility, and blood flow affect absorption.
- Highly soluble and highly concentrated medications are absorbed faster.

(Eliopoulos, 2001; Reuben et al., 2005).

Distribution is affected by the following:
- Circulation, body mass, body temperature, tissue composition, and membrane permeability.
- Ratio of adipose tissue to lean body mass that increases with aging; thus lipid soluble agents will have greater concentration in tissues.
- Reduced cardiac output can result in increased plasma levels of medications, especially water soluble meds.

- Lower serum albumin levels cause reduced efficiency of protein-bound medications, especially when more than one is taken (i.e., nortripyline and salicylates).
- Dehydration and hypoalbuminemia can cause less distribution, resulting in higher plasma levels of medications; dosing needs to be adjusted accordingly.

(Eliopoulos, 2001; Reuben et al., 2005).

METABOLISM AND ELIMINATION

- Medication metabolism can be decreased by sluggish hepatic blood flow or reduced liver mass; thus lower doses than expected may be effective.
- Reduced kidney function significantly affects excretion; medications remain in the body longer, extending medication half-life.
- Enzymes needed for medication metabolism may not be secreted.
- Decreased metabolism caused by dehydration, increased body temperature, reduced mobility, or liver disease can result in buildup of medications at toxic levels.
- Reductions in muscle mass can result in reduced production of creatinine.
- Creatinine clearance is more reliable than serum creatinine levels to assess ability to clear medications; it should be monitored to assess toxic accumulations of medications.
- Doses lower than those generally recommended may be therapeutic and appropriate for older adults.

(Eliopoulos, 2001; Reuben et al., 2005).

General Pharmacokinetics information, about older adults, which is evidence based is scarce. Older adults often have altered responses

Pearls	Every aspect of medication processing can be altered in older adults. It is always best to start treatment using the medication with the fewest and least troublesome possible side effects, via the least invasive route, in the lowest effective dose. **Start low and go slow!**

to medications at recommended adult doses, and older adults often have prolonged analgesic effects at lower than usual adult doses (Eliopoulos, 2001; Reuben et al., 2005).

The World Health Organization (WHO) Pain Relief Ladder is considered by many pain management professionals to be a good foundation for deciding which analgesic medications are appropriate for the older adult patient (D'Arcy, 2010). Although the WHO Ladder was originally designed to guide the management of pain in cancer patients (Mercadante & Fulfaro, 2005; WHO, 2009), it has proven to be effective in guiding the management of chronic noncancer pain as well (Barakzoy & Moss, 2006; Kumar, 2007). When using the WHO Ladder with older adults who have chronic nonmalignant pain, it is important to remember that *lower* doses of opioids are generally indicated and the lowest dose of nonselective nonsteroidal anti-inflammatory drugs (NSAIDs) are recommended (America Pain Society [APS], 2003; Herr, Bjoro, Steffensmeier, & Rakel, 2006; Kumar, 2007).

A good axiom to remember when working to manage pain in older adults is to *Start low and go slow!*

The WHO Ladder is divided into three rungs or levels that list oral medication categories in the order they are recommended (WHO, 2009). On each level, the advisement "with or without (±) adjuvant medications" is included. The adjuvant medications are

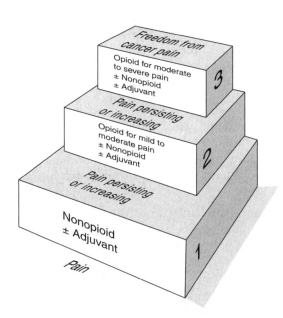

discussed in Chapter 8. This chapter is presented in accordance with analgesic medications on the three levels.

The WHO Ladder Level One Medications for Pain That Is Mild, Persisting, or Increasing are nonopioid analgesics ± adjuvant medications. Mild pain is either described as such using a descriptive assessment tool or rated as 1 to 3 on the numeric rating scale (NRS) (D'Arcy, 2009).

Aspirin is not recommended for analgesic use in older adults and should be avoided. Despite the use of daily low-dose aspirin as a cardioprotective agent, there are many negative effects, including GI irritation, ulceration, and bleeding; extended bleeding times; hypersensitivity reactions; and toxicity (APS, 2003; Herr, et al., 2006).

Acetaminophen is often the first analgesic initiated by older people who use this over-the-counter product for pain, discomfort, sleep, or anxiety. As an initial medication, it may be effective for mild to moderate pain. In fact, most older adults with mild to moderate musculoskeletal pain treated with scheduled, around the clock doses of acetaminophen respond well to it (AGS Panel, 2002).

■ *Mechanism of action* appears to be of a weak and nonspecific cyclooxygenase (COX) inhibitor, but the exact mechanism of action is not known.

■ *Generally it is considered prudent to start acetaminophen at 325 mg every 6 hours with older adults* (AGS, 2009).

The Food and Drug Administration (FDA) reevaluates safe dosing and publishes periodic updates.

■ *Ofirmev*™ is an IV form of acetaminophen. During clinical testing, 15% of the subjects were 65 or older and no differences were noted between older and younger patients. Sensitivity in older adults may occur (Cadence Pharmaceuticals, 2011). As this medication provides a new route of administration, clinical use has not been well documented; however, the safety seems good.

Pharmacokinetic and administration Information are in Tables 7.1 and 7.2.

Safety concerns and cautions are that

■ Total daily dose of acetaminophen *from all sources* should NEVER exceed 4 g per day *when* the older adult has:
  ■ normal renal and hepatic function and
  ■ no history of alcohol abuse (AGS Panel, 2002; Freedman, 2002).

■ Further caution is for frail older adults, for whom the maximum daily dose of acetaminophen should be 3 g per day.

Table 7.1 ■ *Pharmacokinetic Considerations of Analgesic Medications Commonly Used in Older Adults*

Medication	Absorption	Metabolism	Half-life[a]	Elimination	Cautions
2-Acetaminophen	Good orally in healthy older adults; Rectal absorption is limited; IV absorption is good	Primarily via liver	2–3 h	Excreted in urine/stool	*Avoid in hepatic disease or alcohol*
Nonselective NSAIDs	Good orally in healthy older adults	Primarily via liver	1.5–69 h depending upon the NSAID	Excreted in urine/stool	GI irritation; Renal toxicity; Alteration in platelet aggregation; CNS affects; Ceiling effect for each NSAID
Celecoxib	Good orally with peak plasma level in about 3 h	Primarily via liver	11 h	Excreted in urine/stool	
Choline magnesium (Tricosal, Trilisate)			Permits dosing 1–2 times per day after steady state		
Salsalates (Disalcid, Salflex, Mono-Gesic)			Permits dosing 1–2 times per day after steady state		

[a]Half-life of most medications may be prolonged in older adults, particularly when renal function is impaired.

Sources: Based upon information in AGS, 2009; D'Arcy, 2010; Freedman, 2002; Hanlon et al., 2005; Herr et al., 2006; McNeil, 2002; USFDA, 2009; Waknine, 2010.

Table 7.2 ■ *Common Anti-inflammatory Medications with Recommended Daily Doses, Effectiveness, Advantages, and Cautions*

Medication	Routes	Recommended Daily Dose	Effectiveness	Advantages	Cautions
Acetaminophen	PO (tablet, capsule, elixir) PR, IV	Start with 325 mg every 6 h; *Total daily dose from ALL sources Not to exceed 4 g/day and with frail elders, it should not exceed 3 g/day*	Good for mild to moderate pain; arthritis; low back pain; first line of therapy on WHO Ladder	Few adverse effects; less GI side effects; accessible OTC; inexpensive	Recommend lower doses in older adults; Avoid in hepatic disease or alcohol
Nonselective NSAIDs	PO, IV, PR, T	Dosing is specific to the NSAID; Start with lowest possible dose; Use the lowest possible dose for the shortest possible time	No evidence indicates that one NSAID is more effective than others; bur effectiveness is variable among older adults. If one is not effective, another may be effective.		Monitor renal function; may cause GI irritation; alteration of platelet aggregation; ceiling effects with each NSAID
Ibuprophen	PO, IV	200 mg 3 × day	As above		May inhibit antiplatelet effect of aspirin when used together
Ketorolac	PO, IV	Reduce dose by 50% in elders; Not to exceed 60 mg/day for no longer than 48 h	As above		Monitor BUN and creatinine

Naproxen	PO	220 mg 2 × day	As above	Fewer GI and CV side effects than most other NSAIDs; Better tolerated by elders	Preferred in older adults
Ketoprophen	PO	12.5 mg 4 × day	As above		Educate elders not to exceed RDD
Diclofenac	PO, IR, ER	25–50 mg 3 × day	As above	Available in topical agents	May have greater CV risk
Diclofenac	T				
Celecoxib	PO	100 mg daily starting dose	Reported similar to diclofenac; mixed anecdotal reports		
Choline magnesium (Tricosal, Trilisate)	PO, PR, topical	500–750 mg every 8 h	Good	Reportedly safe in older adults; minimal effect on platelets	Monitor levels in frail elders and those with hepatic or renal impairment
Salsalates (Disalcid, Salflex, Mono-Gesic)	PO, PR, topical	500–750 mg every 12 h	Good	Reportedly safe in older adults; minimal effect on platelets	Monitor levels in frail elders and those with hepatic or renal impairment

Ep, Epidural; h, hours; IT, intrathecal; IV, intravenous; mg, milligrams; PO, oral; PR, rectal; RDD, recommended daily dose; SR, sustained release; T, topical; TD, transdermal

Sources: Half-life of most medications can be prolonged in older adults.

Sources: AGS Panel, 2002; AGS, 2009; APS, 2003; APS, 2006; D'Arcy, 2010; FDA, 2005; Gleason et al., 2011; Hanlon et al., 2005; Harder & An, 2003; Herr et al., 2006; King Pharmaceutical, 2010; Kingdon et al., 2010; Kurth et al., 1998; McNeil, 2002; Mercadante & Fulfaro, 2005; Munir et al., 2007; Pfizer, 2002; USFDA, 2009.

The 4 g limit is a particular concern when older people use combination medications and may not realize the combination includes acetaminophen. Education is imperative (Herr et al., 2006).

Additional safety concerns are for elders with

- renal dysfunction
- concomitant warfarin therapy (more than 2 g of acetaminophen per day may increase the INR)
- hepatic dysfunction/damage (through excess of a toxic metabolite)
- risky alcohol consumption or abuse
- frail health and multiple comorbidities
- risk for GI irritation or bleeding

Individuals in these groups should either not take acetaminophen or doses should be reduced by 50%–75%.

If it is essential to use acetaminophen with older people at risk for GI issues, concomitant prescription of a mediating medication, such as proton pump inhibitor (PPI), should be considered; however, the cost may be prohibitive (AGS Panel, 2002; APS, 2003; D'Arcy, 2010; USFDA, 2009).

Miscellaneous Note

Many older adults use acetaminophen routinely to manage usual "aches and pains." When they are admitted to the hospital, acetaminophen often is not ordered or is ordered as "prn for fever." The usual dose of acetaminophen should be included in the total hospital pain management plan of care unless contraindicated.

NONSTEROIDAL ANTI-INFLAMMATORY DRUGS

- With older adults, all NSAIDs need to be used with respect, caution, and in recommended dosages or less.
- Administer the lowest dose possible for the shortest duration possible in acute care situations (Herret al., 2006).
- There are three categories of NSAIDs:
  - nonselective NSAIDs,
  - COX-2 selective NSAIDs, and
  - the salicylates.

Mechanism of action is through inhibition of the COX enzyme, thus hindering the formation and synthesis of prostaglandins. This in turn results in less sensitivity of both the peripheral nerves and the central neurons to pain stimuli (APS, 2003). NSAIDs interfere with the inflammatory cascade through inhibition of prostaglandin synthesis and inhibition of the COX-2 enzyme (Harder & An, 2003).

Pharmacokinetic and administration information are in Tables 7.1 and 7.2.

Selection of an NSAID needs to be based upon
- comorbid illness that may contradict use (i.e., cardiac or renal pathology)
- undesirable or unacceptable side effects
- personal history of effectiveness (what has worked for the person in the past)
- cost

A Good Rule of Thumb	*"NSAIDs should be used at the lowest effective dose for the shortest time they are needed"* with older adults (APS, 2003).

General safety concerns with NSAIDs include the following:

- *Caution older adults not to exceed the recommended or prescribed daily dose of NSAIDs, including those available OTC.*(FDA, 2009; King Pharmaceutical, 20l0; Lionberger, Joussellin, Lanzarotti, Yanchick, & Magelli, 2011).
- *GI irritation*, ulcer, or bleeding. Advise patients to eat, not fast, when taking NSAIDs; adding a PPI may be helpful.
- *Renal toxicity* may occur with frequent or long-term use. Elders with congestive heart failure, chronic renal disease, lupus, and atherosclerotic disease are particularly vulnerable to renal toxicity. Carefully monitor renal function (creatinine and blood urea nitrogen [BUN]) of older adults receiving NSAIDs, especially IV ketorolac.
- *Alteration in platelet aggregation* occurs in nonspecific NSAIDs through inhibition of COX-1 enzyme function.
- *NSAIDs are contraindicated* in situations where there is anticoagulation, coagulopathy, thrombocytopenia, and concomitant use of anticoagulants.
- Orthopedic surgeons generally are opposed to using nonselective NSAIDs immediately postoperatively due to concern for platelet aggregation and inhibition of the inflammatory response necessary for bone healing. This is important for older adults who have surgery related to osteoarthritis.
- *Central nervous system (CNS) affects* include dizziness, decreased attention, drowsiness, impaired short-term memory, anxiety, confusion, and difficulty with cognitive calculations.

- *Respiratory problems* are rare but bronchospasm may occur.
- There is a *ceiling effect* for each NSAID, above which occurrence of adverse effects increases. It is important to check the product information of each NSAID before prescribing and administering the medication.
- Nonselective NSAIDs should be discontinued prior to surgery. If not contraindicated (see section below), a COX-2 NSAID can be substituted.
- *Urological* — A recent study of 80,966 men between 45 and 69 years of age reported that men who use NSAIDs have an increased risk of developing erectile dysfunction. The men who took NSAIDs three times per day for 3 or more months were 2.4 times more likely to have dysfunction even after controlling for race, smoking, and comorbidities.
- *NSAID interaction with aspirin* is of concern with older adults. Regular NSAID use over time inhibits the cardioprotective effects of low- dose aspirin.

(APS, 2003; AGS, 2009; Gleason et al., 2011; Harder & An, 2003; Herr et al., 2006; Kingdon et al., 1998; Kurth et al., 2003; Mercadante & Fulfaro, 2005).

Pearls	The *lowest dose* of nonselective NSAID is recommended in older adults. A good axiom with older adults is to *Start low and go slow!*

COX-2 selective NSAIDs were developed with the intention of providing the efficacy of nonselective NSAIDs without the GI risks associated with them. They have been referred to as COX-2 inhibitors but that is a misnomer because they are not specific but rather selective in their action (APS, 2003). The only COX-2 selective NSAID that is currently available in the United States is Celecoxib (US DHHS, 2005).

The *mechanism of action* of COX-2 selective NSAIDs is inhibition of prostaglandin synthesis by inhibiting the COX-2. They do not inhibit COX-1 that is involved in platelet inhibition (APS, 2003; APS, 2006; Hanlon, Guay, & Ives, 2005; McNeil, 2002; Pfizer, 2002).

Pharmacokinetic and administration information are in Tables 7.2 and 7.3.

General safety concerns include the following:

- There is a concern for increased cardiovascular (CV) risk in all NSAIDs, including COX-2 (USDHHS, 2005).

Table 7.3 ■ *Nonselective NSAID Medications*

Generic Name	Brand Names	Cautions	Comments
Ibuprophen	Motrin	May inhibit antiplatelet effect of aspirin when used concurrently	
Ketaprophen	Actron, Orudis	Not recommended for elders with chronic pain due to GI and renal toxicity	Available in SR form
Ketorolac	Torodol		
Meloxicam	Mobic		
Nabumetone	Relafen		Reported to have minimal effect on platelets
Naproxen	Aleve, Anaprox	Fewer GI and CV side effects than most other NSAIDs; better tolerated by elders	Preferred in older adults
Diclofenac sodium (oral)	Voltaren®	May pose greater CV risk	FDA recommends monitoring trans-aminase every 4–8 weeks with long-term use
Diclofenac sodium (Topical)	FLECTOR® Patch (topical) Voltaren® (topical gel) PennSAID® (topical liquid)	Voltaren gel risk of hepatotoxicity	Absorbed via the skin rather than through the GI tract, thus avoiding GI disturbance
	Lodine (etodolac)		
	Celebrex	Concern for increased CV risks	

Sources: (Information based upon D'Arcy, 2009; FDA, 2005; FDA, 2009; King Pharmaceutical, 2010; Lionberger et al., 2011).

- Doses greater than 100 mg are associated with more GI and CV problems (Herr et al., 2006).
- In older adults weighing 50kg or less, it is recommended to use the lowest recommended dose (Pfizer, 2002; Savage, 2006).
- *Contraindicated* in older adults with
  - CV disease, including stroke
  - postcardiac surgery
  - per the FDA: "Celebrex should *not* be used in patients who are immediately postoperative from CABG surgery." (U.S. Department of Health and Human Services, 2005)
    - contraindicated in patients receiving warfarin and ACE inhibitors.

(D'Arcy, 2009; Herr et al., 2006; USDHHS, 2005; Savage, 2006).

Miscellaneous Note

It is now believed that COX-2 selective NSAIDs do not provide a GI protective benefit any better than taking a PPI medication along with a nonselective NSAID (APS, 2003; Savage, 2006).

Salicylates

The most common of the salicylates, aspirin, is not recommended for analgesia use in older adults. The remaining salicylate salts fall into two categories:

- *Choline magnesium trisalicylates* (Tricosal and Trilisate)
- *Salsalates* (Disalcid, Mono-Gesic, and Salflex)

Mechanism of action is through inhibition of prostaglandin synthesis *(AGS Panel, 2002; AGS, 2009*; APS, 2003; Munir, Enany, & Zhang, 2007).

Pharmacokinetic and Administration information are in Tables 7.1 and 7.2

Pearls
> NSAIDs should be used with caution in older adults.
> When NSAIDs are prescribed for older adults, monitor renal function, GI status, and potential side effects.
> Use lowest effective dose for the shortest possible time.
> Topical NSAIDs have greater local effect, less GI effects, and good patient approval.

The WHO Ladder Level Two Medications for Pain That Is Mild to Moderate are considered weak opioids ± adjuvants. The weak opioids are short acting and indicated to treat mild to moderate pain, which can be pain that is described as such by the older adult or it can be pain that is rated as being 4 to 6 on the NRS (D'Arcy, 2009).

The medications included in this group are as follows:

- Hydrocodone (Vicodin, Lortab, and Narco)
- Tramadol (Ultram)
- Tramadol with acetaminophen (Ultracet)
- Tapentadol (Nucynta)

MECHANISM OF ACTION

The primary mechanism of action of this group of medications is binding with mu-opioid receptors.

- *Lortab/Vicodin* and *Ultracet* are hydrocodone and tramadol, respectively, with the addition of acetaminophen.
- *Tapentadol,* in addition to binding with the mu-opioid receptor, is a selective norepinephrine (NE) reuptake inhibitor. It is similar to tramadol but is a class II controlled substance.
- *Tramadol* inhibits serotonin and NE reuptake, in addition to binding with the mu-opioid receptor.

(AGS, 2009; Herr et al., 2006; McPherson & Uritsky, 2011).

Pharmacokinetic and administration information are in Tables 7.4 and 7.5.

Miscellaneous Note

Compared with other opioids, *tramadol* may have less abuse potential. It has lower rate of constipation that can be particularly troublesome in older adults with sluggish GI tracts and those who are less active (APS, 2006; Fine, 2004; McPherson & Uritsky, 2011).

Oxycodone 5mg has been listed in some sources as an opioid for use with moderate pain (the second level of the WHO Ladder) (APS, 2008). As oxycodone is listed as a Step 3 opioid in the recent consensus statement (Pergolizzi et al., 2008) and considered to have

---

Pearls

Each of these weaker opioids has strengths and each has potential for adverse reactions.

Selection must be made considering the pain situation and comorbidities of the individual older adult.

Start low and go slow!

Table 7.4 ◼ *Pharmacokinetic Considerations of Opioid Medications*

Medication	Absorption	Metabolism	Half-life	Peak Level	Elimination	Cautions[a]
Hydrocodone with acetaminophen (Vicodin, Lortab, Narco)	Via GI tract	Liver	2.5–4.5 h		Urine	Commercially available in only combination with acetaminophen or ibuprophen (see Table __ cautions)
Tramadol (Ultram)	Via GI tract	Liver	2–5 h	2–3 h	Urine	
Tramadol with acetaminophen (Ultracet)	Via GI tract; about 75% available orally	Liver	2–5 h	2–3 h	Urine	
Tapentadol (Nucynta)	Via GI tract	Extensive first pass metabolism	4 h	1.25 h	Urine	Caution with respiratory problems, obesity; confusion reported
Oxycodone		Liver	3.5 h		Urine	
Oxycontine		Liver	4.5–8 h		Urine	
Morphine		Liver with metabolite cleared in kidneys	1.5–4.5 h		Urine	Accumulation can occur with impaired renal or hepatic function

Fentanyl	Age-related changes on absorption are variable; not well absorbed orally	Liver	3.65 h IV; 7 h via transmucosal; 17 h via transdermal (however, half-life may be up to 3 times this in older adults)		Since fentanyl is lipophilic and older adults have greater body fat, half-life is expected to be up to 3 times longer
Hydromorphone		Liver where it is metabolized to generally inactive metabolites	2.5 h	Urine	
Methadone	Good in older adults	Biphasic in the liver	30 h average; the half-life is expected to be extended in older adults	Urine	Methadone is lipophilic and older adults have greater body fat, so half-life is expected to be longer

[a]All opioid medications have potential side effects of somnolence, sedation, respiratory depression, and constipation.

Sources: APS, 2003; APS, 2006; Grond & Sablotzki, 2004; Hanlon et al., 2005; Herr et al., 2006; Kharasch, Hoffer, Whittington, & Sheffels, 2004; Ortho-McNeil-Janssen Pharmaceutical, 2010; McPherson & Uritsky, 2011; Pergolizzi et al., 2008; Zydus Pharmaceuticals, 2011.

Table 7.5 ■ *Common Opioid and Opioid-like Medications with Recommended Daily Doses, Effectiveness, Advantages, and Caution*

Medication	Routes	Recommended Daily Starting Dose	Effectiveness	Cautions[a]
Hydrocodone with acetaminophen (Vicodin, Lortab, Narco)	PO (also in elixir)	5–10 mg every 4–6 h	Effective for mild to moderate pain; similar in effect to tramadol	Dose is restricted by amount of acetaminophen or ibuprophen, which differs by product
Tramadol (Ultram)	PO	25 mg every 6 h; Max daily dose 300 mg in those > 75 y	Effective for mild to moderate pain; similar in effect to hydrocodone; effective with arthritis, back pain, diabetic neuropathy, fibromyalgia	Titrate slowly over several weeks Seizures, serotonin syndrome in high doses or when prone to developing Dizziness, asthenia, somnolence, nausea and vomiting are reported; discontinuation must be gradual
Tramadol with acetaminophen (Ultracet)	PO	25 mg every 6 h	Effective for mild to moderate pain; similar in effect to hydrocodone	Dose is restricted by acetaminophen Titrate slowly over several weeks Seizures, serotonin syndrome in high doses or when prone to developing Dizziness, asthenia, somnolence, nausea and vomiting are reported; discontinuation must be gradual

Tapentadol (Nucynta)	PO	50 mg every 6 h	Effective for mild to moderate pain; effectiveness of 50 mg is similar to oxycodone 10 mg when prescribed every 4–6 h	Contraindicated with MAO inhibitors Contraindicated with severe renal or hepatic pathology
Oxycodone	PO (pills, elixir)	2.5–5 mg every 4–6 h	Considered safe and highly effective in older adults; no appreciable difference in pharmacokinetics in young vs. older adults	When in combination with acetaminophen the dose is limited by the acetaminophen
Oxycontin	PO (pills)	10 mg every 12 h	New formulation is tamper resistant	The 12-h effect may be extended to 14–24 h in older adults requiring dosing adjustments Extended-release formulations are available for both 8-h and 24-h administration
Morphine	PO (IR and ER), PR, IV, IT Epidural	IR oral 2.5–10 mg every 4 h; ER oral 15 mg every 8–24 h	Effective for moderate to severe pain; often considered the "gold standard" of opioid analgesia	Safe and effective in older adults
Fentanyl	IV; transdermal; transmucosal IT, epidural	Transdermal 12–25 mcg every 72 h; Transmucosal 100 mcg to be titrated for BTP *Dosing is in micrograms not milligrams*	Safe and effective in older adults	*Approximately 80–100 times the potency of morphine* *Transdermal is not indicated for acute pain*

(continued)

Table 7.5 ■ *(continued)*

Medication	Routes	Recommended Daily Starting Dose	Effectiveness	Cautions[a]
Hydromorphone	PO (IR and ER) IV, IT, epidural	IR oral 1–2 mg every 3–4 h	Safe and effective; Preferred in older adults with renal impairment	*Approximately 5–8 times the potency of morphine; ER formulation is indicated only for opioid-tolerant patients; older adults are considered at risk for overdose*
Methadone	PO, IV, IT	Dosing should be determined and supervised by a pain management specialist	Research is needed to determine effectiveness in older adults	Very long half-life that is most likely extended in older adults

[a]All opioid medications have potential side effects of somnolence, sedation, respiratory depression, and constipation.

Sources: AGS, 2009; APS, 2003; D'Arcy, 2009; Fine, 2004; Freedman, 2002; Hadjistavropoulos & Fine, 2006; Herr et al., 2006; Kharasch, Hoffer, Whittington, & Sheffels, 2004; King Pharmaceutical, 2010; Mallinckrodt Inc., 2011; McPherson & Uritsky, 2011; Pergolizzi et al., 2008; Reuben et al., 2005.

equivalent or more potency than morphine (APS, 2003), it is discussed in the next section, with the third level of the WHO Ladder. *The WHO Ladder Level Three Medications for Pain That Is Moderate to Severe* are opioids that are considered potent opioids ± nonopioids They are indicated to treat moderate to severe pain, which can be pain that is described as such by the older adult or it can be considered pain that is rated as "severe" or being 5 or greater on the NRS (D'Arcy, 2009). These opioids may be available in either short-acting, sustained-release, or long-acting preparations. Some may also be available alone or in combination with other medications.

Opioids can be used safely and effectively with older adults. Start low and go slow is the key to this. With opioid naïve older adults, it is recommended to reduce the initial dose by 25% to 50% to avoid side effects such as sedation or respiratory depression. When monitoring for side effects, it is important to assess for signs of decreased elimination (D'Arcy, 2010; Herr et al., 2006). After initiation, opioids can be increased using a titration of about 25% until the older adult is comfortable or the pain is reduced by approximately 50% (Herr et al., 2006).

When selecting the appropriate opioid medication for older people, it is important to remember that each older person is unique. In general, it is best to select opioids with a shorter half-life (i.e., morphine, hydromorphone, and oxycodone) (Herr et al., 2006). When selecting an opioid, the following factors are to be considered:
- Comorbid illnesses
- General health
- Current essential medications
- Unacceptable side effects (nausea/vomiting, pruritus, and confusion).
- Cost of the medication
- Effects of using multiple opioids at the same time
  - If side effects develop, it is difficult to identify the source if more than one opioid is used.
  - Incidence of side effects, including delirium, increases with multiple medications.

(Herr et al., 2006).
The mu-agonist opioids are considered to be "the first-line opioid analgesics." Medications in this group include
- **Morphine**
  - Immediate-release as MSIR, Roxanal
  - Sustained-release as MS contin
  - Sustained-release 24-hour dosing as Avinza, Kadian

Combination extended-release morphine with naltrexone hydrochloride (Embeda) is considered to be an abuse-deterrent product with 12- to 24-hour dosing.

- **Oxycodone**
  - Immediate-release as Oxycodone, Roxicet, Oxyfast
  - Combination as Percocet, Percodan, Oxyfast
  - Sustained-release as Oxycontin
- **Hydromorphone**
  - Immediate-release as Dilaudid
  - Extended-release as Exalgo
- **Fentanyl**
  - Immediate-release as Actiq, Fentora, Onsolis.
  - Sustained-release as Duragesic transdermal.

(AGS, 2009; APS, 2003; Herr et al., 2006; McPherson & Uritsky, 2011).

Mechanism of action for most opioids is through binding with CNS mu-receptors (Hanlon et al., 2005; McPherson & Uritsky, 2011).

Pharmacokinetic and administration information are in Tables 7.4 and 7.5.

One study investigating the effect of transmucosal fentanyl reported decreased oxygen saturation in 9 of 12 older adults; however, no other untoward side effects were reported in that small sample (Kharasch, Hoffer & Whittington, 2004).

General considerations of opioid dosing

- Opioids can be used safely and effectively with older people. Starting low and going slow is key.
- With opioid naïve older adults, it is recommended to reduce the initial dose by 25% to 50% to avoid side effects such as sedation or respiratory depression.
- When monitoring for side effects, it is important to assess for signs of decreased elimination.
- After initiation, opioids can be increased using a titration of about 25% until the older person is comfortable or pain is reduced by approximately 50%.
- With older adults, titration should allow for the opioid to achieve steady-state serum level prior to escalation.
- As a general rule, there is usually a greater peak followed by a then longer period of action of opioids in older adults.

■ There is no maximum dose for opioids; however, doses may be limited by side effects.

(D'Arcy, 2010; Fine, 2004; Herr et al., 2006).

Specific recommendations for starting doses of opioids with older adults are in Table 7.4

Equianalgesic dosing must be considered when changing from one opioid to another. That may be necessary because of either inadequate analgesia or unacceptable side effects. Morphine is considered the "gold standard" for *equianalgesic dosing* of other opioids (McPherson & Uritsky, 2011). When changing from one opioid to another, a standard equianalgesic table should be used for conversion. Initially, it may be prudent to reduce the equianalgesic dose by 50% when converting to a new opioid in patients with well-controlled pain. Careful titration is important to ensure safety. Adjust the doses according to patient response, pain score, and ability to function.

When short-acting opioids are used in conjunction with long-acting or sustained-release opioids, the recommended dose is

■ With oral opioids, 10%–15% of the total daily dose

■ With IV or intraspinal 25%–50% of the total daily dose.

(Arnold & Weissman, 2009; Herr et al., 2006).

General consideration of opioid administration

■ Short-acting oral opioids used for breakthrough pain (BTP) may be administered every hour or two.

■ IV or intraspinal opioids used for BTP may be administered every 30–60 min as needed.

(Herr et al., 2006).

Patient controlled analgesia (PCA) use with older adults can be safe and effective. IV or epidural PCA commonly are used with morphine, hydromorphone, or fentanyl. The decision of the individual opioid should be made considering the pharmacokinetics and side-effect profile for the individual opioids. Additional things to consider include the following:

■ Need for opioids through a route other than oral

■ Cognitive ability to understand the PCA concept

■ Physical ability to use the equipment

■ Usual lock out time between patient administered boluses is 5 to 10 minutes.

(Reuben et al., 2005)

ADMINISTRATION OF ANALGESIA VIA EPIDURAL AND REGIONAL INFUSIONS

Epidural Administration

Smaller doses of opioids are needed via the epidural route because the medication is delivered close to the receptors in the spinal cord. Local anesthetic (LA) can be used in addition to opioids via the epidural route, resulting in even lower doses of opioids to be needed. It is anticipated that with less opioid required, side effects would be less as well, which is most desirable in older adults.

Continuous epidural infusions can be used postoperatively for acute pain and as a palliative measure for chronic pain at the end of life. In either situation, the continuous infusion can be via either the IV or the SC route. It can be a fixed infusion or it can be patient controlled epidural analgesia.

Advantages

Some studies report better pain relief in older adults with epidural analgesia compared to IV; however, more research is needed.

Cautions

Risk of falling is related to:

- motor blockade that can cause weakness and inability to use the area or limb affected
- hypotension, including orthostatic hypotension
- LA toxicity.

(Fong, Sands, & Leung, 2006)

Continuous regional analgesia is also called *continuous peripheral nerve blocks* or *perineural analgesia* and is generally used to manage postoperative pain. LA (i.e., bupivocaine or ropivocaine) are continuously infused in immediate proximity to a peripheral nerve through a catheter inserted by an anesthesiologist or a certified registered nurse anesthetist.

Advantages

- Excellent analgesia without the side effects associated with NSAIDs and opioids.
- Analgesia is specific to nerves innervating the area of pain.

Cautions

Risk of falling is related to:

- motor blockade that can cause weakness and inability to use the area or limb affected,

- hypotension, including orthostatic hypotension, and
- LA toxicity

(Arnstein, 2010; Banks, 2007).

SAFETY CONCERNS WITH OPIOIDS IN OLDER ADULTS

Neurological concerns include sedation, dizziness, and ataxia. Confusion and delirium are rare when dosing is started low and dose escalation is slow.

Respiratory concerns include respiratory depression and increased risk and possible complications in patients with asthma and obstructive sleep apnea.

GI concerns include nausea, vomiting, and constipation.

- Caution must be observed in treating nausea and vomiting to include medications (i.e., phenergan) that may have synergistic effect of increased sedation.
- All patients receiving opioids need to have education and orders for appropriate bowel management to prevent constipation.

(Fine, 2004).

Patient and family education should include the following:

- Caution to never cut or crush sustained-release preparations.
- Never cut fentanyl transdermal patch.
- *Never* apply heat directly to fentanyl transdermal patch, or the person can inadvertently receive a significant overdose of medication.

DISCONTINUATION OF OPIOID MEDICATIONS

As some degree of physical dependence occurs with opioid analgesia, it is important to avoid sudden withdrawal by carefully weaning the person to discontinuation (Fine, 2004).

MONITORING AND REASSESSMENT OF OLDER ADULTS

It is imperative to monitor older adults receiving analgesia for pain management. Assessment and reassessment should include

- effectiveness of the medication in achieving pain control
- possible side effects of analgesic medications
- untoward symptoms related to the analgesia

Table 7.6 ■ *Analgesic Medications to Avoid with Older Adults*

Medication	Reason	Possible Substitutes
Aspirin	Bleeding risk	Acetaminophen
Indomethacin	Adverse effects	Other NSAIDS
Amitryptiline	potential for hypotension	gabapentin or pregabalin
Meperidine	Metabolite normeperidine can cause seizures, tremors, and delirium	Oxycodone, morphine, hydromorphone, fentanyl
Methadone	Very long half-life can result in accumulation and side effects	Oxycodone, morphine, hydromorphone, fentanyl
Pentazocine	Significant side effects, may cause delirium	
Butorphanol	Significant side effects, may cause delirium	

Sources: (Information based on APS, 2008; D'Arcy, 2010; Herr et al., 2006 ; Kharasch, Hoffer, Whittington, & Sheffels, 2004).

■ need for titration of medication (upward or downward) depending upon effectiveness and side effects.

(AGS Panel, 2002; Fine, 2004) (see Table 7.6).

Pearls

> Opioids are good choices for the management of moderate and severe pain in older adults.
>
> Start low and go slow—generally 25% to 50% is the recommended starting dose for adults.
>
> Choose an opioid with a short half-life whenever possible.
> Do not use multiple opioids simultaneously.
>
> Monitor older adults for side effects, accumulation, and tolerance.
>
> For most older adults, morphine is the opioid of choice.
> Take precautions to prevent opioid-related constipation.

Some opioids are NOT recommended for use in OLDER adults

Methadone (Dolophin and Methadose) has a mechanism of action on the mu-receptor. Although it is recommended whenever possible to avoid using *methadone* in older adults, chronic pain of some older adults may necessitate treatment with methadone. It is recommended that older adults receiving methadone for chronic pain be supervised by a pain management specialist and titration be done very slowly and carefully. Methadone is lipophilic and has a very long half-life that may result in accumulation and toxicity (respiratory depression and sedation) in older adults (Fine, 2004; Herr et al., 2006; Kharasch, Hoffer, Whittington, & Sheffels, 2004).

Meperidine (Demerol) is no longer recommended for use as an analgesic medication due to the toxic metabolite normeperidine that can cause seizures, tremors, and delirium. It is contraindicated in patients with renal impairment and those using mono-amine oxidase (MAO) inhibitors (APS, 2008; D'Arcy, 2010; Herr et al., 2006).

Pentazocine (Talwin) and *Butorphanol* (Stadol) are not recommended for use with older adults because of the significant side effects (D'Arcy, 2010). They result in psychotomimetic effects and may result in delirium (Herr et al., 2006).

Multimodal pain management is the practice of using multiple medications and nonpharmacological interventions to help older adults control their pain. The intention is twofold. First, using more than one appropriate medication and intervention, less of each medication can be used, thus reducing the potential side effects of any one medication. Second when there are multiple factors contributing to the pain, using medications that are most appropriate for each factor increases the analgesic benefit.

Multimodal analgesia can be considered akin to making a soup that satisfies the needs and tastes of the individual. A plain chicken broth can be nutritious but bland. When relatively small amounts of celery, onions, carrots, parsley, and so forth are added, it increases both the flavor and the nutritional value. This is similar to the benefits that are obtained using a multimodal analgesia.

When an older adult has chronic low back pain with sciatic nerve impingement, it may be most appropriate and effective to manage the pain with an NSAID, a medication for neuropathic pain (see Chapters 8 and 17) and physical or movement therapy. It may also be appropriate to add an as needed opioid.

Pearls	Medications should be administered by the least invasive route. Start low and go slow using one medication at a time. Monitor carefully for toxicity and side effects. Educate patients and families regarding realistic expectations and safety issues. Equianalgesic charts are a guide; know dosages in the elderly with well-controlled pain should initially be reduced by 50%.

RESOURCES/GUIDELINES

Acute pain management in older adults. Herr, K., Bjoro, K., Steffensmeier, J., & Rakel, B. (2006, July). *University of Iowa Gerontological Nursing Research Center.* http://www.guideline.gov/database

Consensus Statement: Opioids and the management of chronic severe pain in the elderly: Consensus statement of an international expert panel with focus on the six clinically most often used World Health Organization step III opioids (buprenorphine, fentanyl, hydromorphone, methadone, morphine, oxycodone). Pergolizzi, J., Boger, R. H., Budd, K., Dahan, A., Erdine, S., & Hans, G. (2008). *Pain Practice, 8,* 287–313.

Pharmacological Management of Persistent Pain in Older Adults. American Geriatrics Society. (2009). *Journal of the American Geriatrics Society, 57,* 1331–1346.

The management of persistent pain in older persons. American Geriatrics Society Panel. (2002). *Journal of the American Geriatrics Society, 50,* S205–S224.

World Health Organization Guidelines on Pain Management (2007). http://www.who.int/medicines/areas/quality_safety/delphi_study_pain_guidelines.pdf

Case Study

Mr. Ray is an 82-year-old active man who is recovering on day 4 from a thoracotomy in the postsurgical unit. When you brought Mr. Ray his dose of coumadin after he ate dinner, he reported his pain as 6/10 at the surgical site and complained of 8/10 pain with the chest tubes. He also tells you that his lower back hurts more than usual. Upon questioning he tells you that he takes 1000 mg of Tylenol four times a day at home for his back and knee pain. He also tells you that the medicine he was getting (ketorolac) really helped.

1. What are the best medication options to treat the postoperative pain?
2. Is the same medication indicated for all the sites of pain reported by Mr. Ray?
3. What factors need to be considered in choosing medications for Mr. Ray?
4. What education is indicated for Mr. Ray?

REFERENCES

American Geriatric Society. (2009). Pharmacological management of persistent pain in older adults. *Journal of the American Geriatric Society, 57,* 1331–1346.

American Geriatric Society Panel. (2002). The management of persistent pain in older persons. *Journal of the American Geriatrics Society, 50,* S205–S224.

American Pain Society. (2003). *Principles of analgesic use in the treatment of acute pain and cancer pain* (5th ed.). Glenview, IL: Author.

American Pain Society. (2006). *Pain: Current understanding of assessment, management, and treatments.* Glenview, IL: Author.

American Pain Society. (2008). *Principles of analgesic use in the treatment of acute pain and cancer pain* (6th ed.). Glenview, IL: Author.

Arnold, R., & Weissman, D. E. (2009). *Calculating opioid dose conversions* (2nd ed). *Medical College of Wisconsin End of Life/Palliative Education Resource Center, 36.* Retrieved January 12, 2011, from http://www.mcw.edu/fastFact/ff_36.htm database

Arnstein, P. (2010). *Clinical coach for effective pain management.* Philadelphia, PA: F. A. Davis Company.

Banks, A. (2007). Innovations in postoperative pain management: Continuous infusion of local anesthetics. *AORN Journal, 85,* 904–914.

Barakzoy, A. S., & Moss, A. H. (2006). Efficacy of the World Health Organization Analgesic Ladder to treat pain in end-stage renal disease. *Journal of the American Society of Nephrology, 17,* 3198–3203.

Cadence Pharmaceuticals, Inc. (2011, November). Ofirmev™ (acetaminophen) Injection. *Highlights of Prescribing Information.* Retrieved March 27, 2011, from http://www.ofirmev.com/pdf/OFIRMEVPrescribingInformation.pdf database

D'Arcy, Y. (2009). Overturning barriers to pain relief in older adults. *Nursing, 39* (10), 32–38.

D'Arcy, Y. (2010). *Compact clinical guide to chronic pain management: An evidence based approach for nurses.* New York, NY: Springer.

Eliopoulos, C. (2001). *Gerontological nursing* (5th ed., Rev.). Philadelphia, PA: Lippincott.

Endo Pharmaceutical. (2010). *LIDODERM® (Lidocaine Patch 5%).* Retrieved March 26, 2011, from http://www.lidoderm.com/pdf/lidoderm_pack_insert.pdf database

FDA. (2009). *Voltaren Gel – (diclofenac sodium topical gel) 1% – Hepatic effects labeling changes.* Retrieved from http://www.fda.gov/default.htm database

Fine, P. (2004). Pharmacological management of persistent pain in older adults. *Clinical Journal of Pain, 20,* 220–226.

Fong, H. K., Sands, L., & Leung, J. M. (2006). The role of postoperative analgesia in delirium and cognitive decline in elderly patients: A systematic review. *Anesthesia and Analgesia, 102,* 1255–1255.

Freedman, G. M. (2002). Clinical management of common causes of geriatric pain. *Geriatrics, 57,* 35–41.

Gagliese, L., & Melzack, R. (2003). Age-related differences in the qualities but not the intensity of chronic pain. *Pain, 104,* 597–608.

Gleason, J. M., Slezak , J. M., Jung, H., Reynolds , K., Van Den Eeden, S. K., Haque, R., Jacobsen, S. J. (2011). Regular nonsteroidal anti-inflammatory drug use and erectile dysfunction. *The Journal of Urology, 185,* 1388–1393.

Green, C. R., Ndao-Brumblay, K., Nagrant, A. M., Baker, T., & Rothman, E. (2004). Race, age, and gender influences among clusters of African American and White patients with chronic pain. *The Journal of Pain, 2004,* 171–182.

Grond, S., & Sablotzki, A. (2004). Clinical pharmacology of tramadol. *Clinical Pharmacokinetics, 43,* 879–923.

Hadjiistavropoulos, T., & Fine, P. G. (2006). Chronic pain in older adults: Prevalence, assessment and management. *Reviews in Clinical Gerontology, 16,* 231–241.

Hanlon, J. T., Guay, D. R., & Ives, T. J. (2005). Oral analgesics: Efficacy, mechanism of action, pharmacokinetics, adverse effects, drug interactions, and practical recommendations for use in older adults. In S. J. Gibson & D. K. Weiner (Eds.), *Pain in older persons* (pp. 205–237). Seattle, WA: IASP Press.

Harder, A. T., & An, Y. H. (2003). The mechanisms of the inhibitory effects of nonsteroidal anti-inflammatory drugs on bone healing: A concise review. *The Journal of Clinical Pharmacology, 43,* 807–815.

Herr, K., Bjoro, K., Steffensmeier, J., & Rakel, B. (2006, July). Acute pain management in older adults. *University of Iowa Gerontological Nursing Research Center: Research Dissemination Core.* Retrieved March 10, 2011, from http://www.guideline.gov/database

Kharasch, E. D., Hoffer, C., Whittington, D. (2004). Influence of age on the pharmacokinetics and pharmacodynamics of oral transmucosal fentanyl citrate. *Anesthesiology, 101,* 738–743.

Kharasch, E. D., Hoffer, C., Whittington, D., & Sheffels, P. (2004). Role of hepatic and intestinal cytochrome P450 3A and 2B6 in the metabolism, disposition, and miotic effects of methadone. *Clinical Pharmacology & Therapeutics, 76,* 250–269.

King Pharmaceutical. (2011). What is FLECTOR® Patch? *FLECTOR® Patch.* Retrieved March 20, 2011, from http://www.flectorpatch.com/What-Is-FLECTOR-Patch.cfm database

Kingdon, R. T., Stanley, K. J., & Kizior, R. J. (1998). *Handbook for pain management.* Philadelphia, PA: W. B. Saunders.

Kumar, N. (2007, June). Report of a delphi study to determine the need for guidelines and to identify the number and topics of guidelines that should be developed by WHO. *WHO normative Guidelines on Pain Management.* Retrieved March 11, 2011, from http://www.who.int/medicines/areas/quality_safety/delphi_study_pain_guidelines.pdf database

Kurth, T., Glynn, R. J., Walker, A. M., Chan , K. A., Buring, J. E., Hennekens, C. H., & Gaziano, J. M. (2003). Inhibition of clinical benefits of aspirin on first myocardial infarction by nonsteroidal anti-inflammatory drugs. *Circulation Journal of the American Heart Association, 108,* 1191–1195.

Lionberger, D. R., Joussellin, E., Lanzarotti, A., Yanchick, J., & Magelli, M. (2011). Diclofenac epolamine topical patch relieves pain associated with ankle sprain. *Journal of Pain Research, 4,* 47–53.

Mallinckrodt Inc. (2011). *NDA 21-217 EXALGO™ (hydromorphone hydrochloride) extended release tablets CII.* Retrieved March 26, 2011, from *http://www.accessdata.fda.gov/drugsatfda_docs/label/2010/021217s001REMSExalgo.pdf*

McNeil. (2002). Executive summary. *McNeil Executive Summary Report.* Retrieved March 19, 2011, from http://www.fda.gov/ohrms/dockets/ac/02/briefing/3882B1_13_McNeil-Acetaminophen.pdf database

McPherson, M. L., & Uritsky, T. L. (2011). Pharmacotherapy of pain in older adults: Opioid and adjuvant. In F. M. Gloth (Ed.), *Aging medicine: Handbook of pain relief in older adults* (pp. 83–104). Totowa, NJ: Humana Press.

Mercadante, S., & Fulfaro, F. (2005). World health organization guidelines for cancer pain: A reappraisal. *Annals of Oncology, 16,* iv132–iv135.

Munir, M. A., Enany, N., & Zhang, J. M. (2007). Non-opioid analgesics. *Anesthesiology Clinics, 25,* 761–774.

Ortho-McNeil-Janssen Pharmaceuticals. (2010). Highlights of prescribing information. *Nucynta Product Information.* Retrieved March 20, 2010, from http://www.nucynta.com/sites/all/themes/nucynta/pdf/Nucynta-PI.pdf database

Pergolizzi, J., Boger, R. H., Budd, K., Dahan, A., Erdine, S., & Hans, G. (2008). Opioids and the management of chronic severe pain in the elderly: Consensus statement of an international expert panel with focus on the six clinically most often used World Health Organization step III opioids (buprenorphine, fentanyl, hydromorphone, methadone, morphine, oxycodone). *Pain Practice, 8,* 287–313.

Pfizer. (2002). CELEBREX U.S. Physician Prescribing Information. *Pfizer Product Finder*. Retrieved March 20, 2011, from http://www.pfizer.com/products/rx/rx_product_celebrex.jsp database

Reuben, D. B., Herr, K. A., Pacala, J. T., Pollock, B. G., Potter, J. F., & Semla, T. P. (2005). *Geriatrics at your fingertips* (7th ed.). New York, NY: American Geriatric Society.

Savage, R. (2006). Cyclo-oxygenase-2 inhibitors: When should they be used in the elderly. *Drugs Aging, 2005,* 185–200.

U.S. Food and Drug Administration. (2009). Use caution with pain relievers. *FDA U.S. Food and Drug Administration - Drugs*. Retrieved March 18, 2011, from http://www.fda.gov/Drugs/EmergencyPreparedness/BioterrorismandDrugPreparedness/ucm133425.htm database

U.S. Department of Health and Human Services. (2005). Information for Healthcare Professionals: Celecoxib (marketed as Celebrex). *FDA U.S. Food and Drug Administration: Drugs*. Retrieved March 20, 2011, from http://www.fda.gov/Drugs/DrugSafety/PostmarketDrugSafetyInformationforPatientsandProviders/ucm124655.htm database

Waknine, Y. (2010). FDA approves first intravenous formulation of acetaminophen. *Medscape Medical News, November 4, 2010*. Retrieved March 19, 2011, from http://www.medscape.com/viewarticle/731994

World Health Organization. (2009). WHO's pain ladder. *World Health Organization – Cancer*. Retrieved March 16, 2011, from http://www/who.int/cancer/palliative/painladder/en/database

Zacharoff, K. L., Zeis, J., Frayjo, K., Chiauzzi, E., & Reznikova, M. (2009). *Cross-cultural pain management*. Newton, MA: Infexxion.

Zydus Pharmaceuticals. (2011, February). Tramadol tablets description. *Tramadol Tablets*. Retrieved from http://www.drugs.com/pro/tramadol-tablets.html database

8

Adjuvant Analgesic Medications

Adjuvant analgesics or *coanalgesics* are a varied group of medications that were originally developed to treat conditions other than pain; however, they also have analgesic properties that are effective in some pain conditions (National Pharmaceutical Council & American Pain Society [NPC APS], 2006). Principles of multimodal analgesia encourage using adjuvant medications to improve analgesia while minimizing the side effects of any one medication (American Society of Anesthesiologists Task Force on Acute Pain Management, 2004; Kehlet & Dahl, 1993). As many side effects are dose related and problematic for older adults, this is an important benefit when considering how best to manage pain in older adults. At the same time, each adjuvant has side effects and cautions with older adults that must also be carefully considered.

This chapter provides an overview of representative adjuvant or coanalgesic medications, including anticonvulsants, antidepressants, corticosteroids, muscle relaxant groups, and topical agents. A few infrequently used adjuvant medications are also mentioned. Additional agents used for specific pain conditions are discussed in the pertinent chapters.

ANTICONVULSANT OR ANTIEPILEPTIC MEDICATIONS FOR COANALGESIA

Although other anticonvulsant medications have been effective in managing some neuropathic pain (NP), gabapentin and pregabalin are the anticonvulsant medications that are best tolerated when used for NP in older people (American Pain Society [APS], 2003).

Gabapentin (Neurontin)

Gabapentin (Neurontin) is an antiepileptic/anticonvulsant medication that is considered the "first-line off-label treatment for NP" (NPC APS, 2006, p. 42).

Indications are for NP related to a variety of disorders, including peripheral diabetic neuropathy (PDN) and postherpetic neuralgia (PHN) (see Chapter 17). Gabapentin is also effective in regional sympathetic dystrophy or complex regional pain syndrome, HIV-related neuropathy, phantom limb pain (PLP), migraine prophylaxis, thalamic pain, and deafferentation pain.

Mechanism of action is not fully known, but it affects the calcium channel. It is believed to, at least in part, inhibit substance P release on glutamate (Maneuf, Hughes, & McKnight, 2001; McCleane, 2009).

Pharmokinetic and administration information are given in Tables 8.1 and 8.2.

Safety concerns in older adults

- Side effects of somnolence, dizziness, fatigue, and ataxia, which can increase the risk of falling in older adults who may be at increased risk for falling.
- Assessment of gait and ambulation should be considered.
- Education to patient and family regarding symptoms that may increase the risk of falling is important.

Caution

With renal impairment, plasma concentration is elevated and elimination half-life is prolonged (APS, 2003; Blum et al., 1994; NPC APS, 2006; PDR, 2011).

Pregabalin (Lyrica)

Indication is treatment of NP of PDN, PHN, and fibromyalgia.

Mechanism of action is through an analog of gamma-amino butyric acid (GABA); it binds to calcium channels in the central nervous system and modulates the calcium influx. Although the exact mechanism of action is not known, this process results in analgesia, as well as anxiolytic and anticonvulsant effects (Roe, Velez, & Rey, 2006).

Pharmokinetic and administration information are given in Tables 8.1 and 8.2.

Safety concerns

- Concern in older adult is possible increased risk of falling related to dizziness and blurred vision.
- As equivalent effects to gabapentin were demonstrated with pregabalin at lower doses than needed with gabapentin, dose-related adverse events are expected to be less with pregabalin (American Geriatric Society Panel [AGS], 2009; APS, 2003, 2005; Gilron, Wajsbrot, Therrien, & Lemay, 2011; PDR, 2011).

Table 8.1 ■ *Pharmacokinetic Considerations of Anticonvulsant or Antiepileptic Medications Commonly Used in Older Adults*

Medication	Absorption	Metabolism	Half-life[a]	Elimination	Cautions
Gabapentin (Neurontin®)	Via GI tract	Very limited Bioavailability is approximately 60% but is not dose related	5–7 h	Urine basically unchanged	Plasma concentration is elevated and elimination half-life prolonged with renal impairment SE: dizziness, somnolence, fatigue, ataxia, risk of falling
Pregabalin (Lyrica®)	Good via the GI tract	Negligible with 90% bioavailable with onset of action 48–72 h	6.3 h	Urine with 90% unchanged	SE: dizziness, somnolences, sedation, weight gain, blurred vision
Carbamazepine (Tegretol®)	Via GI tract	Liver	Variable: 35–65 h with initial dosing; 12–17 h with repeated dosing	72% urine; 28% feces	Common side effects include sedation, mental clouding, dizziness, nausea

SE, side effects.

[a]Half-life of most medications may be prolonged in older adults particularly when renal function is impaired (AGS, 2009; APS, 2003; Blum et al., 1994; Gilron et al., 2011; NPC APS, 2006; PDR, 2011).

Table 8.2 ■ *Common Anticonvulsant or Antiepileptic Medications with Recommended Daily Doses, Effectiveness, Advantages, and Cautions*

Medication	Routes	Recommended Daily Dose	Effectiveness	Advantages	Cautions*
Gabapentin (Neurontin®)	Oral: tablets, capsules, elixir	Recommended starting dose for older adults is 100 mg at HS; can be titrated up to 2,400–3,600 mg daily in three divided doses	Similar to TCAs in doses of 2,400–3,600 mg/day; effectiveness in NP is related to being administered in 3 divided doses	Effective for NP; generally well-tolerated in older adults	Plasma concentration is elevated and elimination of half-life prolonged with renal impairment SE: dizziness, somnolence, fatigue, ataxia, risk of falling
Pregabalin (Lyrica®)	Oral: capsules	Recommended starting dose for older adults is 25 mg daily at HS; can be titrated up to 300 mg/day in 2 or 3 divided doses	Demonstrated in diabetic peripheral neuropathy, fibromyalgia, and other NP conditions	Effective for NP and fibromyalgia	SE: dizziness, somnolences, sedation, weight gain, blurred vision
Carbamazepine (Tegretol®)	Oral: tablets	Recommended starting dose for older adults is 25% reduction of recommended daily dose of 100 mg/day	NP related to TGN, glossopharyngeal neuralgia, dysesthesia, migraine prophylaxis	Effectiveness with TGN is reportedly superior	Aplastic anemia and agranulocytosis risk is 5–8 × greater; toxic epidermal necrolysis; Stevens–Johnson syndrome; SE: sedation, mental clouding, dizziness, nausea; close monitoring is needed

HS, hours of sleep or bedtime; SE, side effects; TCA, tricyclic antidepressants

Source: AGS, 2009; APS, 2003; Blum et al., 1994; Gilron et al., 2011; NPC APS, 2006; PDR, 2011.

*Half-life of most medications can be prolonged in older adults.

Carbamazepine (Tegretol)

Carbamazepine (Tegretol) is effective for NP related to trigeminal neuralgia (TGN), PDN, and migraine prophylaxis, glossopharyngeal neuralgia, spinal cord injury (dysesthesia), post-laminectomy pain, and PLP (APS, 2003, National Pharmaceutical Council & American Pain Society, 2006).

Mechanism of action in TGN is not known.

Pharmokinetic and administration information are given in Tables 8.1 and 8.2.

Safety concerns

In older adults, initially and periodically *monitor* the following:

- Liver function/damage via hepatic transaminases
- Thrombocytopenia via complete blood count
- Creatinine and blood urea nitrogen
- Hyponatremia via electrolytes
- Serum carbamazepine levels
- Interactions with other medications

Cautions

- *Aplastic anemia/Agranulocystosis* risk is 5 to 8 times greater than among normal adults. Baseline and close monitoring of platelets and WBC is required.
- *Toxic dermatological* side effects, including toxic epidermal necrolysis and Stevens–Johnson syndrome. Close monitoring is needed (AGS, 2009; APS, 2006; Epocrates, 2011; PDR, 2011).

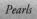 *Pearls*

Anticonvulsant medications are effective in managing NP in older adults.

The choice of the anticonvulsant medication in older adults is often limited by the side-effect profile.

Careful monitoring of side effects is imperative.

ANTIDEPRESSANTS USED FOR COANALGESIA

Tricyclic Antidepressants

Tricyclic antidepressants (TCAs) have a primary indication for depression; however, they are recognized by the International Association for the Study of Pain (IASP) as first-line therapy (desipramine and nortriptyline) for treating NP (McPherson & Uritsky, 2011).

However, the AGS (2009) *cautioned* that there are significant risks of adverse effects in older adults. Anticholinergic side effects can range from annoying to morbidity.

Using TCAs with Older Adults Is Discouraged

If it is necessary to use medications in this category, it is recommended to:

- slowly titrate using "very low doses"
- use TCAs with fewer anticholinergic effects, such as nortriptyline or desipramine
- carefully monitor older adults for side effects (AGS, 2009; Fine, 2004, p. 224)

Note

Amitryptiline, imipramine, and doxepine are *not* recommended for use in older adults (McPherson & Uritsky, 2011). Amitryptiline is considered a high severity medication by the Centers for Medicare & Medicaid Services (CMS) and inappropriate for use in older adults (Reuben et al., 2005).

Doses of TCAs for NP are less than those indicated for antidepressant treatment. If the older adult also needs pharmacological treatment for depression in addition to TCA treatment for NP, it is recommended for him or her to be under the care of a mental health professional who has experience in geriatric psychiatry.

The three most common TCAs are discussed in detail. Although desipramine and nortriptyline are the preferred TCAs for use with older adults, and amitryptiline is *not* recommended in older adults, discussion of amitryptiline is included for two reasons. First, so that the reader has adequate information about the concerns for use with older adults. Second, some older adults may be treated by another provider with amitryptiline, and it is important to understand the issues and concerns.

Desipramine (Norpramine)

Mechanism of action of this agent is believed to be by blocking the reuptake of serotonin and norepinephrine, thus inhibiting the nociceptive pain pathway.

Pharmokinetic and administration information are given in Tables 8.3, 8.4, and 8.5.

Table 8.3 ■ *Pharmacokinetic Considerations of TCA Used for Coanalgesia with Older Adults*

Medication	Absorption	Metabolism	Half-life[a]	Elimination	Cautions
Desipramine	Rapid via GI tract	Liver with wide variation of rate		70% in urine	Anticholinergic SE (see Table 8.5)
Nortriptyline Pamelor® Aventyl®	Via GI tract	Extensively in the liver	18–44 h	Primarily urine, some via feces	Anticholinergic SE (see Table 8.5)
Amitriptyline	Via GI tract	Liver Active metabolites include nortriptyline	10–26 h	Urine and feces	Severe anticholinergic SE (see Table 8.5)

Sources: AGS, 2009; APS, 2003; Fick et al., 2008; McPherson & Uritsky, 2011; PDR, 2011; Sanofi-Aventis, 2009.

[a]Half-life of most medications may be prolonged in older adults, particularly when renal function is impaired. TCAs are *not* recommended in older adults but if needed, preferred agents are nortriptyline or desipramine. Using TCAs with older adults is *discouraged.*

Significant risks and anticholinergic side effects can occur. These side effects include visual disturbances, ataxia, sedation, confusion, cognitive impairment, urinary retention, orthostasis, arrythmias, AV block

Table 8.4 ■ *Common TCA Used for Coanalgesia with Older Adults with Recommended Daily Doses, Effectiveness, Advantages, and Cautions*

Medication	Routes	Recommended Daily Dose	Effectiveness	Advantages	Cautions
Desipramine	Oral: tablets	Recommended to start at 10 mg at HS. May be titrated slowly as tolerated	NP	SE are less intense than with amitriptyline. Inexpensive	Anticholinergic SE (see Table 8.5)
Nortriptyline Pamelor® Aventyl®	Oral: tablets, elixir	Recommended to start at 10 mg at HS	NP	Considered first-line therapy for NP by IASP** Better tolerated than amitriptyline; inexpensive	Anticholinergic SE (see Table 8.5)
Amitriptyline	Oral: tablets	Not recommended for older adults. Recommended to start at 10 mg at HS	Wide range of NP conditions	Effective for NP. Inexpensive	Not recommended for use in older adults; Significant safety concerns; severe anticholinergic SE (as in Table 8.5)

HS, hours of sleep; bedtime; SE, side effects

Sources: (AGS, 2009; APS, 2003, 2006; D'Arcy, 2010; Epocrates, 2011; Fick et al., 2008; McPherson & Uritsky, 2011; PDR, 2011).

*Half-life of most medications can be prolonged in older adults.

** International Association for the Study of Pain.

Table 8.5 ■ *Anticholinergic Side Effects That May Occur with TCAs*

- Dry mouth
- Visual disturbances
- Urinary retention
- GI
- Constipation
- Ataxia
- Sedation
- Confusion
- Cognitive impairment
  - Cardiovascular
  - Orthostasis
  - Arrhythmias
  - Atrioventricular blockade

Safety concerns

■ Anticholinergic side effects noted previously.

■ Fall risk related to the potential side effects of ataxia, confusion, and orthostatic hypotension.

Cautions

■ Start with low dose and titrate slowly.

■ Monitor for anticholinergic side effects.

■ Educate patients and family of risk of falling (AGS, 2009; APS, 2003; Epocrates, 2011; McPherson & Uritsky, 2011; PDR, 2011; Sanofi-Aventis, 2009).

Nortriplyline (Pamelor, Aventyl)

Indications are for depression and PDN and mixed NPs

Mechanism of action of this agent is believed to be by blocking the reuptake of serotonin and norepinephrine, thus inhibiting the nociceptive pain pathway

Pharmokinetic and administration information are given in Tables 8.3, 8.4, and 8.5.

Safety concerns

■ Anticholinergic side effects noted previously.

■ Risk of falling related to the potential side effects of ataxia, confusion, and orthostatic hypotension.

■ In addition, insomnia is a potential problem, therefore it should be administered during the day rather than at night.

Cautions
- Start with low dose and titrate slowly.
- Monitor for anticholinergic side effects.
- Educate patients and family of risk of falling.

Older adults with comorbid depression may experience worsening of the depression and suicide ideation (Mallinckrodt, 2009); however, suicide ideation appears to be less common among those older than 65 years (AGS, 2009; APS, 2003, 2006; D'Arcy, 2010; Epocrates, 2011; Fine, 2004; Mallinckrodt, 2009; McPherson & Uritsky, 2011; PDR, 2011).

Amitryptiline (Elavil) is not recommended in older adults

Indication is for depression and various NP conditions that affect older adults, including chronic facial pain, PHN, PDN, fibromyalgia, and chronic low back pain.

Despite the indications for use in conditions from which older adults may suffer, *it is not recommended for use with older adults* because of the significant anticholinergic and sedating side effects. It is rated as a high severity concern on the updated Beers criteria for potentially inappropriate medications in older adults (Fick et al., 2008).

Mechanism of action of this agent is believed to be by blocking the reuptake of serotonin and neurepinephrine, thus inhibiting the nociceptive pain pathway.

Pharmokinetic and administration information are given in Tables 8.3, 8.4, and 8.5.

Safety concerns are significant. There are significant risks in older adults for developing adverse effects that include the following:
- Anticholinergic effects, including visual, urinary, and gastrointestinal (GI) symptoms
- Cardiovascular (CV) effects, including orthostasis and AV blockade

Cautions
Side effects are intense.

Particular caution is needed when administered concurrently with opioids (AGS, 2009; APS, 2003, 2006; D'Arcy, 2010; Epocrates, 2011; Fick et al., 2008; McPherson & Uritsky, 2011; PDR, 2011).

> *Pearls*
>
> TCAs can be effective in treating NP.
> Amitryptiline is *not indicated* for NP in older adults.
> Desipramine and nortriptyline can be used in older adults,
> but it is important to monitor for anticholinergic side effects.

Serotonin–Norepinephrine-Reuptake Inhibitor Antidepressant Medications

Duloxetine (Cymbalta)

Indication is primarily for the treatment of major depression, but it has been approved for treatment of NP related to diabetic peripheral fibromyalgia and chronic musculoskeletal pain.

Mechanism of action is as a serotonin–norepinephrine reuptake inhibitor (SNRI); however, the exact mechanism is not known.

Pharmokinetic and administration information are given in Tables 8.6 and 8.7.

Cautions
- Monitor blood pressure.
- Doses need to be reduced in older adults with renal insufficiency.
- Use with caution in older adults with hepatic insufficiency.
- Use with caution in older men with prostatic hypertrophy due to reported urinary retention.

Miscellaneous Note
No greater benefit was noted when dosing exceeded 60 mg/day (AGS, 2009; APS, 2003, 2005; Epocrates, 2011; Hadjistavropoulos & Fine, 2007; McPherson & Uritsky, 2011; PDR, 2011).

Venlafaxine (Effexor)

Indication is primarily for depression; however, it has been effective with NP.

Mechanism of action is through inhibition of serotonin reuptake when low doses are prescribed and inhibition of both serotonin and norepinephrine when higher doses are prescribed. It is reported to inhibit dopamine reuptake.

Pharmokinetic and administration information are given in Tables 8.6 and 8.7.

Table 8.6 ■ *Pharmacokinetic Considerations of Antidepressants Used for Coanalgesia with Older Adults*

Medication	Absorption	Metabolism	Half-life[a]	Elimination	Cautions
Duloxetine (Cymbalta®)	Via GI tract	Extensively via liver	12 h	70% urine; 20% feces	SE: dizziness, fatigue, memory impairment, somnolence, suicidality but less over 6 years, *serotonin syndrome*, extrapyramidal symptoms, hepatotoxicity, fatigue
Venlafixine (Effexor®)	Via GI tract	Extensively via liver	5 h; (the metabolite desmethylvenlafaxine is 11 h)	87% via urine with 5% unchanged	Concern for increased heart rate and increased blood pressure that are considered dose related. Must taper to discontinue
Minacipran (Savella®)	Via GI tract	Minimally via liver; Metabolism is largely unknown	6–8 h	Primarily via urine with 55% unchanged	*Contraindicated in older adults who have narrow angle glaucoma, end-stage renal disease, or who use MAO inhibitors. Caution with renal insufficiency;* SE: Hypertension, palpitations, constipation, hyperhidrosis, hot flashes. Must taper dose to discontinue

Sources: AGS, 2009; APS, 2003; Fick et al., 2008; McPherson & Uritsky, 2011; PDR, 2011; Sanofi-Aventis, 2009.

[a]Half-life of most medications may be prolonged in older adults, particularly when renal function is impaired.

Table 8.7 ■ *Common SNRI Antidepressants Used for Coanalgesia with Older Adults with Recommended Daily Doses, Effectiveness, Advantages, and Cautions*

Medication	Routes	Recommended Daily Dose	Effectiveness	Advantages	Cautions
Duloxetine (Cymbalta®)	Oral: capsules	Recommended to start with 20 mg in older adults and increase as tolerated	NP and fibromyalgia	Fewer anticholinergic effects than TCAs	SE: dizziness, fatigue, memory impairment, somnolence, suicidality but less over 6 years, *serotonin syndrome*, extrapyramidal symptoms, hepatotoxicity, fatigue
Venlafixine (Effexor®)	Oral: immediate and extended release	37.5 mg/day *Recommended to take with food*	Treatment of DN when doses are 150–225 mg/day *Not FDA approved for this use as of 6/2011*	Side effect profile is safer than TCAs Extended release allows for once per day dosing	Concern for increased heart rate and increased blood pressure that are considered dose related; Must taper to discontinue
Minacipran (Savella®)	Oral	12.5 mg/day; increase dose slowly	Primarily for treatment of fibromyalgia	Effective for fibromyalgia	*Contraindicated in older adults who have narrow angle glaucoma end-stage renal disease or who use MAO inhibitors Caution with renal insufficiency;* SE: hypertension, palpitations, constipation, hyperhidrosis, hot flashes; Must taper dose to discontinue

SE, side effects

Sources: AGS, 2009; APS, 2003, 2005; Epocrates, 2011; Hadjistavropoulos & Fine, 2007; McPherson & Uritsky, 2011; PDR, 2011.

*Half-life of most medications can be prolonged in older adults.

- *Safety concerns* are primarily for increased heart rate and blood pressure that are considered to be dose related.
- **Cautions**
  - Monitor pulse and blood pressure.
  - Taper doses to discontinue (AGS, 2009; Epocrates, 2011; McPherson & Uritsky, 2011; PDR, 2011).

Minacipran (Savella®)

Indication is primarily for depression; however, it is indicated for the pain of fibromyalgia (see Chapter 21).

Mechanism of action is through the inhibition of norepinephrine and serotonin reuptake.

Pharmokinetic and administration information are given in Tables 8.6 and 8.7.

- **Cautions**
  - *Contraindicated* in older adults who
    - have narrow angle glaucoma
    - use monoamine oxidase (MAO) inhibitors
    - have end-stage renal disease
  - *Use caution* and reduce dose by 50% in older adults with renal insufficiency and those with a creatinine clearance below 30 mL/min.
  - It is necessary to taper doses when the medication is *discontinued* (Forest Laboratories, 2009; McPherson & Uritsky, 2011; PDR, 2011; US Federal Drug Administration, 2010).

Pearls | Duloxetine and Minacipran are antidepressants that are effective in managing the symptoms of fibromyalgia.
When initiating medications with older adults, it is important to start low and go slow.

STEROIDS USED FOR COANALGESIA

Corticosteroids include the following:

Dexamethasone (Decadron®)
Methylprednisolone (Medrol®)

Indications include the following:

- Rheumatological conditions and arthralgias

- Inflammatory reactions
- Treatment of acute nerve compression
- Spinal cord compression
- Increased intracranial pressure
- Superior vena cava syndrome
- Lymphedema
- Pain due to bone metastases
- Sympathetic pain syndromes
- Additive to opioid analgesia

Mechanism of action for anti-inflammatory properties is not exactly known; however, they are known to inhibit a variety of inflammatory cytokines and prostaglandin synthesis. They are also reported to decrease spontaneous discharge from nerves that have been injured.

Pharmacokinetic considerations

- *Absorption* of oral preparations is via the GI system.
- *Metabolism* is via the liver.

Half-life

  - for *dexamethasone*, 1.8 to 3.5 hours (plasma half-life), 36 to 54 hours (biological half-life)
  - for *methylprednisolone*, 18 to 36 hours
- *Elimination* is via the urine.
- *Effectiveness* is reported for a variety of pain situations.
- *Advantages* in older adults are that they tend to
  - increase appetite
  - decrease nausea
  - improve mood

Recommended dosing

  - Use the lowest possible dose and titrate slowly.
  - Specific dosing depends upon the indication.

Administration

  - Dexamethosone can be given orally and intravenously.
  - Methylprednisolone can be given orally.
- *Safety concerns* are for the numerous side effects, including:
  - fluid retention and edema
  - glycemic alterations/hyperglycemia
  - vertigo
  - muscle weakness
  - osteoporosis with prolonged use
  - insomnia
  - nervousness

- mood swings
- euphoria, and
- delirium

Cautions
- *in elderly patients* for any indication
- in the presence of immunosuppression
- in those with osteoporosis
- when renal impairment is present
- with diabetes mellitus
- with seizure disorder
- with congestive heart failure and hypertension (APS, 2003; Kelly, 2010; Kingdon, Stanley, & Kizior, 1998; Vanni & Rehm, 2010)

MUSCLE RELAXANTS USED FOR COANALGESIA

Skeletal muscle relaxants include the following:
- Carisprodol (Soma)
- Cyclobenzaprine (Flexeril)
- Orphenadrine (Norflex)
- Tizanidine (Zanaflex)
- Methocarbamol (Robaxin)

Indications are to alleviate pain in muscles.

Mechanism of action varies by the particular medication.

Pharmacokinetic considerations vary by medication.

Effectiveness, recommended dosing, and administration vary by medication; evidence regarding effectiveness is mixed.

Advantage is that they are effective for some pain situations.

Recommended dosing depends upon the individual medication.

Administration is oral or parenteral.

Safety concerns are risk of dependency after 1 to 2 weeks.

Caution
- CMS classifies the following medications as potentially inappropriate in treating older adults (Reuben et al., 2005).

This same list of medications is listed as high severity for potential problems in older adults related to the anticholinergic effects (Fick et al., 2008) (see Table 8.5).

CMS recommended that if used, they should only be used for short times (less than 1 week) and not more frequently than every 3 months.

- Carisprodol (Soma)
- Cyclobenzaprine (Flexeril)
- Orphenadrine (Norflex)
- Metaxalone (Skelaxin)
- Methocarbamol (Robaxin) (Reuben et al., 2005)

Miscellaneous note

The AGS (2009) stress the following:

- These medications do *not* relax muscles and are *not* indicated for muscle spasms.
- If muscle spasms are present, *baclofen* or one of the benzodi-azepines is the medication of choice (AGS, 2009; APS, 2003; Epocrates, 2011; Fick et al., 2008; Reuben et al., 2005).

ANTI-SPASMOTIC MEDICATION USED FOR COANALGESIA

Baclofen

Indication is only for TGN as a pain condition.

Mechanism of action is through inhibiting the release of presyn-aptic excitatory amino acids.

Pharmacokinetic considerations

- *Absorption* of oral preparation is via the GI tract.
- *Metabolism* is in the liver of the oral form.
- *Half-life* is variable due to autoinduction but ranges from 2.5 to 7 hours with initial doses and 12 to 17 hours with subsequent doses.
- *Elimination* is 72% in the urine and 28% in the feces.

Effectiveness

- reportedly less than carbamazepine
- considered a second-line therapy because of challenges with toler-ating it

Advantages

- Effective for TGN
- *Recommended dosing* is 5 to 10 mg three times daily.
- *Administration* is oral (can also be used intrathecally).
- *Safety concerns* focus on the side effects:
  - dizziness
  - drowsiness
  - ataxia
  - confusion
  - nausea and vomiting

- cardiac arrhythmias
- urinary frequency

Caution

Use with caution with central nervous system (CNS) depressants (opioids, alcohol, and antihistamines).

Gradually titrate when discontinuing this medication, because abrupt withdrawal can result in hallucinations, rhabdomyolysis, seizures, anxiety, and tachyarrhythmia that may persist for as long as 2 months (Epocrates, 2011; Ghafoor & St. Marie, 2010; Hanlon, Guay, & Ives, 2005; PDR, 2011).

LOCAL ANESTHETICS USED AS COANALGESIA

Lidocaine Transdermal Patch

Mechanism of Action appears to be in the sodium channels of peripheral nerves.

Absorption is dependent upon the number of patches applied; however, only 3% ± 2% of the amount of lidocaine in each patch is designed to be absorbed.

Distribution is via plasma protein, with peak plasma level achieved after 9.25 hours.

Metabolism of lidocaine is in the liver; it is not known if there is metabolism in the derma. Older adults with severe liver disease should be monitored carefully for toxic blood levels.

Elimination of lidocaine is through the kidneys.

Dosing and administration

- Available in 5% strength via transdermal patch.
- Apply up to 3 patches to intact skin 12 hours on and 12 hours off during each 24-hour interval.
- These patches may be cut to fit the affected area.

Safety data is that it is relatively safe and has an excellent safety profile, with the only side effects noted as local skin irritation. Patches should be applied to intact skin.

Indications include PHN, neuropathic conditions, low back pain, joint pain, and chest tube sites.

Caution

Contraindicated in patients who are being treated with Class 1 antiarrhythmic medications and those with severe hepatic dysfunction

(AGS, 2009; APS, 2003; Endo Pharmaceutical, 2010; Fine & Herr, 2009; Gammaitoni, Alvarez, & Galer, 2003; Hadjistavropoulos & Fine, 2007; McPherson & Uritsky, 2011).

Mexiletine (Mexitil)

Mexiletine is an oral congener of lidocaine

Indications are for NP (DN and central poststroke pain) and refractory pain.

Mechanism of action is through stabilization of membranes.

Pharmacokinetic considerations

■ *Absorption* is via the GI tract.
■ *Metabolism* is via the liver.
■ *Half-life* is 10 to 12 hours but longer with creatinine clearance less than 10 and with severe hepatic impairment.
■ *Elimination* is via urine with 10% unchanged.
■ *Effectiveness* in older adults with TGN and poststroke pain has been positive.

Advantages

　　■ It is effective for refractory and poststroke pain.
　　■ Pharmacokinetics are reportedly not changed in older adults.

Recommended dosing in older adults is to start at 50 mg daily, possibly increasing to two or three times per day after 2 or 3 days *under the supervision of a pain management specialist.*

■ *Administration* is oral via capsules.
■ *Safety concerns* in older adults are for side effects and the consequential increased falling risk. Side effects include the following:
　　■ Dizziness
　　■ Irritability/nervousness
　　■ Tremor
　　■ Coordination problems
　　■ Headache

Caution is to *avoid* this medication in older adults who have bradyarrhythmia and conduction block (2nd or 3rd degree). Older adults with other cardiac pathologies should be cleared by a cardiologist.

　　Monitor electrocardiograms (ECGs).

　　There is a *black box warning* of excessive mortality or nonfatal cardiac arrest (AGS, 2009; Hanlon et al., 2005).

> *Pearls*   Local anesthetics can be effective as an adjuvant to opioids in managing acute and chronic pain.
>
>   The pain situation and comorbidities of the individual older adult must be considered.

ADDITIONAL MEDICATIONS USED FOR COANALGESIA

Capsaicin (Zostrix) (Qutenza)

Indication is for pain related to rheumatoid arthritis, osteoarthritis, DN, postmastectomy pain, PHN, and other neuropathic conditions.

Mechanism of action is not exactly known. It is believed that there is binding with nerve membrane receptors by initially stimulating and then desensitizing. It also degenerates cutaneous nociceptive neurons. A reduction in the secretion of substance P may decrease the transmission of the pain impulse to the CNS (Epocrates, 2011).

Pharmacokinetic considerations

- *Absorption* is transdermal.
- *Metabolism* is not known; reportedly there is minimal systemic absorption.
- *Half-life* is not known.
- *Elimination* is not known.

Effectiveness has been seen in reducing both neuropathic and non-NP; however, several weeks of consistent application may be required before effectiveness is seen.

- *Advantage* is that there are no known systemic side effects.

Recommended dosing

- 0.025% to 0.75% cream is applied 3 to 4 times/day.
- Patch is 8% after local anesthetic (LA) application.
- *Administration* is topical either via cream or topical patch.

- **Safety concerns are generally minimal.**
  - neurotoxicity (only reported serious reaction)
  - burning
  - erythema
  - thermal hyperalgesia
- **Cautions**
  - Apply only to intact skin.

- Educate patients prior to first use that
  - application will initially cause a burning sensation at the site of application
  - patients need to wear gloves when applying cream
  - patients should not touch other parts of the body especially the eyes
- Initial burning sensation may persist for an extended period of time
- Prior to applying the patch, LA must be applied to the area. (AGS, 2009; APS, 2003; D'Arcy, 2010; Epocrates, 2011; PDR, 2011).

Ropinirole (Requip)

Indication is for restless leg syndrome.

Mechanism of action is through the stimulation of dopamine receptors.

Pharmacokinetic considerations

- *Absorption* is rapid via the GI tract, with peak levels being reached in 1 to 2 hours.
- *Metabolism* is extensively in the liver.
- *Half-life* is 6 hours.
- *Elimination* is via urine with 10% unchanged with some reduced clearance noted in older adults.
  - *Effectiveness* with restless leg syndrome was demonstrated in randomized double-blind, placebo-controlled studies.

Advantages

- It is effective for restless leg syndrome.
- *Recommended dosing* is 0.25 mg at hour of sleep. This may be titrated to 4 mg/day maximum.
- *Administration* is oral via tablets, either immediate or sustained release.
- *Safety concerns* are for dopaminergic effects.

Assess for

- sedation
- orthostatic hypotension
- dyskinesia
- syncope
- confusion
- hallucinations (more common in older adults with Parkinson's disease)
- exacerbation of parkinsonism

Caution

- in elderly patients
- in comorbid CV disease patients
- *Avoid stopping abruptly,* taper gradually (Epocrates, 2011; Glaxo SmithKline, 2009; Hadjistavropoulos & Fine, 2007).

NMDA RECEPTOR BLOCKERS

(Ketamine, Dextromethorphan, and Dronabinol) are *not* recommended as first-line medications for treatment of pain in older adults. They should be used only with refractory pain and under the supervision of a pain management specialist.

Indications are for hyperalgesia, centrally mediated NP, and refractory pain when all analgesic options have been ineffective or are inappropriate. These medications are **not** indicated as either first-line or second-line analgesia and should be used only under supervision of someone with experience using them.

Cautions are that these medications have significant side effects and adverse reactions associated with them.

Ketamine side effects include hallucinations and memory impairment. A significant abuse potential is associated with ketamine.

Dronabinol side effects include cognitive changes, psychosis, and sedation

Dextromethorphan side effects include dizziness, insomnia, as well as nausea. (D'Arcy, 2010; Epocrates, 2011; PDR, 2011).

GUIDELINES AND RESOURCES

Acute pain management in older adults. Herr, K., Steffensmeier, J., & Rakel, B. (2006, July). *University of Iowa Gerontological Nursing Research Center.* http://www.guideline.gov/database

American Society of Anesthesiologists Task Force on Acute Pain Management. (2004). Practice guidelines for acute pain in the perioperative setting. *Anesthesiology, 100,* 1573–1581.

Consensus statement: Opioids and the management of chronic severe pain in the elderly: Consensus statement of an International Expert Panel with focus on the six clinically most often used World Health Organization Step III opioids (buprenorphine, fentanyl, hydromorphone, methadone, morphine, oxycodone). Pergolizzi, J., Boger, R. H., Budd, K., Dahan, A., Erdine, S., Hans, G., Sacerdote, P. (2008). *Pain Practice, 8,* 287–313.

National Pharmaceutical Council & The Joint Commission. (2005, May). Special update to: Pain: Current understanding of assessment, management, and treatments. Retrieved from http://www.APSnow.org/App_Themes/Public/pdf/Issues/pub_related_research/pub_quality_care/Pain Addendum.pdf database.

Pharmacological management of persistent pain in older adults. American Geriatrics Society. (2009). *Journal of the American Geriatrics Society, 57,* 1331–1346.

The management of persistent pain in older persons. American Geriatrics Society Panel. (2002). *Journal of the American Geriatrics Society, 50,* S205–S224.

World Health Organization Guidelines on pain management. (2007). http://www.who.int/medicines/areas/quality_safety/delphi_study_pain_guidelines.pdf

Case Study

Mrs. Davis is a 68-year-old woman who was admitted to the hospital for repair of a fractured wrist sustained during a fall in her home. She also sustained three rib fractures. She reports 10/10 pain "everywhere." She says that she has chronic pain related to fibromyalgia, TGN, and injuring her back 30 years ago when working as a nursing assistant. At home she treats the pain with Oxycontin 40 mg twice daily, Percocet 5/325 two every 4 hours, amitryptiline 10 mg twice a day, and carbamazepine 100 mg three times per day.

Questions

1. What are the best options for managing the pain Mrs. Davis is experiencing?
2. Should all of her home medications be continued?
3. What home medications may need to be adjusted?
4. What education regarding pain medications should be provided to Mrs. Davis?

REFERENCES

American Geriatric Society Panel. (2009). Pharmacological management of persistent pain in older adults. *Journal of the American Geriatric Society, 57,* 1331–1346.

American Pain Society. (2003). *Principles of analgesic use in the treatment of acute pain and cancer pain* (5th ed.). Glenview, IL: Author.

American Society of Anesthesiologists Task Force on Acute Pain Management. (2004). Practice guidelines for acute pain in the perioperative setting. *Anesthesiology, 100,* 1573–1581.

Blum, R. A., Comstock, T. J., Sica, D. A., Schultz, R. W., Keller, E., Reetze, P., Sedman, A. J. (1994). Pharmacokinetics of gabapentin in subjects with various degrees of renal function. *Clinical Pharmacology & Therapeutics, 56,* 154–159.

D'Arcy, Y. (2010). *Chronic pain management: An evidence-based approach for nurses.* New York, NY: Springer.

Epocrates. (2011). *Drug reference.* Retrieved from http://www.epocrates.com database.

Fick, D. M., Cooper, J. W., Wade, W. E., Waller, J. L., Maclean, J. R., & Beers, M. H. (2008). Updating the Beers criteria for potentially inappropriate medication use in older adults. *Archives of Internal Medicine, 163,* 2716–2724.

Fine, P. G. (2004). Pharmacological management of persistent pain in older adults. *Clinical Journal of Pain, 20,* 220–226.

Fine, P. G., & Herr, K. (2009). Pharmacologic management of persistent pain in older persons. *Clinical Geriatrics, 17,* 25–32

Forest Laboratories. (2009). Savella (milnacipran HCl) tablets: Prescribing information [Brochure]. St. Louis, MO: Author.

Gammaitoni, A. R., Alvarez, N. A., & Galer, B. S. (2003). Safety and tolerability of the lidocaine patch 5%, a targeted peripheral analgesic: A review of the literature. *The Journal of Clinical Pharmacology, 43,* 111–117.

Ghafoor, V. L., & St. Marie, B. (2010). Overview of pharmacology. In B. St. Marie (Ed.), *Core curriculum for pain management nursing* (Rev. ed., pp. 235–305). Dubuque, IA: Kendall Hunt.

Gilron, I., Wajsbrot, D., Therrien, F., & Lemay, J. (2011). Pregabalin for peripheral neuropathic pain: A multicenter, enriched enrollment randomized withdrawal placebo-controlled trial. *Clinical Journal of Pain, 27,* 185–193.

GlaxoSmithKline. (2009, April). Requip® (ropinirole tablets). Product information. Retrieved from http://us.gsk.com/products/assets/us_requip.pdf database.

Hadjistavropoulos, T., & Fine, P. G. (2007). Chronic pain in older persons: Prevalence, assessment and management. *Reviews in Clinical Gerontology, 16,* 231–241.

Hanlon, J. T., Guay, D. R., & Ives, T. J. (2005). Oral analgesics: Efficacy, mechanism of action, pharmacokinetics, adverse effects, drug interactions, and practical recommendations for use in older adults. In S. J. Gibson & D. K. Weiner (Eds.), *Pain in older adults* (pp. 205–222). Seattle, WA: IASP Press.

Kehlet, H., & Dahl, J. B. (1993). The value of "multimodal" or "balanced analgesia" in postoperative pain treatment. *Anesthesia and Analgesia, 37,* 1048–1056.

Kelly, A. M. (2010). Gerontology pain management. In B. St. Marie (Ed.), *Core curriculum for pain management nursing* (2nd ed., Rev., pp. 573–586). Dubuque, IA: Kendall Hunt.

Kingdon, R. T., Stanley, K. J., & Kizior, R. J. (1998). *Handbook for pain management.* Philadelphia, PA: W. B. Saunders Company.

Mallinckrodt (2009, June). Pamelor™: (nortriptyline HCl) capsules USP; (nortriptyline HCl) oral solution USP. Retrieved from http://imaging.mallinckrodt .com/imageServer.aspx?doc191777.pdf?contentID=18704&contenttype= application/pdf database.

Maneuf, Y. P., Hughes, J., & McKnight, A. T. (2001). Gabapentin inhibits the substance P-facilitiate K^+-evoked release of [^{3}H]glutamate from rat caudal trigeminal nucleus slices. *Pain, 93,* 191–196.

McCleane, G. (2009). Antiepileptic drugs. In H. S. Smith (Ed.), *Current therapy in pain* (pp. 458–465). Philadelphia, PA: Saunders Elsevier.

McPherson, M. L., & Uritsky, T. J. (2011). Pharmacotherapy of pain in older adults: Opioid and adjuvant. In F. M. Gloth (Ed.), *Aging medicine: Handbook of pain relief in older adults.* Totowa, NJ: Humana Press.

National Pharmaceutical Council & American Pain Society. (2006). Pain: Current understanding of assessment, management, and treatments. Retrieved from http://www.APSnow.org/App_Themes/Public/pdf/Issues/pub_related_ research/pub_quality_care/Pain-Current-Understanding-of-Assessment-Management-and-Treatments.pdf database.

PDR. (2011). *Nurse's drug handbook.* Montvale, NJ: PDR Network, L.L.C.

Roe, J. N., Velez, E. M. & Rey, J. A. (2006). Pregabalin (Lyrica): a new treatment option for neuropathic pain

Reuben, D. B., Herr, K. A., Pacala, J. T., Pollock, B. G., Potter, J. F., & Semla, T. P. (2005). *Geriatrics at your fingertips* (7th ed., Rev.). New York, NY: American Geriatrics Society.

Sanofi-Aventis. (2009). Nonprime: Desipramine hydrochloride tablets USP. Product information. Retrieved from http://products.sanofi-aventis.us/norpramin/ norpramin.pdf database.

US Federal Drug Administration. (2010, February). Savella (milnacipran HCl) tablets: Safety labeling changes approved. Retrieved from http://google2.fda. gov/search?q=milnacipran+hcl&x=5&y=12&client=FDAgov&proxystyleshe et=FDAgov&output=xml_no_dtd&sort=date%253AD%253AL%253Ad1& site=FDAgov-MedWatch-Safety

Vanni, L., & Rehm, M. N. (2010). Cancer pain management. In S. St. Marie (Ed.), *Core curriculum for pain management nurses* (2nd ed., pp. 461–479). Dubuque, IA: Kendall Hunt.

9

Managing Medication Side Effects and Specific Recommendations for Using Medications with Older Patients

I. SPECIFIC RECOMMENDATIONS FOR USING MEDICATIONS WITH OLDER PATIENTS

Managing pain in older adults can be challenging. As with any individual experiencing pain, in the older adult pain is a multifaceted experience involving physical, emotional, cognitive, functional, and experiential factors. In the older person, this is often complicated by comorbid illnesses and the medications needed to manage them. All of this must be considered when using analgesic and adjuvant medications (American Geriatric Society [AGS], 2009).

Medication management is generally an important component of a multidisciplinary plan. Despite the challenges, analgesic and adjuvant medications can be used safely and effectively with older adults, when the benefits are balanced with the risks and careful consideration is given to several factors (AGS, 2009; Hadjistavropoulos & Fine, 2007).

Effective pain management of older adults begins with *screening,* followed by a thorough *multidimensional pain assessment* and setting *realistic/reasonable goals.* Reasonable goals must balance achieving optimal function and quality of life (AGS, 2009) for the older adult while ensuring safety.

CONSIDER BENEFITS AND RISKS OF MEDICATIONS

Managing pain in the older adult requires considering and balancing the desired benefits with the risks of the analgesic and adjuvant medications. This necessitates a thorough knowledge of the older adult and the medications involved. This chapter will provide information to help guide decisions regarding the analgesic and adjuvant medications.

AGE-RELATED PHYSIOLOGICAL CHANGES THAT AFFECT MEDICATION ABSORPTION, METABOLISM, AND ELIMINATION

Gastrointestinal (GI) absorption must be considered because the oral route is the first option for administration of analgesic medications in the majority of older adults. There are several age-related factors to consider with oral analgesia:

- Swallowing can be slowed to twice the time of younger adults.
- GI blood flow is reduced.
- Motility of the esophagus and stomach is decreased.
- GI transit time may be increased.
- Esophageal emptying is slower.
- Gastric emptying may be slower but is not necessarily a part of normal aging.
- Less gastric acid secretion can result in reduced absorption and changes in breakdown of pills and capsules.
- Gastric pH is generally increased.
- Some chronic conditions may alter pH, resulting in decreased absorption.
- Intestinal atrophy occurs throughout the small and large intestines.
- Absorbing cells on the intestinal wall surface are reduced in number.
- Fat absorption is slower.
- Consequences of previous GI surgeries may reduce absorption.
- Older adults may have a history of colostomy, short bowel, or gastric bypass surgery (AGS, 2009; Benjamin & Fletcher, 2006; Eliopoulos, 2001; Ghafoor & St. Marie, 2010; Wold, 2008; Zwicker & Fulmer, 2008).

The GI tract is also involved with *elimination* of some analgesic and adjuvant medications. Although there is decreased mucous secretion and elasticity in the large intestines, with aging, there is not a reduction in motility. Normal aging does not cause constipation; however, it may occur as a result of chronic illnesses (Eliopoulos, 2001). A common side effect of opioids is constipation, and the related dysmotility may be greater in older adults (AGS, 2009).

Transmucosal absorption is increasingly seen as an alternate route of medication administration (Hadjistavropoulos & Fine, 2007). This can be an option for older adults. When considering this route, it is important to remember that with aging saliva becomes more viscous with approximately one-third of the amount produced in younger adults (Eliopoulos, 2001).

Absorption via the integumentary system can be an important consideration. *Transdermal topical or* suicide completion (SC) routes provide an alternative for administration in older adults for whom oral medication is contraindicated. When considering the administration of analgesics or adjuvants via these routes, it is important to evaluate the condition of the skin in the older person. With aging, skin becomes thinner, dryer, more fragile, less vascular, and less elastic with less subcutaneous fat. Although not common, these factors may affect the absorption of medications through the transdermal or topical route in older adults. Body temperature may be lower in older adults, and that may affect absorption of medications through some transdermal systems (AGS, 2009; Eliopoulos, 2001).

There are important changes that occur in the *musculoskeletal system*. With aging, muscle mass generally atrophies to some degree, fibrous tissue increases, and muscle activity often lessens. Absorption and distribution of medication via muscle tissue is generally slower, even less predictable than in younger adults (Herbert, 2006).

Additional factors to consider regarding *absorption* of medications in older adults include the following:

■ Reduction in intracellular fluid can reduce medication absorption.
■ Cardiac output and circulation may be reduced.
■ Body metabolism is generally slower.
■ Effects of many age-related chronic illnesses alter absorption of medications with
  ■ increased absorption in older adults with diabetes mellitus and hypokalemia
  ■ slowed absorption with pain and edema of the mucosa (Benjamin & Fletcher, 2006)

Distribution of medication in older people is highly variable. In general there is increase in adipose tissue compared with lean body mass that may lead to an increased volume of the distribution of lipid-soluble medications. Obesity may lead to a prolonged medication half-life. When distribution is decreased, serum levels increase, thus, lower doses of medication may be warranted. Other factors that may affect distribution of analgesic or adjuvant medications are as follows:

■ Body temperature
■ Circulatory function
■ Alterations in the vasculature
■ Alterations in plasma protein
■ Reduction in the serum albumin level
■ Membrane permeability
■ Tissue structure changes

Reduced cardiac output can lead to increased plasma levels and reduced deposition of medications in reservoirs. Reduced total water volume can result in a higher concentration of hydrophilic medications. Competition of protein-bound medications for protein-binding sites may displace one or more medication (i.e., nortriptyline, phenytoin, and salicylates). Dehydration decreases distribution. Hypoalbuminemia decreases distribution (AGS, 2009; Benjamin & Fletcher, 2006; Eliopoulos, 2001; Wold, 2008; Zwicker & Fulmer, 2008).

Metabolism of most analgesic medications and adjuvants is via the *liver* (see Chapters 7 and 8). Although oxidation is variable, it may decline with aging. It can be affected by cirrhosis, hepatitis, or other pathology resulting in prolonged half-life of medications. With aging, the liver usually

■ preserves normal conjugation
■ continues with usual first-pass effect that is not altered
■ decreases in size
■ has less blood flow
■ loses the secretion of some enzymes
■ is not as efficient in regenerating damaged cells
■ has prolongation of the multistage metabolism

Although the specific effects of these changes have not been established, it is known that detoxification of medications may be markedly decreased, resulting in elevated serum levels of medications (Eliopoulos, 2001). In addition, many older adults have chronic illnesses that affect hepatic function, and some hepatic enzymes may be affected by genetic enzyme polymorphisms. Reduced hepatic circulation and less active hepatic enzymes can increase the first-pass effect with a lower metabolic rate and resultant accumulation of the medication (AGS, 2009, Eliopoulos, 2001; Gould, 2006; Zwicker & Fulmer, 2008).

Elimination of many analgesic and adjuvant medications is via the kidneys (see Chapters 7 and 8). *Renal function* becomes less proficient with aging. With normal aging, the renal blood flow rate declines. The glomerular filtration rate declines by up to 50% in those who are 90 years and older. With the resulting decrease in renal tubular function, the exchange of substances and excretion is less efficient. The half-life of medications can increase up to 40% with resultant accumulation and risk of adverse reactions. Chronic renal disease increases the propensity of renal toxicity. This can be a concern in medications with side effects of respiratory depression and sedation (i.e., opioids) (AGS, 2009; Eliopoulos, 2001; Zwicker & Fulmer, 2008).

As the aging changes are unique to each older adult, it is recommended to calculate the creatinine clearance rather than the serum creatinine level, which is not an accurate assessment of renal function. It is recommended to assess renal function in older adults using the Cockroft–Gault serum creatinine concentrations with the formula (Benjamin & Fletcher, 2006; Wold, 2008; Zwicker & Fulmer, 2008):

Cockroft–Gault Serum Creatinine Clearance Formula

Men	$\text{Creatinine clearance} = \dfrac{(140 - \text{age in years} \times \text{weight in kg}}{72 \times \text{serum creatinine (mg/dL)}}$
Women	$\text{Creatinine clearance} = \dfrac{(140 - \text{age in years} \times \text{weight in kg}}{72 \times \text{serum creatinine (mg/dL)} \times 0.85}$

With older women, the calculated creatinine clearance value needs to be multiplied by 0.85.

Sources: From *Gerontologic Nursing* (3rd ed., pp. 447–467), by C. Benjamin and K. Fletcher, 2006, St. Louis, MO: Mosby Elsevier; *Basic geriatric nursing* (4th ed., Rev.), by G.H. Wold, 2008, St. Louis, MO: Mosby Elsevier; and *Evidence-based geriatric nursing protocols for best practice* (3rd ed., Rev., pp. 257–308), by D. Zwicker and T. Fulmer, 2008, New York, NY: Springer. Adapted with permission.

Pearls	Medications that are more soluble are absorbed faster than less-soluble medications.
	Older adults are a heterogeneous population and each needs to be assessed considering the specific conditions affecting absorption.
	Longer half-life, less effective metabolism, and slower excretion can lead to adverse effects of medications in older adults.

CONSIDER THE ROUTES OF ADMINISTRATION

Always start with the least intrusive route of administration of analgesic medication.

Generally the *oral* route is the least intrusive route. Benefits of oral administration are that it is convenient and results in steady blood levels. The major disadvantage of oral analgesia is that medications administered via this route can take 30 to 120 minutes before being effective. Although older adults with chronic pain can be taught how best to use oral medications to manage their pain, the longer time frame needed for oral medications to be effective may not be reasonable in acute pain situations. It is imperative to teach older adults, caregivers, and family members never to cut or crush extended release or sustained release pills. Crushing or chewing can result in overdose due to extremely rapid absorption of the entire dose of medication (AGS, 2009; Fine, 2004).

Transdermal, topical, oral transmucosal, and rectal routes can be effective for older adults who have difficulties swallowing (AGS, 2009), are at increased risk for aspiration, or have an aversion to swallowing pills or capsules. It is important to assess the condition of the mucosa, skin, and underlying SC tissue in the older adult for age-related changes to determine if these are viable routes. Another important consideration is how the medication is absorbed and the duration of action. Although these routes can be good alternatives to oral analgesia, it is imperative to review the product information and cautions (Louis & Meiner, 2006).

Parenteral (intravenous, intramuscular [IM], and SC) routes are appropriate in acute pain situations or when other routes are not available. IM and SC routes of administration have the disadvantages of unreliable absorption and "more rapid fall-off of action than the oral route" (AGS, 2009, p. 1333). In addition, IM administration is painful and can result in the older adult choosing pain over the pain of the IM injection.

SCHEDULING OF MEDICATION ADMINISTRATION

Around the Clock Scheduled Administration

For most older adults who live with continuous chronic pain, it is best to schedule around the clock medication to maintain a concentration of the analgesia in the blood (AGS, 2009) to optimize comfort and function. The medication can be in the form of long-acting, sustained-release or short-acting medications that are taken on a scheduled basis. For many older adults, it is easier to remember to take medication at the same time every day rather than having to decide if their pain is "bad enough" to take the pain medicine. Using scheduled analgesic medication is particularly important when managing pain in older adults who experience confusion or dementia (AGS, 2009).

As Needed or PRN Administration of Analgesia

When *chronic pain* in older adults is managed with scheduled around the clock analgesia, short-acting analgesia needs to be prescribed on an as need basis for the following:

- *Breakthrough pain (BTP)* that may occur as the effectiveness of the dose of medication wanes or the pain is more severe than usual.
- *Incident pain* involved with activities that are known to cause additional pain, such as wound care procedures or physical therapy (PT).
- *Spontaneous pain,* such as the fleeting pain that may occur with chronic neuropathic pain (NP).
- *End of dose failure* can occur when the scheduled medication is no longer effective. If this occurs on a consistent basis, the dose and time interval of the scheduled medication needs to be reevaluated and adjusted (AGS, 2009).

PRN analgesic medications are also indicated in older adults with *acute pain.*

Patient controlled analgesia (PCA) is a delivery system of medication through which the older adult can self-administer medications (opioid and/or local anesthetic) as needed via the IV, SC, or epidural routes.

Indications for PCA are as follows:

- Acute pain (postoperative, trauma, sickle cell crisis, and changes in chronic pain)
- Inability to tolerate oral analgesia
- Ability to comprehend and remember PCA concepts
- Ability to physically use the PCA device

Cautions regarding the use of PCA include the following:

- Use in older adults must be cautious.
- Only the patient can use the PCA device.
- Family members and visitors must be educated *not* to use the PCA device.

■ Start with low doses and titrate upward based upon patient use and patient response (Reuben et al., 2005).

> *Pearls*
>
> In general, medications administrated via intravenous, inhaled, and topical routes are absorbed most efficiently (Eliopoulos, 2001).
>
> Persistent pain is best managed with scheduled medications.
>
> It is imperative to remember that older adults are unique individuals with unique responses to medications.
>
> The golden rule of medication management is to start with a low dose and titrate slowly.

II. SPECIFIC RECOMMENDATIONS FOR USING MEDICATIONS WITH OLDER PATIENTS

SELECTING ANALGESIC AND ADJUVANT MEDICATIONS

Selection of the most appropriate analgesic and adjuvant medications for the individual older adult can be a complex process that requires many considerations. The WHO ladder can be used as a general guideline, knowing that modifications may need to be made based upon the needs and circumstances of the individual older adult. Some of the things to consider are as follows:

■ Types of pain (somatic, visceral, neuropathic, and mixed)
■ Pain and analgesic history
■ Comorbidities and concurrent medications
■ Intensity of pain
  ■ Generally mild pain should be managed with a nonopioid analgesic unless contraindicated.
  ■ Moderate pain should be managed with the nonopioid analgesic plus a mild opioid (tramadol or hydrocodone or 5 mg oxycodone).
  ■ Moderate to severe pain generally requires strong opioid analgesia (morphine, oxycodone, hydromorphone, fentanyl, and methadone) plus a nonopioid unless contraindicated.
■ Frequency of pain (constant, chronic/persistent, intermittent, episodic, and acute) indicates if short-acting or sustained release medications are most appropriate
■ Interference of pain with function and usual activities
■ Previous experiences with analgesic and adjuvant medications

■ Medication allergies
■ GI, hepatic, and renal function and concerns
■ Factors that affect absorption, metabolism, and excretion of medications

The opioids of choice with older adults with hepatic insufficiency are hydromorphone and morphine. The opioids of choice with older adults with renal insufficiency are fentanyl, hydromorphone, methadone, and oxycodone.

■ Interference of pain with function and usual activities
■ Cognitive abilities to manage different medication regimens
■ Cost of medications and the older adults' ability to afford them (Ghafoor & St. Marie, 2010; Herr, Bjoro, Steffensmeier, & Rakel, 2006; Reuben et al., 2005)

Some *cautions* to remember when selecting analgesic and adjuvant medications for use in older adults are as follows:

■ Nonsteroidal anti-inflammatory drugs (NSAIDs) are not indicated for long-term use (COX-2 medications may be a better choice).
■ Whenever possible use one type of opioid (sustained-release with short-acting morphine for BTP or sustained release with short-acting oxycodone for BTP).
■ Use long-acting medications (i.e., methadone, levorphanol, and transdermal fentanyl) with caution with reduced metabolism and excretion (Reuben et al., 2005).

COORDINATION WITH APPROPRIATE SPECIALISTS

The multifaceted qualities of pain often require a multidisciplinary approach to pain management. With their significant comorbidities, this is often particularly important in older adults (AGS, 2009) to ensure that the most appropriate and safest medications are selected considering how the body of the individual older adult is functioning. Among the specialist who may need to be included in developing a plan for pain management are

■ cardiologist
■ gastroenterologist
■ geriatrician
■ home health nurse
■ internist
■ neurologist
■ occupational therapist

- orthopedist
- PT
- psychiatrist
- pulmonologist
- social worker

III. MANAGING MEDICATION SIDE EFFECTS

All medications have side effects. The *best* way to manage the side effects is, whenever possible, to prevent or minimize them. As many side effects of analgesic and adjuvant medications are dose related, it is important to initiate medications at low doses and slowly titrate the dose to achieve optimal, but safe, analgesia (AGS, 2009; American Pain Society [APS], 2003; Herr et al., 2006; Strassels, McNicol, & Suleman, 2008).

It is beyond the scope of this chapter to address all potential side effects of all analgesic and adjuvant medications or to discuss in-depth management of side effects. The most common and serious side effects are identified, along with a brief description of management options. For detailed descriptions of all side effects for any analgesic or adjuvant medication, it is recommended to consult the product information or a reputable pharmaceutical guide.

GENERAL PRINCIPLES OF MANAGING ANALGESIC AND ADJUVANT-RELATED SIDE EFFECTS

As a result of physiological changes affecting metabolism, distribution, and elimination of medications, older adults are at particular risk for experiencing side effects of medications. Although there are innumerable side effects related to these medications, there are some general guidelines for managing side effects. These include the following:

- Start with the lowest reasonable dose and titrate slowly to the most effective and best tolerated dose.
- Multimodal analgesia that includes using multiple medications and nonpharmacological interventions provides for lower doses, with fewer side effects, of any one medication (Ghafoor & St. Marie, 2010).
- Some side effects, such as nausea, may be controlled by reducing the dose by 25% to 50% (if necessary to maintain adequate analgesia,

the dosing interval can also be reduced, i.e., to every 3 hours rather than every 4 hours).

■ Peaks in serum level may cause side effects; the side effects may be avoided using a long-acting or sustained-release medication.

■ Older adults have individual reactions to specific medications, even though medications in one class have similar side effects, the individual older adult may be able to tolerate one medication better than another (ASP, 2003; Benjamin & Fletcher, 2006; Herr et al., 2006).

RESPIRATORY EFFECTS

Respiratory depression is considered the most serious side effect of opioids, and older adults are considered at increased risk for this adverse effect. Opioids depress respiration by shifting the CO_2 response curve requiring an increased amount of CO_2 to stimulate respirations. When respiratory depression occurs, opioids should immediately be discontinued and avoided or used with extreme caution (Herr et al., 2006).

Respiratory depression occurs rapidly in individuals who are opioid naïve (no or little prior experience with receiving opioid analgesia) and with individuals receiving lipid-soluble medications (Strassels et al., 2008).

Assessment and monitoring of respiratory function and sedation are important. During hospitalization, older adults who are started on opioid therapy should be assessed for the initial 24 hours of therapy every 1 to 2 hours (Herr et al., 2006; Pasero, Portenoy, & McCaffery, 1999). The respiratory rate alone and pulse oximetry level are not adequate to identify evolving respiratory depression. Monitoring should include assessment of

■ sedation
■ respiratory rate
■ respiratory quality (depth of respirations)

Pearls
Snoring does not indicate the person is sleeping well.
Breathing is impaired when snoring.
Snoring is an indicator that respiratory quality is impaired.
All people who snore should be evaluated for obstructive sleep apnea.

The assessment tool that is most specific to assessing opioid induced sedation is the Pasero opioid-induced sedation scale. This tool is very useful because it guides assessment of sedation and guides follow-up actions.

Pasero Opioid-Induced Sedation Scale with Interventions[a]

S = Sleep, easy to arouse
Acceptable; no action necessary; may increase opioid dose if needed
1 = Awake and alert
Acceptable; no action necessary; may increase opioid dose if needed
2 = Slightly drowsy, easily aroused
Acceptable; no action necessary; may increase opioid dose if needed
3 = Frequently drowsy, arousable, drifts off to sleep during conversation
Unacceptable; monitor respiratory status and sedation level closely until sedation level is stable at less than 3 and respiratory status is satisfactory; decrease opioid dose 25%–50%[b] or notify primary[c] or anesthesia providers for orders; consider administering a nonsedating, opioid-sparing nonopioid, such as acetaminophen or an NSAID, if not contraindicated; ask patient to take deep breaths every 15–30 min.
4 = Somnolent, minimal or no response to verbal and physical stimulation
Unacceptable; stop opioid; consider administering naloxone[d,e]; call Rapid Response Team (Code Blue), if indicated by patient status; stay with patient; stimulate and support respiration as indicated by patient status; notify primary care or anesthesia providers for orders; monitor respiratory status and sedation level closely until sedation level is stable at less than 3 and respiratory status is satisfactory.

Source: *Pain Assessment and Pharmacologic Management* (p. 510), by C. Pasero and M. McCaffery, 2011, St. Louis, MO: Mosby. Adapted with permission

[a]Appropriate action is given in italics at each level of sedation.
[b]Opioid analgesic orders or a hospital protocol should include the expectation that a nurse will decrease the opioid dose if a patient is excessively sedated.
[c]For example, the physician, nurse practitioner, advanced practice nurse, or physician's assistant responsible for the pain management prescription.
[d]For adults experiencing respiratory depression, mix 0.4 mg of naloxone and 10 mL of normal saline in syringe and administer this dilute solution very slowly (0.5 mL over 2 min) while observing the patient's response (titrate to effect). If sedation and respiratory depression occur during administration of transdermal fentanyl, remove the patch; if naloxone is necessary, treatment will be needed for a prolonged period, and the typical approach involve a naloxone infusion. Patient must be monitored for at least 24 h after discontinuation of the transdermal fentanyl.
[e]Hospital protocols should include the expectation that a nurse will administer naloxone to any patient suspected of having life-threatening opioid-induced sedation and respiratory depression.

Recommended interventions:

Immediate intervention for respiratory depression is administration of naloxone (Narcan®). It is important to understand that naloxone is an opioid agonist that is used to reverse the action of opioids. The dose should be adjusted to ensure controlled reversal to avoid sudden antagonizing (withdrawal) effects. It is recommended to dilute one 0.4 mg ampule of naloxone in 10 mL normal saline and administer it at 1 mL intervals observing the effect on the person.

After reversal is complete, it is important to monitor the older adult, remembering that naloxone is a short-acting medication. If the opioid that was administered is long acting, it may be advisable to initiate a low-dose continuous IV naloxone infusion (Strassels et al., 2008).

CENTRAL NERVOUS SYSTEM SIDE EFFECTS

Central nervous system (CNS) side effects are of particular concern in older adults who are at increased risk for confusion and falling as part of the aging process. In general it is prudent to restrict driving of motor vehicles by older adults with new prescriptions of analgesia or adjuvants, until the effect of the medications and dose are adjusted for optimal cognitive functioning (Fine, 2004).

ATAXIA

Ataxia or gait disturbance is a side effect of many medications (AGS, 2009) and is of concern with older adults who are at increased risk for falling and at increased risk for sustaining life-threatening fractures. Prevention through assessment, careful choice of analgesia, and patient/family education is imperative. It is prudent to refer older adults who are known to have mobility challenges or a history of frequent falling for PT evaluation and possible use of assistive devices. A caution is that older adults who use assistive devices may be at increased risk for falling (Quinlan-Colwell & Taylor, 2006).

CONFUSION

Although confusion can be a side effect of analgesics or adjuvants, it can also result from inadequately managed pain (Herr & Decker 2004). It is therefore imperative to fully assess and determine the cause of confusion and treat the cause appropriately (Esterowicz, Quinlan-Colwell, Vanderveer, & Menez, 2010).

DELIRIUM

Delirium may be caused by analgesia (NSAIDs, anticholinergeic medications, pentazocine, and meperidine) or their side effects, or by other causes (i.e., electrolyte abnormalities, infection, sleep disturbances, environmental changes, and sensory deprivation) (Eliopoulos, 2001) particularly during hospitalization. *Since postoperative delirium also develops as a result of unrelieved pain, it is important to ensure adequate analgesia prior to reducing analgesic doses* (Pasero & McCaffery, 2010).

Possible *interventions* for delirium are as follows:
- Ensure safety of the older adult.
- Differentiate between delirium and dementia; identify the cause of delirium and treat accordingly and provide psychological support and reassurance.
- Provide a calm environment.
- Ensure adequate oxygenation.
- Haloperidol may be effective as a short-term intervention for delirium; however, it is important to be aware that it may mask pain and has a risk of QT prolongation (Ghafoor & St. Marie, 2010; Herr et al., 2006).

Interventions should be done early. If the cause is determined to be opioid related, there are two primary options: decreasing the dose of opioid and utilizing other multimodal options. Another option is to switch to another opioid, such as fentanyl, hydromorphone, or oxycodone (Eliopoulos, 2001; Esterowicz et al., 2010; Ghafoor & St. Marie, 2010; Herr et al., 2006; Kelly, 2010).

DIZZINESS

Dizziness is an episode of lightheadedness that occurs within 30 minutes of standing that can last for a few seconds to several minutes (Reuben et al., 2005). It is listed as a side effect for many of the analgesic and adjuvant medications used to treat pain in older adults. It is a particular concern for older adults who may have an impaired sense of balance.

Interventions are to either decrease the dose of the medication or change to another medication. It is also always important to educate older adults, their families, and their caregivers about dizziness as a potential side effect.

MYOCLONUS

Myoclonus involves sudden, generally brief, involuntary muscle contractures that can range from mild twitching to generalized muscle spasms that frequently occur with drowsiness or falling to sleep (McNicol et al., 2003; Pasero & McCaffery, 2010). Although myoclonus can occur during treatment with any opioid, it is most common when meperidine is used (McMichael et al., 2003). Generally myoclonus is related to large doses of opioids, is mild, and is self-limiting but at times can become severe and cause increased pain (Pasero & McCaffery, 2010).

Interventions to manage myoclonus are as follows:

- Reduce the dose of the opioid and add adjuvant medications.
- If the opioid is meperidine, it is recommended to immediately stop that to prevent further accumulation of normeperidine.
- Switch to another opioid (i.e., hydromorphone).
- Hydrate to encourage elimination of metabolites.

When myoclonus is not responsive to these conservative measures, treatment with a benzodiazepine (i.e., clonazepam and midazolam) or a skeletal muscle relaxant (i.e., dantrolene and baclofen) may be effective (Ghafoor & St. Marie, 2010; McMichael et al., 2003; Pasero & McCaffery, 2010).

It is important to note that most cases of myoclonus resolve with reduction or change in opioid (McMichael et al., 2003). Treatments with carbamazeprine, phenytoin, valproic acid, and high-dose valium are of either *little* or *no effect* in efforts to manage myoclonus (Pasero & McCaffery, 2010).

SEDATION

Sedation is common during the initiation of opioid therapy and when there are significant increases in dose (McMichael et al., 2003; Pasero & McCaffery, 2010).

Interventions

- Educating older adults, family, and caregivers that sedation is a potential side effect of medications but that it is generally short-lived.

- Reassure and educate that tolerance generally develops to sedation.
- Educate to avoid driving and the use of alcohol.
- Avoid concurrent use of medications that are known to cause sedation (i.e., promethazine, muscle relaxants, and hypnotics).
- It may be necessary to reduce the dose of medication or change to a different medication.
- If an opioid is involved, it may be appropriate to switch to tramadol (Ghafoor & St. Marie, 2010; McMichael et al., 2003; Pasero & McCaffery, 2010).

It is important to remember that sedation is the earliest indicator of opioid-induced respiratory distress and must be assessed accordingly (Pasero & McCaffery, 2010).

GI TRACT SIDE EFFECTS

GI bleeding is a potential complication of NSAIDs, which should never be used in older adults with a history of peptic ulcers or in those otherwise at risk for GI bleeding (Herr et al., 2006). In older adults who may be at risk for GI bleeding, concurrent administration of a proton pump inhibitor with the NSAID may provide some protection (Herr et al., 2006; Sturkenboom et al., 2003).

Although their occurrence is somewhat less common in older adults (Herr et al., 2006), *nausea and vomiting* are common side effects of NSAIDs or opioid medications and occur as a result of

- irritation
- direct stimulation of the chemoreceptor trigger zone
- depression of the vomiting center
- slowing of GI motility
- gastroporesis

INTERVENTIONS

Reducing the dose or changing to a different medication in the same class may be effective if the medication is considered causative. As they have anticholinergic effects to which older adults may be particularly sensitive, antiemetic medications need to be used cautiously in older adults. Medications to counteract the nausea/vomiting are as follows:

- Ondansetron (Zofran)
- Transdermal scopolamine (if there is a motion sickness component to the nausea/vomiting)

- Metoclopramide (Reglan)
- Misoprostol (Cytotec)
- Prochlorperazine (oral, rectal, or IV)
- Transdermal scopolamine (if there is a motion sickness component to the nausea/vomiting)
- Meclizine (Antivert)
- Dimenhydrinate (Dramamine) (APS, 2003; Herr et al., 2006; Strassels et al., 2008)

Older adults who are scheduled for surgery and have two or more risk factors for postoperative nausea and vomiting (PONV), female, nonsmoker, history of PONV, history of motion sickness, and opioids used preoperatively, may benefit from prophylactic administration of ondansetron or dexamethasone preoperatively (Gan et al., 2003).

CONSTIPATION

Constipation is a very common side effect of opioid analgesia and is twice as common in older adults as among younger adults. It is caused through opioid effects that result in diminished peristalsis and intestinal secretions, resulting in dry stools that are difficult to eliminate. This can be complicated by immobility, diet, and dehydration (APS, 2003; Esterowicz et al., 2010; Strassels et al., 2008).

As tolerance to the constipating effects of opioids may never fully develop, it is imperative to regularly assess for constipation and to ensure that all older adults receiving opioids also take prophylactic laxatives. Stool softeners are helpful to keep the stools soft; however, they do not counteract the effect of diminished peristalsis. It is important that both a stool softener and a stimulant laxative (i.e., senna products) be taken on a regular basis (APS, 2003; Herr et al., 2006; Strassels et al., 2008).

Intervention is ideally through preventive education to the older adult, family, and caregivers and should include the following:

- Relationship of opioid therapy with constipation
- Importance of taking stool softeners and stimulants on a regular basis
- Need to be as active as possible
- Importance of being well hydrated
- Dietary needs for fiber

GENITOURINARY SYSTEM SIDE EFFECTS

Urinary Retention

The side effect of opioids relaxing the detrusor muscle and relaxing sphincter tone of the bladder, resulting in bladder spasms or urinary retention, is common and occurs more frequently in older adults. It is important to assess for this and intervene to avoid catheterization. Measurement of intake and output may be necessary to accurately assess for this, particularly in older males who have comorbid prostate disorders.

Interventions include changing to a different opioid or adding a medication to contract the bladder (i.e., bethanechol chloride) (Esterowicz et al., 2010; Herr et al., 2006; Strassels et al., 2008).

INTEGUMENTARY SYSTEM SIDE EFFECTS

Pruritus

Pruritus (itching) occurs with opioid use, but the relationship is not fully understood. It is believed that histamine release contributes and opioids may cause a relaxation of the inhibition of neurons that are specific for itching. Itching without rash is not an allergy; however, it may be advisable to reduce the dose and if necessary add a nonopioid or change to a different opioid to see if the itching subsides (Herr et al., 2006; Strassels et al., 2008).

The side effect of itching can be particularly troublesome for older adults who tend to have itchy skin as a result of less sebum being produced. As older skin tends to be thinner, it is more easily damaged by scratching (Herbert, 2006).

Interventions for pruritus include
■ stopping the opioid
■ changing to a different opioid
■ treating pharmacologically with antihistamines
■ using antihistamines that have the least sedating effects (i.e., hydroxyzine and cyproeptadine)
■ using low-dose nalbuphine
■ using low-dose naloxone infusions for older adults who are hospitalized (Esterowicz et al., 2010; Gan et al., 1997; McMichael et al., 2003; Strassels et al., 2008)

> *Pearls*
>
> With older adults it is essential to balance the benefit of medications with the potential side effects both, of the medication and as a result of physiological aging changes.
>
> Assess for side effects often and intervene early.
>
> Stool softeners are not sufficient in managing opioid-related constipation. Prophylactic stimulants must be used with stool softeners.

GUIDELINES AND RESOURCES

American Academy of Pain Management at http://www.aspainmanage.org/literature/publications.php

American Academy of Pain Medicine at http://www.painmed.org/clinical_info/guidelines.html

American Geriatric Society. (2009). Pharmacological management of persistent pain in older adults. *Journal of the American Geriatrics Society, 57,* 1331–1346.

American Pain Society at http://www.ampainsoc.org/pub/cp_guidelines.htm

http://www.ampainsoc.org/links/clinician1.htm

Federation of State Medical Boards at http://www.fsmb.org/RE/PAIN/resource.html

Merk Manual Online http://www.merk.com/mmpe/sec20/ch306/ch306b.html

Case Study

Mr. Harris is an 82-year-old man who plays golf three times per week. He was recently diagnosed with prostate cancer and urinary retention. He is concerned that he will need to stop taking the ibuprophen he uses to manage the arthritis in his knees to play golf. During the pain assessment he reports that he has "pretty strong" pain in his lower back "most of the time" but he does not like to take medications and has some heart burn on a regular basis. He further relays that he is "afraid of getting hooked" on pain medicine.

1. What additional assessment questions should be asked of Mr. Harris?
2. What changes may be appropriate in his analgesic regimen?
3. What medication side effects need to be considered when adjusting the analgesic regimen?
4. What education is needed with Mr. Harris?
5. What additional specialist should be consulted?

REFERENCES

American Geriatric Society. (2009). Pharmacological management of persistent pain in older adults. *Journal of the American Geriatrics Society, 57,* 1331–1346.

American Pain Society. (2003). *Principles of analgesia use in the treatment of acute pain and cancer pain* (5th ed.). Glenview, IL: Author.

Benjamin, C., & Fletcher, K. (2006). Pharmacologic management. In S. Meiner & A. Lueckenotte (Eds.), *Gerontologic nursing* (3rd ed., pp. 447–467). St. Louis, MO: Mosby Elsevier.

Eliopoulos, C. (2001). *Gerontological nursing* (5th ed., Rev.). Philadelphia, PA: Lippincott Williams & Wilkins.

Esterowicz, N., Quinlan-Colwell, A., Vanderveer, B., & Menez, J. A. (2010). Acute pain management. In B. St. Marie (Ed.), *Core curriculum for pain management nursing* (2nd ed., Rev., pp. 329–379). Dubuque, IA: Kendall Hunt.

Fine, P. G. (2004). Pharmacological management of persistent pain in older adults. *Clinical Journal of Pain, 20,* 220–226.

Gan, T. J., Ginsberg, B., Glass, P., Fortney, J., Jhaveri, R., & Perno, R. (1997). Opioid-sparing effects of low-dose infusion of naloxone in patient administered morphine sulfate. *Anesthesiology, 87,* 1075–1081.

Gan, T. J., Meyer, T., Apfel, C. C., Chung, F., Davis, P. J., Eubanks, S., Watcha, M. (2003). Consensus guidelines for managing postoperative nausea and vomiting. *Anesthesia and Analgesia, 1,* 62–71.

Ghafoor, V., & St. Marie, B. (2010). Overview of pharmacology. In B. St. Marie (Ed.), *Core curriculum for pain management nurses* (2nd ed., Rev., pp. 235–306). Dubuque, IA: Kendall Hunt.

Gould, D. (2006). Drugs and older people. In S. J. Redfern & F. M. Ross (Eds.), *Nursing older people* (4th ed., pp. 583–600). London, UK: Churchill Livingston Elsevier.

Hadjistavropoulos, T., & Fine, P. G. (2007). Chronic pain in older persons: Prevalence, assessment and management. *Clinical Gerontology, 16,* 231–241.

Herbert, R. A. (2006). The biology of human ageing. In S. J. Redfern & F. M. Ross (Eds.), *Nursing older people* (pp. 57–81). Edinburgh, UK: Churchill Livingstone Elsevier.

Herr, K., Bjoro, K., Steffensmeier, J., & Rakel, J. (2006). *Acute pain management in older adults. Gerontological nursing interventions research center: Research translation and dissemination core.* Iowa City, IA: University of Iowa.

Herr, K. & Decker, S. (2004). Assessment of pain in older adults with severe cognitive impairment. *Annals of Long-Term Care: Clinical Care and Aging, 12*(4), 46–52.

Kelly, A. M. (2010). Gerontology Pain Management. In B. St. Marie (Ed.), *Core curriculum for pain management nursing* (2nd ed., pp. 573–586). Dubuque, IA: Kendall Hunt.

Louis, M., & Meiner, S. E. (2006). Pain. In S. Meiner & A. Lueckenotte (Eds.), *Gerontologic nursing* (3rd ed., pp. 304–327). St. Louis, MO: Mosby Elsevier.

McMichael, E., Horowicz-Mehler, N., Fisk, R. A., Bennett, K., Gialeli-Goudas, M., Chew, P. W., Carr, D. (2003). Management of opioid side effects in cancer-related and chronic noncancer pain: A systematic review. *The Journal of Pain, 4,* 231–256.

McNicol, E., Horowicz-Mehler, N., Fisk, R. A., Bennett, K., Gialeli-Goudas, M., Chew, P. W., Lau, J. & Carr, D. et. al. (2003). Management of opioid side effects in cancer related and chronic noncancer pain: a systematic review. *Journal of Pain, 5,* 231–256.

Pasero, C., & McCaffery, M. (2010). *Pain assessment and pharmacologic management.* St. Louis, MO: Elsevier Mosby.

Pasero, C., Portenoy, R. K., & McCaffery, M. (1999). Opioid analgesics. In C. Pasero & M. McCaffery (Eds.), *Pain: Clinical manual* (2nd ed., pp. 161–299). St. Louis, MO: Mosby.

Quinlan-Colwell, A., & Taylor, C. (2006, May). *Relationship of falling with the use of assistive devices: A secondary analysis of the LSOA.* Paper presented at the University of North Carolina at Greensboro Doctoral Program Statistical Analysis Presentations. Greensboro, NC.

Reuben, D. B., Herr, K. A., Pacala, J. T., Pollock, B. G., Potter, J. F., & Semla, T. P. (2005). *Geriatrics at your fingertips* (7th ed.). New York, NY: American Geriatrics Society.

Strassels, S. A., McNicol, E., & Suleman, R. (2008). Pharmacotherapy of pain in older adults. *Clinics in Geriatric Medicine, 24,* 275–298.

Sturkenboom, M. C., Burke, T. A., Tangelder, M. J., Dieleman, J. P., Walton, S., & Goldstein, J. L. (2003). Adherence to proton pump inhibitors or H_2-receptor antagonists during the use of non-steroidal anti-inflammatory drugs. *Alimentary Pharmacology and Therapeutics, 18,* 1137–1147.

Wold, G. H. (2008). *Basic geriatric nursing* (4th ed., Rev.). St. Louis, MO: Mosby Elsevier.

Zwicker, D., & Fulmer, T. (2008). Reducing adverse drug events. In E. Capezuti, D. Zwicker, M. Mezey, & T. Fulmer (Eds.), *Evidence-based geriatric nursing protocols for best practice* (3rd ed., Rev., pp. 257–308). New York, NY: Springer.

10

Interventional Options Such as Vertebroplasty for Compression Fractures, Nerve Blocks, and Acupuncture

To manage pain in older adults, the least invasive method of analgesia is always recommended. Yet, pharmacological therapy can be challenging with many older adults who are particularly sensitive to side effects of medications and those being treated with a variety of medications for comorbid illnesses (American Geriatrics Society [AGS], 2009). Avoiding problematic side effects of medicines while trying to control pain can be particularly challenging. In those instances, interventional techniques *may* be a good treatment choice for elders (Bernstein, Lateef, & Fine, 2005; Sharma, Staats, & Luthardt, 2004).

This chapter will provide an overview of the most common interventional options used with older adults. If assessment and discussion with the elder indicate that an interventional method may be helpful, referral to an health care provider who is experienced in performing the technique with older adults is needed.

Nursing care of the patient following any interventional procedures must include monitoring for the following:
- Hemodynamic changes
- Signs of infection
- Neurological changes
- Unexpected pain
- Complications specific to the procedure
- Side effects specific to the medications used

INTERVENTIONS FOR MYOFASCIAL PAIN SYNDROMES

Trigger point injection are fairly common in the treatment of myofascial pain syndromes. The injection of local anesthetic (LA) or saline

167

is done into the "knots" in the taut muscle and fascia from which irritated nerves radiate pain. Reviews have found little and weak evidence of benefit of trigger point injections with LA and/or steroids.

Advantages

■ Temporary relief of pain has been reported

Cautions

■ Effectiveness is questionable.
■ Pain and bruising are common at the site.
■ Temporary paresthesia can occur.
■ Prolonged use of steroids may cause muscle wasting.
■ Syncopal episodes can occur.
■ Particular caution should be used in the thoracic, head, and neck areas (Arnstein, 2010; Bernstein et al., 2005; Chou, Atlas, Stanos, & Rosenquist 2009; Stolker & Groen, 2000).

Botulinum toxin (Botox) injection is an antispasmodic approved by the Federal Drug Administration (FDA) for treatment of cervical dystonia and hemifacial spasm. Botulinum toxin has been studied with success as a treatment with tension headaches, temporomandibular disorders, low back pain (LBP), and poststroke spasticity in older adults, but it is not FDA approved for use in these conditions.

Advantages

■ Isolated studies report success in treating pain associated with cervical dystonia.

Cautions

■ Local weakness can develop.
■ Anaphylaxis has been reported.
■ Long-term effectiveness needs to be determined.
■ Cost is high and may be prohibitive to older adults on fixed incomes (Arezzo, 2002; Brashear et al., 2002; Chou et al., 2009; Difazio & Jabbari, 2002; Freund, Schwartz, & Symington, 2000; Jankovic, 2004; Lew, 2002; Loder & Biondi, 2002; Schmitt, Slowey, Fravi, Weber, & Burgunder, 2001).

NERVE BLOCKS

These can be used for either diagnosis or treatment. They have been used effectively to manage pain in older adults in the outpatient surgery setting and with those who suffer with chronic pain. Blockade can be either temporary or permanent. The type of block is dependent on the location of pain and the area affected. Common blocks are as follows:

- Stellate ganglion block for facial and upper body pain
- Celiac plexus blocks for pancreatitis or cancer-related pain
- Lumbar spinal blocks for pain in the lower extremities

Advantages

- Less opioid is needed to control pain intraoperatively and postoperatively.
- Pain relief is provided when pharmacological options have not been successful.

Cautions

- Complications, which are rare, include bleeding, hematoma, nerve trauma, infection, inadvertent intraarterial or intravenous injection, and epidural, subdural, and subarachnoid spread.
- Use for complex regional pain syndrome (CRPS) needs further investigation (Bernstein et al., 2005; Cepeda, Lau, & Carr, 2002; Collins, Halwani, & Vaghadia, 1999; Manchikanti et al., 2007; Manchikant et al., 2009; Wong, Schroeder, & Carns, 2004).

Interventions for chronic pain related to the spine accounts for the majority of all chronic pain disorders, involving between 54% and 80% of people (Boswell et al., 2007). Chronic low back pain (CLBP) is the most costly and third most common reason for disability in older adults (Chou, Lew, Coelho, & Slipman, 2005). Although 14% of people report high pain and disability related to chronic neck pains, 25% report high pain and disability related to CLBP, with 27% of older adults suffering from CLBP (Manchikanti et al., 2007). The following interventions are options for managing chronic pain related to the spine that can either be used alone or in conjunction with other analgesia (Sehgal, Dunbar, Shah, & Colson, 2007).

Epidural corticosteroid injection using steroids and LA can be used at any point along the spinal column to treat inflamed nerve roots. Different techniques are used in the cervical, thoracic, and lumbar areas. Documented results vary depending on the area injected, etiology of the pathology, technique used, and use of fluoroscopy. Between 1994 and 2001, epidural steroid injections for sciatica, radiculopathy and herniated discs, spinal stenosis, and LBP increased by 271% among older adults receiving Medicare benefits.

Advantages

- Pain relief may last 3 to 12 months.
- Complications are not common.

Cautions

- Epidural injections are *contraindicated* in patients who are coagulo-pathic or have skin infections in the region.
- The procedures can be quite expensive and often require preapproval from insurance carriers.
- Cost effectiveness must be individually evaluated based on the benefit to quality of life.
- Long-term effects have not been documented.
- Complications include pain, epidural hematoma, epidural abscess, and neurological dysfunction. (Bernstein et al., 2005; Friedly, Chan, & Deyo, 2007; Manchikant et al., 2009).

SACROILIAC JOINT INJECTION

Pain associated with the synovial sacroiliac (SI) joint can radiate to the groin, buttocks, and thigh. It is common in older adults and may be the source of pain in 10% to 27% of CLBP cases. LA can be injected into the SI joint.

Advantages

- There is moderate evidence regarding accuracy of LA blocks to the SI for diagnostic purposes and limited evidence as a therapeutic intervention.

Cautions

- There is no clear evidence that supports therapeutic benefit of SI injections (Hansen et al., 2007; Weiner & Cayea, 2005).

FACET JOINT INJECTION

Facet or zygapophysial joints are paired articulations between vertebrae in all segments of the spinal column. For many patients with arthritis or microtrauma, they are the source of neck, thoracic, and LBP. Blocks can be done for diagnosis as well as treatment through blockade of the innervating nerve or injection directly into the joint using fluoroscopy. Longer relief can be achieved through radiofrequency ablation of the medial nerve. Between 1994 and 2001, there was 231% increase in facet injections among older adults receiving Medicare benefits (Bernstein et al., 2005; Boswell et al., 2007; Manchikanti et al., 2004).

Advantages

■ There is good evidence that facet joint injections using LA are useful in diagnosing pain in the neck or lower back regions and moderate evidence in diagnosing pain that originates in facet joints in the thorax.

■ Manchikanti et al. (2007) reported facet injections can be effective in achieving temporary relief (about 3 months) with no difference when LA was used alone or with steroids. This is a potential benefit for elders for whom steroid injections may not be advisable.

Cautions

Complications tend to be infrequent and include

■ hemorrhage
■ dural puncture
■ spinal cord trauma
■ neural trauma, infection
■ intra-arterial injection
■ intravenous injection
■ meningitis
■ pneumothorax, hematoma (Bernstein et al., 2005; Friedly et al., 2007; Manchikanti et al., 2003; Manchikanti et al., 2007; Sehgal et al., 2007)

PERCUTANEOUS THERMOCOAGULATION INTRADISCAL TECHNIQUES

A large number of CLBP cases are the result of disc damage. Discogenic pain is definitively diagnosed through provocative discography and can be treated with percutaneous thermocoagulation intradiscal techniques. These are intradiscal electrothermal therapy (IDET) or annuloplasty and percutaneous intradiscal radiofrequency thermocoagulation (PIRFT).

IDET is performed with the patient under sedation. Using fluoroscopic guidance, a catheter probe with a heating element is placed in the intervertebral disc. The probe conducts electrothermal energy (heat that is electrically generated). When placed between the annulus fibrosus and nucleus pulposus, the temperature is increased. Although there are several theories on how this works, there is no clear evidence (Chou et al., 2005).

PIRFT is a similar procedure that uses radiofrequency generated heat.

Advantages
- These procedures are minimally invasive and can be an alternative to surgical spinal fusion, which is advantageous for older adults.

Cautions
- Needs more evaluation with controlled studies
- No evidence of effectiveness
- Possible complications include
  - catheter breaking
  - injury to the nerve roots
  - herniation of the disc
  - damage to the spinal cord
  - cauda equine syndrome
  - infection, including epidural abscess
- They are contraindicated in patients who have
  - any current infection
  - inflammatory arthritis
  - bleeding disorders
  - cauda equine syndrome
  - vertebral fractures
  - comorbid pathology of the spine (Chou et al., 2005; Mekhail & Kapural, 2004; Raj, 2008; Saal & Saal, 2002; Urrutia, Kovacs, Nishishinya, & Olabe, 2007)

PERCUTANEOUS DISC DECOMPRESSION USING COBLATION (NUCLEOPLASTY)

Coblation is combined with removal of the disc to treat herniated intervertebral discs that are confirmed by magnetic resonance imaging (MRI) to be contained. It is also known as nucleoplasty and is indicated for LBP that has not responded to conservative treatment. This minimally invasive procedure is done under moderate sedation with fluoroscopy.

Advantages
- Because it is a minimally invasive procedure that does not require general anesthesia, it is a good option for older adults with comorbidities that may prohibit invasive surgery.
- Nucleoplasty is a good alternative to surgical discectomies that have a low-success rate.
- In one study the majority of patients (75%) had reduction in the intensity of their pain, and approximately half had functional

improvement for at least 12 months (Singh, Piryani, & Liao, 2003).

Cautions

■ There is little evidence of effectiveness.
■ Contraindications are spinal stenosis, loss of 50% of the disc height, fracture, and tumor (Raj, 2008; Singh et al., 2003).

MORE INVASIVE SPINE-RELATED INTERVENTIONS REQUIRING SURGERY

Implanted Intrathecal (IIT) pumps are small computerized devices that have a reservoir to hold the medication. The pump is inserted into a pocket of subcutaneous (SC) tissue, generally in the abdomen. IIT pumps can be used to manage intractable pain in older adults for whom more conservative therapy has not been effective or side effects were intolerable.

All medications used in IIT therapy must be preservative free. Common medications used include the following:

■ Morphine is the most common and the only FDA approved opioid for use in IIT pumps; however, hydromorphone, fentanyl, and methadone are also used.
■ Bupivacaine and ropivacaine are used but are not FDA approved.
■ Clonidine is also used but is not FDA approved.
■ Baclofen is FDA approved.
■ Prialt is FDA approved.

Common conditions for which IIT can be effective in older adults are spinal disorders, failed back surgery, postlaminectomy syndrome, CLBP, lower extremity pain, CRPS, and neuropathic pain (NP). Many of these conditions are often seen in older adults.

Before implanting an IIT pump, a trial using either multiple intrathecal (IT) injections or a continuous IT infusion is needed. Medication selection for the trial is based on history of previous analgesia use/effectiveness and potential side effects of potential medications. During the trial, older adults should be evaluated for adverse effects for at least 24 hours.

Advantages

■ Evidence is considered to be strong that IIT therapy is effective for improvement (less than a year) of neuropathic or malignant pain, and moderate for managing chronic pain over time (Boswell et al., 2005).

- IIT therapy is reported to improve analgesia, function, and quality of life.
- The IIT pump can be removed if the therapy is not effective.
- IIT therapy can be cost effective when compared with traditional medical management of chronic intractable pain

Cautions

When considering an IIT pump, it is important to evaluate the psychological status of the older adult, previous analgesia therapies, and ability of the older adult (or their caregivers) to maintain and operate the pump

Complications associated with IIT include the following:

- Postdural puncture headache
- Infection
- Medication associated side effects (the greatest concern is for respiratory depression)
- Weight gain
- Granuloma at the insertion site
- Urinary retention
- Pump or catheter failure
- Decreased libido
- Equipment malfunction causing leaking or obstruction (Ahmed, Martin, & Chang, 2005; Boswell et al., 2005; Deer et al., 2007; Giller, 2011; Manchikant et al., 2009)

Spinal Cord Stimulation (SCS) involves catheter-like electrodes being placed within the epidural space in an area adjacent to the region of the spine believed to be the source of pain. Electric current is applied to the area in an effort to inhibit and block pain impulses and perception. Once correct placement is ascertained, the electrodes are connected to a stimulator for a trial period. Once effectiveness is ascertained, the stimulator is permanently placed in a SC pocket.

Indications for SCS include

- LBP that may or may not be associated with failed back surgery
- NP, especially of the legs
- phantom limb pain
- radiculopathies of the extremities
- chronic abdominal pain (pelvic, pancreas)
- CRPS

Advantages

Advantages associated with SCS include the following:

- Reduction in pain—evidence of effectiveness is strong for relief lasting less than 1 year and moderate for relief lasting longer than 1 year
- Improved function and quality of life
- Fewer dose escalations in opioids to control pain
- Fewer subsequent instances of surgery
- Does not alter spinal anatomy or permanently interfere with the pain pathway; therefore is reversible

Cautions

Major concerns when considering SCS therapy for elders are as follows:

- Condition of the spinal column; prior surgery; chronic disease or deformity may contraindicate SCS
- Coagulopathy contraindicates placement of a spinal cord stimulator
- Inability to understand the concept of SCS and use the device appropriately

Potential complications include the following:

- Migration of the electrode
- Infection (at the site or meningitis)
- Skin breakdown at the site of insertion
- Problems with the generator pocket or pump
- Nerve damage or nerve injury (Boswell et al., 2005; Chou et al., 2009; Giller, 2011; Kumar et al., 2007; Mailis-Gagnon, Furlan, & Sandoval, 2008; Neuromodulation Therapy Access Coalition [NTAC], 2008)

Balloon Vertebroplasty/Kyphoplasty for Vertebral Compression Fractures (VCF) are used to treat osteoporosis, which is very common among older adults and affects 2 million women throughout the world (Hulme, Krebs, Ferguson, Berlemann, 2006). Many VCF respond to conservative medical treatment (analgesia, rest, external compression, and rehabilitation therapy); however, for some older adults, this is either not adequate or not appropriate. Surgical intervention often is not successful with osteoporotic bones. Vertebroplasty is an effort to alleviate pain by stabilizing the fracture through injection of percutaneous cement (Depalma, Ketchum, Frankel, & Frey, 2011). Kyphoplasty is a procedure in which a balloon or inflatable bone tamp is used to reduce the fracture and restore height. The balloon is then deflated and the cavity is filled with cement (Chen, Yang, & Tang, 2011).

Advantages

- Indications are that vertebroplasty is effective and safe even in the very old.
- Efficacy of vertebroplasty is between 80% and 100%.
- Kyphoplasty is reportedly effective in alleviating pain and restoring height.

Cautions

- Complications related to moderate sedation or general anesthesia needed for these procedures is possible.
- Complications of vertebroplasty include rib fractures, neuritis, pedicle fracture, and infection.
- Recurrent fracture rates have been reported between 12.4% and 24% with vertebroplasty.
- The relationship of vertebroplasty with new onset fractures is not known.
- There have not been enough comparative, blinded, randomized controlled studies to clearly determine efficacy with either procedure.
- Pulmonary embolism is a possible but not common complication with either procedure. (Depalma et al., 2011; Garfin, Hansen, & Reiley, 2001; Mehbod, Aumoble, & Lehuec, 2003; Taylor, Taylor, & Fritzell, 2004).

Acupuncture is an ancient modality in traditional Chinese medicine (TCM). It works through stimulation of specific points identified in the meridians or pathways of the energetic anatomy. According to TCM, this stimulation corrects imbalances that have occurred in the flow of energy. As the imbalance is corrected, pain is relieved.

The 2007 American Pain Society/American College of Physicians Clinical Practice Guideline classifies acupuncture as a moderately effective intervention for CLBP. Reports noted that acupuncture is more effective than placebo (Chou & Huffman, 2007), particularly when it is integrated with other therapies (Ammendolia, Furlan, Imamura, Irvin, & Van Tulder, 2008). In one study using sham acupuncture, the sham acupuncture was more effective than standard multimodal analgesia (Haake et al., 2007; Shih, Costi, & Teixeira, 2008).

Advantages

- There is fair evidence that acupuncture can be effective to relieve pain and improve function of older adults who live with CLBP and osteoarthritis.

Cautions

■ Long-term effectiveness is not clearly ascertained.

■ Pain from insertion of needles is experienced by up to half of people.

■ Additional research is needed to establish efficacy in a variety of painful conditions.

■ Complications are rare but include bleeding; faintness or syncope (less than 0.5%); pneumothorax is extremely rare (2 of 245 patients); infection that is most often related to technique of individual acupuncturist (Ammendolia et al., 2008; Chou et al., 2007; Chou & Huffman, 2007; Ernst, Lee, & Choi, 2011; Mao & Kapur, 2010; Mamtani & Frishman, 2008).

Chiropractic (Spinal manipulation) is a therapy that involves manipulations by the chiropractor, with the intent of restoring function by restoring the natural alignment of the spine. The vast majority of patients who seek care from a chiropractor do so to relieve pain of the back, neck, or head.

Advantages

■ *Advantages* include at least temporary relief of pain, with some chronic pain patients reporting relief 7 months after manipulation.

■ Spinal manipulation is reported to have good evidence and moderate effectiveness when used for CLBP.

Cautions

■ Soreness after a treatment is the most common adverse reaction.

■ The most severe adverse event noted as a result of chiropractic treatment is a stroke after cervical neck manipulation, which occurs very rarely. (Chou & Huffman, 2007; Ernst, 2002; Jackson & Keegan, 2009; Redwood, 2008).

GUIDELINES

American Society of Anesthesiologists Task Force on Pain management. Practice guidelines for chronic pain management. A report from the American Society of Anesthesiologists Task Force on Pain Management, Chronic Pain Section. *Anesthesiology,* 1997 Apr;86(4): 995–1004.

American Society of Interventional Pain Physicians. http://www.asipp.org

American Society of Interventional Pain Physicians. Interventional techniques in the management of chronic spinal pain: Evidence-based practice guidelines Boswell MV, Shah RV, Everett CR, et al. *Pain Physician,* 2005; 8:1–47.

Polyanalgesic consensus conference 2007: Recommendations for the management of pain by intrathecal (intraspinal) drug delivery: Report of an interdisciplinary expert panel. Deer, T., Krames, E. S., Hassenbusch, S. J., Burton, A., Caraway, D., Dupen, S., et al. (2007). *Neuromodulation, 10,* 300–328.

Case Study

Mr. Jones is a 79-year-old retired bricklayer. He has suffered with CLBP for more than 40 years. He has been treated with a variety of medications, including acetaminophen, nonsteroidal anti-inflammatory drugs, vicodin, oxycodone, morphine, and hydromorphone, with little effect. He reports that his ability to care for himself is limited because he cannot bend to put on socks, or remove clothes from the dryer, and he cannot lift anything heavier than 10 pounds. He worries how he will help his pet cocker spaniel if the dog needed to be moved or lifted. Other than the chronic pain, he takes medications for hypertension, psoriasis, and depression. He arrives in clinic today asking what other options are there for his pain.

Questions

1. What interventional options would be appropriate to manage Mr. Jones' pain?
2. With each of them, what things in Mr. Jones history and life need to be considered?
3. What additional information do you need before referring Mr. Jones for evaluation?

REFERENCES

Ahmed, S. U., Martin, N. M., & Chang, Y. (2005). Patient selection and trial methods for intraspinal drug delivery for chronic pain: A national survey. *Neuromodulation, 8,* 112–120.

American Geriatrics Society (AGS). (2009). Pharmacological management of persistent pain in older persons. *Journal of the American Geriatrics Society, 57,* 1331–1346.

Ammendolia, C., Furlan, A. D., Imamura, M., Irvin, E., & Van Tulder, M. (2008). Evidence-informed management of chronic low back pain with needle acupuncture. *The Spine Journal, 8,* 160–172.

Arezzo, J. C. (2002). Possible mechanisms for the effects of botulinum toxin on pain. *The Clinical Journal of Pain, 18,* S125–S132.

Arnstein, P. (2010). *Clinical coach for effective pain management.* Philadelphia, PA: F. A. Davis Company.

Bernstein, C., Lateef, B., & Fine, P. (2005). Interventional pain management procedures in older adults. In S. J. Gibson & D. K. Weiner (Eds.), *Pain in older adults* (p. 263–283). Seattle, WA: IASP Press.

Boswell, M. V., Shah, R. V., Everett, C. R., Sehgal, N., McKenzie-Brown, A. M., Abdi, S., Manchikanti, L. (2005). Interventional techniques in the management of chronic spinal pain: Evidence-based practice guidelines. *Pain physician, 8,* 1–47.

Boswell, M. V., Trescot, A. M., Datta, S., Schultz, D. M., Hansen, H. C., Abdi, S., Manchikanti, L. (2007). Interventional techniques: Evidence-based practice guidelines in the management of chronic spinal pain. *Pain Physician, 10,* 7–122.

Brashear, A., Gordon, M. F., Elovic, E., Kassicieh, V. D., Marciniak, C., Do, M., Turkel, C. (2002). Intramuscular injection of botulinum toxin for the treatment of wrist and finger spasticity after a stroke. *New England Journal of Medicine, 347,* 395–400.

Cepeda, M. S., Lau, J., & Carr, D. B. (2002). Defining the therapeutic role of local anesthetic sympathetic blockade in complex regional pain syndrome: A narrative and systematic review. *Clinical Journal of Pain, 18,* 216–233.

Chen, L., Yang, H., & Tang, T. (2011). Unilateral versus bilateral balloon kyphoplasty for multilevel osteoporotic vertebral compression fractures. *Spine, 36,* 534–540.

Chou, R., Atlas, S. J., Stanos, S. P., & Rosenquist, R. W. (2009). Nonsurgical interventional therapies for low back pain: A review of the evidence for an American Pain Society clinical practice guideline. *Spine, 10,* 1078–1093.

Chou, C., & Huffman, L. H. (2007). Nonpharmacologic therapies for acute and chronic low back pain: A review of the evidence for an American Pain Society/American College of Physicians clinical practice guideline. *Annals of Internal Medicine, 147,* 493–505, W121–W141.

Chou, L. H., Lew, H. L., Coelho, P. C., & Slipman, C. W. (2005). Intradiscal electrothermal annuloplasty. *American Journal of Physical Medicine & Rehabilitation, 84,* 538–549.

Chou, R., Qaseem, A., Snow, V., Casey, D., Cross, T., & Shekelle, P. (2007). Diagnosis and treatment of low back pain: A joint clinical practice guideline from the American College of Physicians and the American Pain Society. *Annals of Internal Medicine, 147,* 478–491.

Collins, L., Halwani, A., & Vaghadia, H. (1999). Impact of a regional anesthesia analgesia program for outpatient foot surgery. *Canadian journal of anesthesia, 46,* 840–845.

Deer, T., Krames, E. S., Hassenbusch, S. J., Burton, A., Caraway, D., Dupen, S., Ver Donck, A. (2007). Polyanalgesic consensus conference 2007: Recommendations for the management of pain by intrathecal (intraspinal) drug delivery: Report of an interdisciplinary expert panel. *Neuromodulation, 10,* 300–328.

Depalma, M. J., Ketchum, J. M., Frankel, B. M., & Frey, M. E. (2011). Percutaneous vertebroplasty for osteoporotic vertebral compression fractures in the nonagenarians. *Spine, 36,* 277–282.

Difazio, M., & Jabbari, B. (2002). A focused review of the use of botulinum toxins for low back pain. *The Clinical Journal of Pain, 18,* S155–S162.

Ernst, E. (2002). Manipulation of the cervical spine: a systematic review of case reports of serious adverse events, 1995-2001. *Medical Journal of Australia, 176,* 376–380.

Ernst, E., Lee, M. S., & Choi, T. Y. (2011). Acupuncture: Does it alleviate pain and are there serious risks? A review of reviews. *Pain, 152,* 755–764.

Freund, B., Schwartz, M., & Symington, J. M. (2000). Botulinum toxin: New treatment for temporomandibular disorders. *British Journal of Oral & Maxillofacial Surgery, 38,* 466–471.

Friedly, J., Chan, L., & Deyo, R. (2007). Increases in lumbosacral injections in the Medicare population 1994–2001. *Spine, 32,* 1754–1760.

Garfin, S. R., Hansen, A. Y., & Reiley, M. A. (2001). Kyphoplasty and vertebroplasty for the treatment of painful osteoporotic compression fractures. *Spine, 26,* 1511–1515.

Giller, C. A. (2011). The neurosurgical treatment of pain. *Archives of Neurology, 60,* 1537–1540.

Haake, M., Müller, H. H., Schade-Brittinger, C., Basler, H. D., Helmut, C., Basler, H. D., Molsberger, A. (2007). German acupuncture trials (GERAC) for chronic low back pain: Randomized, multi-center, blinded, parallel-group trial with 3 groups. *Archives of Internal Medicine, 167,* 1892–1898.

Hansen, H. C., McKenzie-Brown, A. M., Cohen, S. P., Swicegood, J. R., Colson, J. D., & Manchikanti, L. (2007). Sacroiliac joint interventions: A systematic review. *Pain Physician, 10,* 165–184.

Hulme, P. A., Krebs, J., Ferguson, S. J., & Berlemann, U. (2006). Vertebroplasty and kyphoplasty: A systematic review of 69 clinical studies. *Spine, 31,* 1983–2001.

Jankovic, J. (2004). Botulinum toxin in clinical practice. *Journal of Neurology, Neurosurgery, and Psychiatry, 75,* 951–957.

Kumar, K., Taylor, R. S., Line, J., Eldabe, S., Meglio, M., Molet, J., North, R. B. (2007). Spinal cord stimulation versus conventional medical management for neuropathic pain: A multicentre randomised controlled trial in patients with failed back surgery syndrome. *Pain, 132,* 179–188.

Lew, M. F. (2002). Review of the FDA-approved uses of botulinum toxins, including data suggesting efficacy in pain reduction. *The Clinical Journal of Pain, 18,* S142–S146.

Loder, E., & Biondi, D. (2002). Use of botulinum toxins for chronic headaches: A focused review. *The Clinical Journal of Pain, 18,* S169–S176.

Mailis-Gagnon, A., Furlan, A., & Sandoval, J. A. (2008). Spinal cord stimulation for chronic pain. *The Cochrane Database of Systemic Reviews, 3,* DOI: 10.1002/14651858.CD003783.pub2.

Mamtani, R., & Frishman, W. H. (2008). Acupuncture. In M. I. Weintraub, R. Mamanti, & M. S. Micozzi (Eds.), *Complementary and integrative medicine in pain management* (pp. 215–227). New York, NY: Springer.

Manchikant, L., Boswell, M. V., Singh, V., Benyamin, R. M., Fellows, B., Abdi, S., Hirsch, J. A. (2009). Comprehensive evidence-based guidelines for interventional techniques in the management of chronic spinal pain. *Pain Physician, 12,* 699–802.

Manchikanti, L., Boswell, M. V., Singh, V., Pampati, V., Damron, K., Beyer, K. S., & Beyer, C. D. (2004). Prevalence of facet joint pain in chronic spinal pain of cervical, thoracic, and lumbar regions. *BMC Musculoskeletal Disorders, 204,* 5–15.

Manchikanti, L., Manchikanti, K., Manchukonda, R., Cash, K. A., Damron, K. S., Pampati, V., & McManus, C. D. (2007). Evaluation of lumbar facet joint nerve blocks in the management of chronic low back pain: A preliminary report of a randomized, double-blind controlled trial. Clinical Trial NCT000355914. *Pain Physician, 10,* 425–440.

Manchikanti, L., Staats, P. S., Singh, V., Schultz, D. M., Vilims, B. D., Jasper, J. F., Feler, C. A. (2003). Evidence-based practice guidelines for interventional techniques in the management of chronic spinal pain. *Pain Physician, 6,* 3–80.

Mao, J. J., & Kapur, R. (2010). Acupuncture in primary care. *Primary Care, 37,* 105–117.

Mehbod, A., Aumoble, S., & Lehuec, J. C. (2003). Vertebroplasty for osteoporotic spine fracture: Prevention and treatment. *European Spine Journal, 12,* S155–S162.

Mekhail, N., & Kapural, L. (2004). Intradiscal thermal annuloplasty for discogenic pain: An outcome study. *Pain Practice, 4,* 84–90.

Neuromodulation Therapy Access Coalition [NTAC]. (2008). *Position paper on spinal cord neurostimulation.* Retrieved from http://www.painmed.org/Workarea/DownloadAsset.aspx?id=3263

Raj, P. P. (2008). Intervertebral disc: Anatomy-physiology-pathophysiology-treatment. *Pain Practice, 8,* 18–44.

Redwood, D. (2008). Chiropractic management of chronic low-back pain: commentary on Wilkey et al. *The Journal of Alternative and Complementary Medicine, 14,* 451–452.

Saal, J. A., & Saal, J. S. (2002). Intradiscal electrothermal treatment for chronic discogeneic low back pain: Prospective outcome study with a minimum 2 year follow up. *Spine, 27,* 966–973.

Schmitt, W. J., Slowey, E., Fravi, N., Weber, S., & Burgunder, J. M. (2001). Effect of Botulinum Toxin A Injections in the treatment of chronic tension-type headache: A double-blind, placebo-controlled trial. *Headache: The journal of head and face pain, 41,* 658–664.

Sehgal, N., Dunbar, E. E., Shah, R. V., & Colson, J. (2007). A systematic review of diagnostic utility of facet (zygapophysial) joint injections in chronic spinal pain: An update. *Pain Physician, 10,* 213–228.

Sharma, M. C., Staats, P. S., & Luthardt, F. W. (2004). Interventional strategies for pain management. In F. M. Gloth (Ed.), *Aging medicine: Handbook of pain relief in older adults: An evidence based approach* (pp. 133–164). Totowa, NJ: Humana Press.

Shih, M. L., Costi, J. M., & Teixeira, J. E. (2008). Sham acupuncture is not a placebo. *Archives of Internal Medicine, 168,* 1011.

Singh, V., Piryani, C., & Liao, K. (2003). Evaluation of percutaneous disc decompression using coblation in chronic back pain with or without leg pain. *Pain Physician, 6,* 273–280.

Stolker, R. J., & Groen, G. J. (2000). Medical and invasive management of thoracic spinal pain. In L. G. F. Giles & K. P. Singer (Eds.), *Clinical anatomy and management of thoracic spine pain* (Vol. 2, pp. 205–222). Oxford: Butterworth Heinemann.

Taylor, R. S., Taylor, R. J., & Fritzell, P. (2004). Balloon kyphoplasty and vertebroplasty for vertebral compression fractures: A comparative systematic review of efficacy and safety. *Spine, 31,* 2747–2755.

Urrutia, G., Kovacs, F., Nishishinya, M. B., & Olabe, J. (2007). Percutaneous thermocoagulation intradiscal techniques for discogenic low back pain. *Spine, 32,* 1146–1154.

Weiner, D. K., & Cayea, D. (2005). Low back pain and its contributors in older adults: A practical approach to evaluation and treatment. In S. J. Gibson & D. K. Weiner (Eds.), *Pain in older adults* (pp. 329–354). Seattle, WA: IASP Press.

Wong, G. Y., Schroeder, D. R., & Carns, P. E. (2004). Effect of neurolytic celiac plexus block on pain relief, quality of life, survival in patients with unresectable pancreatic cancer. *Journal of the American Medical Association, 291,* 1092–1099.

11

Complementary Interventions for Pain Management in Older Adults

Often "CAM" is used to describe complementary interventions or modalities. The National Center for Complementary and Alternative Medicine (NCCAM) that is within the National Institutes of Health (NIH), defines "CAM" as "a group of diverse medical and health systems, practices, and products that are not generally considered to be part of conventional medicine" (NCCAM, 2011). NIH further describes that

■ *conventional medicine* is rendered in a traditional manner by physicians and doctors of osteopathy
■ *complementary care* is given **in addition to** conventional medicine
■ *alternative medicine* is provided **instead of** conventional medicine

That difference between complementary and alternative health practices is very important. Complementary interventions *complement* conventional health care, whereas alternative interventions are used as an *alternative* to conventional health care. Because there is no intent to suggest that any of the modalities discussed in this chapter should be used *instead of* or as *alternatives* to conventional health care, all modalities will be discussed from a complementary perspective as part of a multimodal approach to pain management in older adults.

Most complementary interventions are generally safe, when used as part of a multimodal approach to pain; however, they must be evaluated for appropriateness with the individual older adult. It is important to remember that acute or unexpected intensification of pain is a symptom that should always be investigated.

Complementary therapies are commonly used by older adults to help relieve or control pain. In one study, the majority (80%) of the older adults (54 to 92 years of age) used two or more complementary therapies (King & Pettigrew, 2004). This is consistent with the National Health Survey in which it was found the percentage of older adults using at least one CAM intervention actually increased with age:

- 64.8% of those 60 to 69 years of age
- 68.8% of those 70 to 84 years of age
- 70.3% of those 85 years of age and older (Arcury et al., 2006)

In another study of 42 strategies older adults reported using to manage their pain, only 16 could be considered in the realm of traditional Western medicine (Kemp, Ersek, & Turner, 2005). Included in those 16 traditional interventions were psychotherapy, biofeedback, and physical therapy. The majority of interventions used by elders were of a complementary nature.

The American Geriatrics Society (AGS) (2002) guidelines noted that nonpharmacological interventions that increase self-reliance and self-control need to be a central part of coping and managing persistent/chronic pain. In a multimodal approach of controlling pain, complementary interventions serve this purpose and can result in the following:

- Improved control of pain
- Less analgesic medication (with less side effects)
- Improved function
- Greater activity
- Less depression
- Less anxiety
- Improved family involvement (AGS, 2002; Herr, Bjoro, Steffensmeier, & Rakel, 2006; Kemp et al., 2005; Seers, 2006)

Pain is more than a physical experience and affects the mind, body, emotions, and spirit. Augmenting analgesic medication with complementary modalities can reduce the amount of medication needed, thus reducing dose-related side effects (Horgas & Yoon, 2008). This is important with older adults who are sensitive to various side effects (see Chapter 9).

When discussing complementary therapies with older adults, it is important to remember that both older adults and complementary modalities are heterogeneous. It is very important to learn what treatments the individual elder may use; thus it is imperative to approach this topic in an open and nonjudgmental manner. In a large study of older adults, only 53% who used CAM interventions told their primary care providers about the use (Cheung, Wyman, & Halcon, 2007). At a minimum, discussion of pain management must consider culture, personal beliefs, cognitive status, and ability to access (financially and logistically) the particular modalities or interventions (Austrian, Kerns, & Reid, 2005; Herbert, 2006).

Nurses need to be aware of complementary interventions that can be included in multimodal therapy care plans. Aspects of complementary interventions to consider are as follows:

■ Available research done to date
■ Limitations of the available research (generally additional research is needed)
■ Any known potential adverse effects
■ Use of the modality in a complementary rather than alternative manner

IMPROVE COMFORT OF THE OLDER ADULT

Even with the best analgesia, it is very hard for older adults to manage pain when they are not comfortable. The following simple measures are basic to ensuring that older adults are comfortable in the hospital, rehabilitation setting, long-term care facility, or their own homes.

MODIFICATION OF THE ENVIRONMENT

Everyone has preferences about their environment. It is important to ask older adults or their families about their preferences.

Lighting—Although some older adults find bright light to be offensive, others need more light because of waning vision. Because the threshold for light perception increases with age, additional light may be needed intermittently for reading.

Sounds—Some elders like to be in a quiet environment, whereas others find background music, talk radio, or television comforting. Hearing loss is common with aging and many older adults need to use hearing aids. At the same time, it is important to remember that some older adults continue to have acute hearing and are sensitive to noise.

Temperature—As with younger people, some older people prefer warmer temperatures, whereas others prefer it to be cooler. In general, older adults are more sensitive to cold as a result of a lower body temperature and less subcutaneous fat underlying their thinning skin. At the same time, they are not able to modulate their responses to heat as well as younger people.

Position—It is difficult to be comfortable when not in a position that is comfortable. Supportive devices designed to relieve pressure and pillows can help achieve a more desirable position. Assisting elders to reposition as needed can greatly contribute to improved comfort with better pain relief.

Rest and Sleep

Older adults do not require more sleep; however, they frequently experience poorer quality sleep. Good sleep hygiene for older adults includes education to do the following:
- Be active during the day.
- Avoid stimulating foods/beverages (chocolate, coffee, caffeine teas, or sodas) 8 hours before bedtime.
- Eat a light snack 1 or 2 hours before bedtime.
- Arrange a comfortable environment (light, temperature, noise).
- Encourage a relaxing bedtime routine.

Interpersonal Interactions

Some elders are very social and appreciate companionship of others most of the time. Others prefer private and alone time. It is important to identify the preferences of the older adult and advocate for them (Eliopoulos, 2001; Herbert, 2006; Herr et al., 2006; Horgas & Yoon, 2008).

COGNITIVE BEHAVIORAL INTERVENTIONS

Cognitive Behavioral Techniques

Cognitive behavioral techniques are an important part of multimodal analgesia (AGS, 2002) and are frequently used by older adults. Before discussing possible cognitive interventions, it is important to assess the cognitive and physical ability of the older person to actively participate in particular interventions (Herr et al., 2006).

Education

Education is a vital component of pain management and can improve pain management by increasing the sense of control and empowerment of the elder. In this case, knowledge is power. This is enhanced when education includes techniques to cope with and control pain. Often it is advisable for caregivers and family members to attend sessions with the older person to know what is taught and reinforce the education with the older person.

Education can focus on

- The etiology of the pain
- Measures to alleviate pain
- Pharmacological interventions
- Management of side effects
- Comfort measures
- Nonpharmacological interventions
- Muscle relaxation (AGS, 2002; Oliveira, Gevirtz, & Hubbard, 2006)

Distraction

Distraction activities and techniques that divert attention from pain being experienced are used by many adults. Distraction methods may include learning specific techniques, such as imagery, focal point attention, music, or counting. They can involve pleasurable leisure activities, such as cards games, crossword puzzles, word games, watching sports, knitting, scrap booking, and watching television. In one study, the researchers were surprised to find that when a significant amount of attention was required for a task, pain scores decreased (Berman, Iris, Bode, & Drengenberg, 2009; Ersek, Turner, & Kemp, 2006; Veldhuijzen, Kenemans, De Bruin, Olivier, & Volkerts, 2006).

Hypnosis

Hypnosis has been in use since the early 1800s. It is a process that involves increased mental focus and concentration, with expanded awareness, diminishing perception and interest in peripheral sensations, thoughts, and feelings of the external environment (Anselmo, 2009; Fass, 2008). Hypnosis has been effective in alleviating a variety of pain syndromes experienced by older adults, including osteoarthritis (OA), fibromyalgia, cancer, headaches, coronary disease, and sickle cell disease.

Hypnosis is considered a generally safe and effective modality. Caution is needed in elders who have psychiatric illness. Because effectiveness is related to the experience of the hypnotist, it is recommended that elders consult a hypnotist who is reputable and experienced working with older adults in pain (Fass, 2008; Jensen & Patterson, 2006; Montgomery, DuHamel, & Redd, 2000).

Relaxation Techniques

Relaxation techniques combine psychological and physical responses that involve the parasympathetic system as well as visceral and somatic organs, through which cerebral, physical, and emotional tensions are released (Anselmo, 2009). Several techniques can be used to achieve this release of tension.

Imagery

Imagery begins as a cognitive intervention but is one of many techniques used to promote relaxation and is a particular form of distraction. Although the terms imagery and visualization are often used interchangeably, there is a difference. *Imagery* is the "spontaneous flow of thoughts originating from the unconscious mind, whereas *visualization* involves "a conscious choice with intentional instructions" (Seaward, 2004, p. 381). Thus, visualization is a deliberate process of imagining. With imagery, the elder can allow a free flow of thoughts from the unconscious mind that may include day dreaming or reminiscing.

Guided Imagery

Guided imagery adds a coach or guide to the deliberate process. This can either be in person or through audio tapes. Generally deliberate imagery or visualization begins with relaxing. The older adult is then guided to focus on a place of their choice that encourages them to feel safe and relaxed.

Although most studies involving guided imagery are small, the results have been effective in reducing pain as measured with the visual analog scale when guided imagery is used two to three times daily. Additional research is needed with this intervention.

Observe the following cautions when using guided imagery with older adults:

■ Ensure the older person is able to adequately hear the voice guiding the imagery.
■ Always have the elder choose the location for imagery (to ensure that it is comforting and not threatening).

■ Instruct the elder to ensure he or she is in a comfortable and safe location to prevent fall or injury.

■ Guided imagery is not indicated for older adults with cognitive impairment or with psychotic disorders (Herr et al., 2006; Lazarus, 2000; Morone & Greco, 2007; Seaward, 2004).

BREATHING TECHNIQUES

Relaxation Breathing

Relaxation breathing can take a variety of forms (i.e., square, diaphragmatic, conscious, Lamaze, yoga). Awareness of breathing can be practiced to help relieve anxiety and pain. The benefit is that it is simple and portable with no negative effects (Anselmo, 2009; Frey, 2009; Lazarus, 2000).

Diaphragmatic breathing, also called "soft belly breathing," is the process of slowly inhaling, while focusing on bringing the inhaled air down into the abdomen and watching the abdominal area fill with the air. Then while exhaling, focusing on and watching the air leaving the abdomen. This is analogous to watching an imaginary balloon inflate with inhalation and deflate with exhalation (Lazarus, 2000). Benefits are that it is very easy to learn and helps with the relaxation process. There are no known negative consequences to using this technique.

Square breathing is a technique that helps older adults have control over their breathing and relaxation. The elder either looks at a square (Figure 11.1) or imagines a square (four sides):

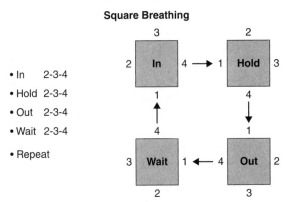

Square Breathing

- In   2-3-4
- Hold 2-3-4
- Out   2-3-4
- Wait 2-3-4
- Repeat

Figure 11.1 ■ Square breathing.

- On the first side, breathe in for 4 seconds.
- On the second side, hold the breath for 4 seconds
- On the third side, breathe out for 4 seconds.
- On the fourth side, wait or pause for 4 seconds.

Although this technique has not been researched, in clinical use, it helps to control rapid breathing, distracts attention, and promotes relaxation. There are no known negative effects (Frey, 2009).

Progressive Muscle Relaxation (PMR)

Progressive muscle relaxation (PMR) was developed to help people relax muscles that become tense because of anxiety, stress, or pain. In traditional PMR, a practitioner instructs the older adult to purposefully tense muscles while inhaling, hold the tension while holding the breath, then slowly relax the muscle while exhaling. Through tensing the muscle the individual learns how tense muscles feel and how to relax them (Anselmo, 2009). Variations of traditional PMR may or may not incorporate tensing of the muscles, color, temperature, or imagery. PMR may be helpful in managing pain of older adults through the relaxation of tense muscles. There are no known adverse effects with PMR.

HEALING ARTS

Music Therapy

Music therapy is the use of "music to address physical, emotional, cognitive, and social needs of individuals of all ages" (AMTA, 2004). It is used to promote wellness and improve health of older adults, including managing stress and pain during activities, at rest, and while preparing for sleep (Herr et al., 2006). It is suggested that beneficial effects of music therapy are related to arousal of emotional responses and distract from the pain experience, thus interrupting pain perception (Kinney & Faunce, 2004).

Music therapy has been shown to be effective in helping individuals better manage pain regardless of age, gender, and duration of the pain. In nearly half the studies reviewed in one meta-analysis, analgesic use was significantly decreased after a music intervention (Nilsson, 2008). In a small study, it was clinically helpful in managing pain when poststroke patients exercised to strengthen the upper body (Kim & Koh, 2005).

PET VISITATION AND ANIMAL ASSISTED THERAPY

At least since the late 18th century, animals have been used for therapy in a variety of ways. Florence Nightingale supported pet animals as companions for chronically ill patients. Therapeutic benefits of animals are based on the bond that occurs between animals and humans. In hospital settings, dogs are most often used because guidelines are well established for dogs in clinical settings.

Pet Visitation

Pet visitation occurs in hospitals, adult day centers, and long-term care facilities, generally with specially trained dogs. The animal can serve as a distraction from pain for older adults who find pet visitation to be a pleasurable experience and benefit in a variety of ways.

Animal assisted therapy (AAT) is a structured intervention involving pets, in treatment to promote physical and cognitive functioning. Goals are established, and the animal works with the older person to achieve them. Often AAT occurs during or in conjunction with pet visitation. Research is inconsistent in reports of benefit. Additional research is needed.

When using animals, cautions must be taken to
- ensure that the animal used for visitation or assistance is certified in those activities
- ensure that the older adult is medically cleared for pet visitation or AAT
- Pet therapy or AAT is contraindicated if the elder
  - has allergies to the type of animal used
  - dislikes or has had negative experiences with animals

Pet ownership involves older adults who live independently and choose to have an animal pet. Some research has indicated that owning a dog buffers stress and that physician visits by people who own dogs are less than among those who do not. It is believed that owning a dog is distracting and encourages exercise, while providing companionship and security (Jorgenson, 2006; Kayes et al. 2009; Nightingale, 1860; Palley, O'Rourke, & Niemi, 2010).

PHYSICAL INTERVENTIONS

Heat and Cold Application

Heat and cold application are used by many older adults.

Superficial heat (heating pads, hot water bottles, poultices, hot compresses/cloths, soft heated packs filled with grain, hot baths, saunas, steam, heat wraps, and infrared heat lamps) to soothe musculoskeletal pain and/or muscle spasms. There is moderate evidence that heat wraps provide some short-term relief for low back pain (LBP) (French, Cameron, Walker, Reggars, & Esterman, 2006; Mayer et al., 2005).

Application of cold (cryotherapy), in the form of ice, cold cloths, cold gel packs, ice packs, or ice massage, is an old and common treatment for acute soft tissue injury, LBP, and postoperative pain. Despite this, there is no sound research to support the effectiveness or to guide treatment protocols for applying cold (Bleakley, McDonough, & MacAuley, 2004; French et al., 2006).

Cautions are important with both heat and cold:

- Limit time and temperature extremes to avoid damaging or burning fragile skin.
- *Never* use heat (heating pad, electric blanket, hot tub, sauna) while using transdermal fentanyl patches; the additional heat will cause increased absorption and accidental overdose.
- Avoid using heat with capsaicin cream (Eliopoulos, 2001; Elliott & Simpson, 2010; FDA, 2005; Jumbelic, 2010; Pedley, 2006).

Therapeutic Massage

Therapeutic massage is one of the most common nonpharmacological interventions for pain management. It is described as "the practice of skilled touch for the purposes of reducing pain brought about by injury, disease or prolonged stress" (Calenda & Weinstein, 2008, p. 144). Haraldsson et al. (2006) reported from their study that they could not make any recommendations regarding the use of massage for neck pain. Massage has been noted as being effective (to varying degrees) for LBP, with benefit increasing when exercise and education were used in addition. Massage, with hand massage in particular, is reported to be beneficial to alleviate agitation in older adults with dementia. There are challenges with assessing the effectiveness of massage on pain in older adults:

- Studies are not generally limited to older adults.
- There are a variety of types of massage.
- Education of massage therapists varies widely.
- Controlled, quality research is needed with older people in particular.

Current data indicate that massage is generally a safe and pleasurable intervention for musculoskeletal pain. Hand massage is a nonintrusive intervention that takes little time and can be beneficial for older adults. The only adverse reactions are that some people report discomfort at points during the massage, and some have topical reactions to oils used during the massage.

Elders who use massage as a treatment for pain, need to

- consult someone experienced in working with elders
- either test the oils on a small area of skin or bring their own oils
- know they should tell the practitioner if they have discomfort or want to stop the session (Calenda & Weinstein, 2008; Furlan, Brosseau, Imamura, & Irvin, 2002; Furlan, Imamura, Dryden, & Irvin, 2008; Hansen, Jørgensen, & Ørtenblad, 2006; Haraldsson et al., 2006).

ENERGY-BASED INTERVENTIONS

Therapeutic Touch

Therapeutic touch (TT) is a contemporary interpretation of ancient healing practices developed in 1973 by Dolores Krieger, PhD, RN, and Dora Kunz. It is the conscious and intentional use of hands to direct human energies with the intent of helping or healing someone through modulation of their energy field (Krieger, 1979; Krieger, 2002).

The process begins with the TT practitioner explaining TT to the person and obtaining permission. This is followed by

- The TT practitioner centers himself or herself.
- The practitioner then makes a conscious intention to help the patient.
- Next, the energy field of the person is assessed for differences. That is done with the hands generally 2 to 4 inches above the patient, moving symmetrically from head to foot.
- Using rhythmic hand motions, the energy is directed in accordance with the assessment findings, working to clear any areas of imbalance.
- The field is reassessed throughout the treatment.

■ The intervention concludes by encouraging the patient to rest, and the response is evaluated and documented (Nurse Healers-Professional Associates International, 2008).

A CINAHL search using "Therapeutic Touch" reveals more than 1,000 references, with many studies involving pain. In 2009, Monroe conducted an integrative literature review that involved five studies in which TT was used to help manage pain in adults with chronic pain and anxiety; older adults with degenerative arthritis; adults with OA of the knee; adults with fibromyalgia; and people with burns. Monroe concluded that TT is effective in relieving pain. Two of the studies in her review were specifically with older adults. Difficulty controlling for placebo effect is a concern of research on touch therapies; however, in one detailed review of TT, Reiki, and Healing Touch, the placebo effect was not statistically significant and pain intensity scores did decrease (So, Jiang & Qin, 2008). In one randomized control study, TT was incorporated with a cognitive behavioral pain treatment program (CBPTP) as the experimental group, compared to patients who received relaxation training. The patients who received TT and attended the CBTPTP had better clinical outcomes and greater group attendance (Woodsmith, Arnstein, Rosa, & Wells-Federman, 2002).

Although anyone can learn TT, many workshops are available for nurses who wish to learn it. There is no certification, but nurses can achieve the status of being qualified (Therapeutic Touch International Association, 2011). TT is a safe and effective intervention that nurses can use for pain. There are no documented adverse effects (Monroe, 2009; Woodsmith, Arnstein, Rosa, & Wells-Federman, 2003).

Reiki

Reiki is a healing energy practice that originated in Japan. The belief is that health and healing can be promoted by accessing the universal energy field. It can be used to achieve relaxation and pain relief either as a self-care technique, or elders can receive a treatment from a reiki therapist acting as a conduit (Chou, 2004; NCCAM, 2009b). When reiki is performed by another person, it can be done either with hands on approach or from a distance (Chou, 2004; NCCAM, 2009b). There is a process for becoming a Reiki practitioner. Although good results have been reported in relieving pain, anxiety, and depression when used with older community-dwelling adults, additional research is needed (Richeson, Spross, Lutz, & Peng, 2010).

Reflexology

Reflexology is a technique using focused pressure on the hands or feet with the intent of stimulating certain reflex areas or zones that correspond to the various body organs. It is believed that stimulation can facilitate an improved flow of energy, promoting healing or achieving homeostasis (Bisson, 2008). There are formal courses and certification available for nurses who are interested in this intervention.

Reflexology is reported to be an effective intervention for nurses to use to help patients manage pain and anxiety (Stephenson & Dalton, 2003; Stephenson, Dalton, & Carson, 2003; Stephenson & Weinrich, 2000). Results in one study were positive when reflexology was used to manage stress in nursing home patients, with early to moderate stage dementia (Hodgson & Andersen, 2007). Rare and mild adverse effects include fatigue, headache, nausea, perspiration, and diarrhea (Bisson, 2008).

MOVEMENT THERAPIES

Movement therapies help the older adult remain active and retain strength, which are important factors in maintaining function and quality of life (Hayden, Van Tulder, & Tomlinson, 2005; Rose & Keegan, 2009). The AGS reported that strong evidence supports that "regular participation in physical activities may help control persistent diseases and lessen the clinical impact of the biological changes of aging" (2002, p. S219).

Exercise

Exercise is central to maintaining physical function, which is integral for successful aging, but function can be severely limited by pain. It is advisable to maintain optimal function in older adults as much as possible. When strength, particularly of the lower extremities, decreases, risk of falls with resultant fractures or other trauma increase

(Rose & Keegan, 2009). Thus exercise can be both a restorative and preventive therapy.

Once pain is controlled enough to allow activity, a vital part of multimodal pain management among older persons is reconditioning exercise (AGS, 2002). There are various types of exercise (stretching, cardiovascular, muscle strengthening) programs that can be done in the home of the older person, at a health club, or in a health care setting. Participation can either be individually or in a group. Hayden et al. (2005) conducted a systematic review of research assessing various exercise programs undertaken by adults who live with chronic nonspecific low back pain (CNLBP). They concluded that individually designed exercise programs, which include supervised stretching and strengthening exercise, may help to improve function and decrease pain in people living with CNLBP. Again, more research with well-designed studies is needed.

Tai Chi

Tai Chi "is a Chinese martial art form that consists of slow, rotational, mutisegmental movements with sequential weight shifting" (Nnodim et al., 2006, p. 1825). Tai chi is a mind-body activity that works to improve strength, balance, posture, and concentration. Achieving these aims, being able to do it any where, and not needing special equipment make it particularly beneficial for elders (Choi, Moon, & Song, 2005; Chou, 2004).

In one research study, 12 forms of tai chi were used to improve function in people living with arthritis. The authors reported improvement in arthritis symptoms, balance, and function of the older female participants (Song, Lee, Lam & Bae, 2003). This was consistent with results of a prior study with older adults who reported lower pain intensity after participating in 10 weekly tai chi classes (Adler, Good, Roberts, & Snyder, 2000). In yet another study with older adults, tai chi was effective in improving strength and reducing the risk of falls in older adults in residential care facilities (Choi et al., 2005). Although this study did not directly assess pain, improving strength and reducing fall risks are important aspects of comprehensive pain management for older adults.

Han et al. (2004) reviewed four research studies involving tai chi used by individuals with rheumatoid arthritis of various ages.

They concluded that although there was no evidence that tai chi affected pain, it did have a positive affect on lower extremity range of motion. The only adverse effects were transient muscle soreness during the initial 3 weeks of the program. Additional research is needed to determine the effect of tai chi on pain, particularly in older adults.

Yoga

Yoga is "a philosophy of living that unites physical, mental, and spiritual health" that involves breathing and stretching exercises (Anselmo, 2009). It is not necessary to adopt the philosophy of yoga to practice it. The postures and breathing exercises were designed to quiet and "cleanse" the mind as well as the body (Cashwell, Bentley, & Yarborough, 2007). Because the exercises can be started very gently, it can be a good exercise to recondition muscles and joints. It is reported to be effective in reducing pain in older adults. Although generally safe, yoga may need to be modified to meet the particular needs of older adults (Morone & Greco, 2007).

Research has reported reductions in stress, depression, anxiety, and muscle tension associated with yoga. Although considered generally safe, it is not recommended for older adults with disc disease (NCCAM, 2009c). It is recommended that elders work with a yoga instructor who understands the needs and limitations of older adults.

SPIRITUALITY AND PRAYER

Spirituality and prayer are the most common CAM interventions used by older adults (King & Pettigrew, 2004). Consistent with earlier reports, Dunn and Horgas (2000) reported 96% of 50 older adults surveyed used prayer to cope with stress.

Centering Prayer

Centering prayer is a meditative practice in the Christian tradition. It focuses on words or sounds and is considered to be nondenominational and appropriate for people of all faiths. The contemplative journey, on which centering prayer is the vehicle, is described as a process of letting go (Keating, 1999).

Loving Kindness Meditation

Loving kindness meditation (LKM) is a type of meditation from the Buddhist tradition with the intent of releasing negative emotion and embracing a sense of love. LKM begins with developing positive feelings and love toward loved ones, then toward self. This is done progressively toward others until positive feelings are for a person who has done harm to the person meditating. Because anger is often related to chronic pain situations, this meditation can be used to help manage pain by managing the anger associated with the pain. Although research is limited, one study using LKM showed improvement in pain and adjustment among people living with chronic low back pain (Carson et al., 2005). There are no negative effects known to embracing a practice of LKM.

Mindfulness Meditation

Mindfulness meditation was introduced by Jon Kabat-Zinn as a clinical intervention for chronic pain. He defined it as "moment-to-moment awareness" that "is cultivated by purposefully paying attention to things we ordinarily never give a thought to" (Kabat-Zinn, 1990, p. 2). An advantage of mindfulness is it can be integrated with daily activities, such as breathing, sitting, walking, washing dishes, or driving. Incorporated with learning and practicing mindfulness are patient, nonjudgmental, accepting, and nonstriving attitudes. It has been effectively used to help manage pain and anxiety in many patients and with older adults in particular. Although there are no adverse effects associated with mindfulness, the initial education does involve a commitment of several weekly classes. This time commitment is a challenge for conducting research studies (Lindberg, 2005; Morone & Greco, 2007; Morone, Greco, & Weiner, 2008).

DEVICES

Transcutaneous electrical nerve stimulations are discussed in Chapter 12.

Magnets have a century-long history of use for controlling pain. Currently magnets are available in patches, bracelets, shoe inserts, and mattress pads. The mechanism of action is not known, but some researchers and manufacturers of magnets propose that, in the affected part of the body, magnets

- change nerve cell processing
- restore the balance between growth and death in cells
- improve blood flow
- improve oxygen and nutrients to tissue
- increase temperature

Additional research is needed. Results of existing studies do not generally support claims that magnets are beneficial in managing pain. Generally magnet therapy appears safe; however, *cautions* are for older adults who have pacemakers or defibrillators (Kuipers, Saunder, & Ray, 2007; NCCAM, 2009a).

ADDITIONAL COMPLEMENTARY MODALITIES

Acupuncture

Acupuncture is discussed in Chapter 10.

Aromatherapy

Aromatherapy is the use of volatile and essential oils of aromatic plants that have been extracted for therapeutic use when inhaled through the olfactory system. It is a relatively new modality in the United States, but it has long been considered an established portion of health care in the United Kingdom, Japan, and Australia, where the majority of research has been done. Lavender oil is well known for relaxing effects and bergamot has uplifting benefits. More research is needed in the area of aromatherapy with pain, but early work is promising (Braden, Reichow & Halm, 2009). In the United States, for nurses interested in aromatherapy, there is certification (Buckle Associates, 2010).

Although this modality seems innocuous, there are cautions. All essential oils can cause skin irritation and some are toxic. Skin patch testing should be done prior to use. Topical use of essential oils should be done only by practitioners trained in their use (Cook & Burkhardt, 2004).

Biofeedback

Biofeedback works to self-regulate physiological processes and gain control over the body. It is an intervention that requires the older adult to be the active participant in the process. Trained biofeedback technicians use concepts of operant conditioning and specially designed equipment that mirrors the autonomic physiological processes to help control these processes to

- reduce tension and stress
- retrain muscles (when muscle tone needs to improve)
- train brain waves (to improve attention and concentration)

As part of a multimodal plan, biofeedback has been effective in managing several types of pain often seen in older adults, including chronic back pain, neck pain, fibromyalgia, temporomandibular disorders, OA, headaches, and sleep disorders. Additional research is needed with biofeedback use among older adults (Goldenberg, Burckhardt, & Crofford, 2004; Jensen, Bergstrom, Ljungquist, & Bodin, 2005; McGrady, 2008; Turner, Mancl, & Aaron, 2006).

Chiropractic

Chiropractic intervention is discussed in Chapter 10.

Mirror Therapy

Mirror therapy is a relatively new intervention to help people who experience phantom limb pain (PLP), complex regional pain syndrome (CRPS), and, more recently, motor limitation as a result of a stroke. In this therapy, a mirror or mirrored box is positioned midline to create the illusion there are two intact limbs (the affected limb is behind the mirror) (Figure 11.2). The illusion facilitates the perception that when the unaffected limb moves or is touched, the touch or movement is experienced in the affected limb as well. The intent is to achieve a functional reorganization of the somatosensory and motor cortex to minimize pain and optimize function. The benefit from mirror therapy has been reported in small studies or case reports with CRPS and PLP.

One study reported side effects of dizziness, confusion, and irritation. Physiological and psychological status of the older adult need to be assessed before initiating mirror therapy (Casale, Damiani, & Rosati, 2009). Additional refinement of the intervention and research into the effects are needed (Brodie, Whyte, & Waller, 2003; Chan et al., 2007; Karmarkar & Lieberman, 2006; MacLauchlan,

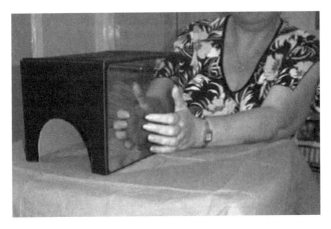

Figure 11.2 ■ Mirror box therapy. Used with permission.
I. Lieberman, Wythenshawe Hospital, Manchester, UK. Mirror box
therapy for regional pain syndrome (2006). *Anesthesia, 61,* 412–413.

McDonald, & Waloch, 2004; Rothgangel, Braun, Beuskens,
Seitz, & Wade, 2011; Selles, Schreuders, & Stam, 2008; Sutbeyaz,
Yavuzer, Sezer, & Koseoglu, 2007).

Nutrition Supplements and Herbal Preparations

Nutrition supplements and herbal preparations are used to help manage pain. It is recommended that all older adults follow dietary
guidelines that provide good nutrition and address the requirements
posed by particular illnesses (i.e., hypertension, diabetes). Herbs and
supplements commonly used to treat particular pain situations are
discussed in those chapters.

Elders need evidence-based information to make informed choices regarding complementary interventions (King &
Pettigrew, 2004). When working with older adults who are using
nutrition supplements and/or herbal preparations to help manage
pain, it is important to consider the following:

■ Potential interactions with the dietary needs
■ Potential interactions with current medication regimen
■ Potential side effects
■ Contraindications

RESOURCES

Academy for Guided Imagery. www.healthy.net/agi
American Cancer Society. www.cancer.org
American Dietetic Association. www.eatright.org
American Heart Association. www.americanheart.org
American Holistic Nurses Association. www.ahna.org
American Institute for Stress. www.stress.org
American Massage Therapy Association. www.amtamassage.org
American Music Therapy Association. www.musictherapy.org
Aromatherapy Associates Ltd. www.aromatherapyassociates.com
Aromatherapy Certification. www.rjbuckle.com
Centers for Disease Control and Prevention. www.cdc.gov
Delta Society (Pet Partners). http://www.deltasociety.org/
Kunz and Kunz Reflexology. www.reflexology-reserach.com
National Center for Complementary and Alternative Medicine. http://
    nccam.nih.gov
Therapeutic Touch International Association. TTIA@therapeutic-touch.org
Therapy Dogs International (TDI). tdi@gti.net

Case Study

Mrs. Cole accompanies her husband for his monthly visit to
assess his progress after surgery and radiation for colon cancer.
Mr. Cole, who is 72, tells you that he is mostly doing all right but
that he continues to have "pretty bad" pain in his hips. He reports
only slight relief from the ibuprofen 400 mg and morphine sulfate extended release 15 mg, both of which he takes three times
per day. Mrs. Cole is very concerned that her husband "is getting
hooked" on the morphine and "it does not seem to do much good
anyway." Mr. Cole agrees but he "needs something to manage this
pain." Mr. Cole says that he will do whatever he needs to do to get
his "life back" and not be "dependent on these meds." He says that
it is bad enough that he has to take pills for his "sugar" (diabetes);
he would rather not have to take them for pain too. The Coles ask
about complementary modalities.

Questions

1. What complementary interventions could you recommend?
2. What things do you need to consider before recommending different modalities?
3. Are there any factors from Mr. Cole's history that would contraindicate any of the modalities?
4. What education will be necessary for the Coles?
5. What role can Mrs. Cole play in a multimodal approach to pain management for her husband?

REFERENCES

Adler, P., Good, M., Roberts, B., & Snyder, S. (2000). The effects of tai chi on older adults with chronic arthritis pain. *Journal of Nursing Scholarship, 32,* 377.

American Geriatrics Society Panel (AGS) (2002). The management of persistent pain in older adults. *Journal of the American Geriatrics Society, 50,* S205–S224.

American Music Therapy Association (AMTA). (2004). *What is music therapy?* Retrieved April 30, 2011, from http://www.musictherapy.org.

Anselmo, J. (2009). Relaxation. In B. M. Dossey & L. Keegan (Eds.), *Holistic nursing: A handbook for practice* (5th ed., Rev., pp. 259–293). Boston, MA: Jones and Bartlett Publishers.

Austrian, J. S., Kerns, R. D., & Reid, M. C. (2005). Perceived barriers to trying self-management approaches for chronic pain in older persons. *Journal of the American Geriatrics Society, 53,* 856–861.

Arcury, T. A., Bell, R. A., Snively, B. M., Smith, S. L., Skelly, A. H., Wetmore, L. K., & Quandt, S. A. (2006). Complementary and alternative medicine use as health self-management: Rural older adults with diabetes. *The Journals of Gerontology Series B Psychological Science and Social Science, 61,* S62–S70.

Braden, R., Reichow, S., & Halm, M. (2009). The use of essential oil lavandin to reduce preoperative anxiety in surgical patients. *Journal of Perianesthesia Nursing, 24,* 348–355.

Berman, R. L., Iris, M. A., Bode, R., & Drengenberg, C. (2009). The effectiveness of an online mind-body intervention for older adults with chronic pain. *The Journal of Pain, 10,* 68–79.

Bisson, D. (2008). Reflexology. In M. I. Weintraub, R. Mamtani, & M. S. Micozzi (Eds.), *Complementary and integrative medicine in pain management* (pp. 201–211). New York, NY: Springer.

Bleakley, C., McDonough, S., & MacAuley, D. (2004). The use of ice in the treatment of acute soft-tissue injury: A systematic review of randomized controlled trials. *The American Journal of Sports Medicine, 32,* 251–261

Brodie, E. E., Whyte, A., & Waller, B. (2003). Increased motor control of a phantom leg in humans results from the visual feedback of a virtual leg. *Neuroscience Letters, 341,* 167–169.

Buckle, R. J. (2010). *Complementary health therapies consulting and education.* R. J. Buckle Associates LLC. Retrieved May 02, 2011, from www.rjbuckle.com

Calenda, E., & Weinstein, S. (2008). Therapeutic massage. In M. I. Weintraub, R. Mamtani, & M. S. Micozzi (Eds.), *Complementary and integrative medicine in pain management* (pp. 139–161). New York, NY: Springer.

Carson, J. W., Keefe, F. J., Lynch, T. R., Carson, K. M., Goli, V., & Fras, A. M. (2005). Loving-kindness meditation for chronic low back pain: Results from a pilot. *Journal of holistic nursing, 23,* 287–304.

Casale, R., Damiani, C., & Rosati, V. (2009). Mirror therapy in the rehabilitation of lower-limb amputation: Are there any contraindications? *American Journal of Physical Medicine and Rehabilitation, 88,* 837–842.

Cashwell, C. S., Bentley, D. P., & Yarborough, P. (2007). The only way out is through: the peril of spiritual bypass. *Counseling and Values, 51,* 139–148.

Chan, B. L., Witt, R., Charrow, A. P., Magee, A., Howard, R., & Pasquina, P. F. (2007). Mirror therapy for phantom limb pain. *New England Journal of Medicine, 357,* 2206–2207.

Cheung, C. K., Wyman, J. F., & Halcon, L. L. (2007). Use of complementary and alternative therapies in community-dwelling older adults. *The Journal of Alternative and Complementary Medicine, 13,* 997–1006.

Choi, J. H., Moon, J. S., & Song, R. (2005). Effects of sun-style tai chi exercise on physical fitness and fall prevention in fall-prone older adults. *Journal of Advanced Nursing, 51,* 14-50-157.

Chou, D. A. (2004). Tai chi, qi gong and reiki. *Physical Medicine and Rehabilitation Clinics of North America, 15,* 773–781.

Cook, A. & Burkhardt, A. (2004). Aromatherapy for self-care and wellness. *Alternative & Complementary Therapies, 10,* 151–155.

Dunn, K. S., & Horgas, A. L. (2000). The prevalence of prayer as spiritual self-care modality in elders. *Journal of Holistic Nursing, 18,* 337–351.

Eliopoulos, C. (2001). *Gerontological nursing* (5th ed., Rev.). Philadelphia, PA: Lippincott.

Elliott, J. E., & Simpson, M. H. (2010). Persistent pain management. In B. St. Marie (Ed.), *Core curriculum for pain management* (2nd ed., Rev., pp. 381–459). Dubuque, IA: Kendall Hunt.

Ersek, M., Turner, J. A., & Kemp, C. A. (2006). Use of the chronic pain coping inventory to assess older adults' pain coping strategies. *The Journal of Pain, 7 (*11) 833–842.

Fass, A. (2008). Hypnosis for pain management. In M. I. Weintraub, R. Mamtani, & M. S. Micozzi (Eds.), *Complementary and integrative medicine in pain management* (pp. 29–40). New York, NY: Springer.

Federal Drug Administration (FDA). (2005, October). Avoiding fatal overdoses with fentanyl patches. *FDA Patient Safety News: Show #44.* Retrieved April 12, 2011, from http://www.accessdata.fda.gov/psn/printer-full.cfm?id=48 database.

French, S. D., Cameron, M., Walker, B. F., Reggars, J. W., & Esterman, A. J. (2006). Superficial heat or cold for low back pain. *Cochrane database for systematic reviews, 2006*(1), CD004750.

Frey, D. (2009). Blending self-esteem, coping skills, and changing cognitive distortions. In A. A. Drewes (Ed.), *Blending play therapy with cognitive behavioral therapy: Evidence based and other effective treatments and techniques* (pp. 373–400). Hoboken, NJ: John Wiley & Sons, Inc.

Furlan, A. D., Brosseau, L., Imamura, M., & Irvin, E. (2002). Massage for low-back pain: A systematic review within the framework of the Cochrane Collaboration Back Review Group. *Spine, 27,* 1896–1910.

Furlan, A. D., Imamura, M., Dryden, T., & Irvin, E. (2008). Massage for low-back pain. *Cochrane Database of Systematic Reviews, 2008*(4), CD001929.

Goldenberg, D. L., Burckhardt, C., & Crofford, L. (2004). Management of fibromyalgia syndrome. *Journal of the American Medical Association, 292,* 2388–2395.

Han, A., Judd, M., Welch, V., Wu, T., Tugwell, P., & Wells, G. A. (2004). Tai chi for treating rheumatoid arthritis. *Cochrane Database of Systematic Reviews, 2004*(3), CD004849.

Hansen, N. V., Jørgensen, T., & Ørtenblad, L. (2006). Massage and touch for dementia. *Cochrane Database of Systematic Reviews, 2006*(4), CD004989.

Haraldsson, B., Gross, A., Myers, C. D., Ezzo, J., Morien, A., Goldsmith, C. H., et al. (2006). Massage for mechanical neck disorders. *Cochrane Database of Systematic Reviews, 2006*(3), CD004871.

Hayden, J. A., Van Tulder, M. W., & Tomlinson, G. (2005). Systematic review: Strategies for using exercise therapy to improve outcomes in chronic low back pain. *Annals of Internal Medicine, 142,* 776–785.

Herbert, R. A. (2006). The biology of human ageing. In S. J. Redfern & F. M. Ross (Eds.), *Nursing older people* (4th ed., pp. 57–82). Edinburgh, UK: Churchill Livingston Elsevier.

Herr, K., Bjoro, K., Steffensmeier, J., & Rakel, B. (2006). *Acute pain management in older adults.* Iowa City, IA: University of Iowa Gerontological Nursing Interventions Research Center, Research Translation and Dissemination Core.

Hodgson, N. A. & Andersen, S. (2007). The clinical efficacy of reflexology with dementia. *The Journal of Alternative and Complementary Medicine, 14,* 1–7.

Horgas, A. L., & Yoon, S. L. (2008). Pain management. In E. Capezuti, D. Zwicker, M. Mezey, & T. Fuller (Eds.), *Evidence-based geriatric nursing protocols for best practice* (3rd ed., pp. 199–222). New York, NY: Springer.

Jensen, I. B., Bergström, G., Ljungquist, T., Bodin, L. (2005). A 3-year follow-up of a multidisciplinary rehabilitation programme for back and neck pain. *Pain, 115,* 273–283.

Jensen, M. P. & Patterson, D. R. (2006). Hypnotic treatment of chronic pain. *Journal of Behavioral Medicine, 29,* 95–124.

Jorgenson, J. (2006). Animal assisted therapy. In M. Snyder & R. Lindquist (Eds.), *Complementary/alternative therapies in nursing* (5th ed., pp. 175–187). New York, NY: Springer.

Jumbelic, M. I. (2010). Deaths with transdermal fentanyl patches. *American Journal of Forensic Medicine & Pathology, 31,* 18–21.

Kabat-Zinn, J. (1990). *Full castrophe living.* NY, NY: Dell Publishing.

Karmarkar, A., & Lieberman, I. (2006). Mirror box therapy for complex regional pain syndrome. *Anesthesia, 61,* 402–414.

Kayes, L., McCarty, R., Walkinshaw, C., Congdon, S., Kleinberger, J., Hartman, V., & Standish, L. J. (2009). Use of complementary and alternative medicine (CAM by Washington State hospices). *American Journal of Hospice and Palliative Care, 25,* 463–468.

Keating, T. (1999). *The human condition: Contemplation and transformation.* Mahwah, NJ: Paulist Press.

Kemp, C. A., Ersek, M., & Turner, J. A. (2005). A descriptive study of older adults with persistent pain: Use and perceived effectiveness of pain strategies. *BMC Geriatrics, 5*(12).

Kim, S. J., & Koh, I. (2005). The effects of music on pain perception of stroke patients during upper extremity joint exercises. *Journal of Music Therapy, 42,* 81–92.

King, M. O., & Pettigrew, A. C. (2004). Complementary and alternative therapy use by older adults in three ethnically diverse populations. *Geriatric Nursing, 25*(1), 30–37.

Kinney, D. T., & Faunce, G. (2004). The impact of group singing on mood, coping, and perceived pain in chronic pain patients attending a multidisciplinary pain clinic. *Journal of Music Therapy, XLI,* 241–258.

Krieger, D. (1979). *The therapeutic touch: How to use your hands to help or heal.* New York, NY: Simon & Schuster.

Krieger, D. (2002). *Therapeutic Touch as transpersonal healing.* New York, NY: Booklight, Inc.

Kuipers, N. T., Saunder, C. L., & Ray, C. A. (2007). Influence of static magnetic fields on pain perception and sympathetic nerve activity in humans, *Journal of Applied Physiology, 102,* 1410–1415.

Lazarus, J. (2000). *Stress relief and relaxation techniques.* Lincolnwood, IL: Keats Publishing.

Lindberg, D. A. (2005). Integrative review of research related to meditation, spirituality, and the elderly. *Geriatric Nursing, 26,* 372–377.

Mayer, J. M., Ralph, L., Look, M., Erasala, G. N., Verna, J. L., Matheson, L. N., & Mooney, V. (2005). Treating acute low back pain with continuous low-level heat wrap therapy and/or exercise: A randomized controlled trial. *Spine Journal, 5,* 395–403.

McGrady, A. (2008). Biofeedback. In M. I. Weintraub, R. Mamtani, & M. S. Micozzi (Eds.), *Complementary and integrative medicine in pain management* (pp. 5–27). New York, NY: Springer.

MacLauchlan, M., McDonald, D., & Waloch, J. (2004). Mirror treatment of lower limb phantom pain: A case study. *Disability and Rehabilitation, 26,* 901–904.

Monroe, C. M. (2009). The effects of therapeutic touch on pain. *Journal of Holistic Nursing, 27,* 85–92.

Montgomery, G. H., DuHamel, K. N., Redd, W. H. (2000). A meta-analysis of hypnotically induced analgesia: how effective is hypnosis? *International Journal of Clinical and Experimental Hypnosis, 48,* 138–153.

Morone, N. E., & Greco, C. M. (2007). Mind–body interventions for chronic pain in older adults: A structured review. *Pain Medicine, 8,* 359–375.

Morone, N. E., Greco, C. M., & Weiner, D.K. (2008). Mindfulness meditation for the treatment of chronic low back pain in older adults: a randomized controlled pilot study. *Pain, 134,* 310–319.

National Center for Complementary and Alternative Medicine (NCCAM). (2009a). *Magnets for pain.* Retrieved April 30, 2011, from http://nccam.nih.gov/health/magnet/magnetsfor pain.htm.

National Center for Complementary and Alternative Medicine (NCCAM). (2009b). *Reiki: An introduction.* Retrieved May 1, 2011, from http://nccam.nih.gov/health/reiki.htm.

National Center for Complementary and Alternative Medicine (NCCAM). (2009c). *Yoga for health: An introduction.* Retrieved May 1, 2011, from http://nccam.nih.gov/health/yoga/D412_BKG.pdf.

National Center for Complementary and Alternative Medicine (NCCAM). (2011). *What is complementary and alternative medicine?* Retrieved September 30, 2011, from http://nccam.nih.gov/health/whatiscam/.

Nightingale, F. (1860). Chattering hopes and advices. In: *Notes on Nursing: What it is, and what it is not (P. 103 footnote).* New York, NY: D. Appleton and Company. Retrieved May 27, 2011, from http://digital.library.upenn.edu/women/nightingale/nursing/nursing.html.

Nilsson, U. (2008). The anxiety- and pain- reducing effects of music interventions: A systematic review. *AORN Journal, 87,* 780–807

Nnodim, J. O., Strasburg, D., Nabozny, M., Nyquist, L., Galecki, A., Chen, S., & Alexander, N. B. (2006). Dynamic balance and stepping versus tai chi training to improve balance and stepping in at-risk older adults. *Journal of the American Geriatrics Society, 54,* 1825–1831.

Nurse Healers-Professional Associates International (NH-PAI). (2008). *Therapeutic touch policy and procedure for health care professionals.* Retrieved April 30, 2011, from http://www.therapeutic-touch.org/newsarticle.php?newsID=6.

Oliveira, A., Gevirtz, R., & Hubbard, D. (2006). A psycho-educational video used in the emergency department provides effective treatment for whiplash injuries. *Spine, 31,* 1652–1657.

Palley, L. S., O'Rourke, P., & Niemi, S. M. (2010). Mainstreaming animal-assisted therapy. *ILAR Journal, 51,* 199–207.

Pedley, G. E. (2006). Maintaining healthy skin. In S. J. Redfern & F. M. Ross (Eds.), *Nursing older people* (4th ed., pp. 373–412). Edinburgh, TX: Churchill Livingstone Elsevier.

Richeson, N. E., Spross, J. A., Lutz, K., & Peng, C. (2010). Effects of Reiki on anxiety, depression, pain, and physiological factors in community-dwelling older adults. *Research in Gerontological Nursing, 3,* 187–199.

Rose, B. H., & Keegan, L. (2009). Exercise and movement. In B. M. Dossey & L. Keegan (Eds.), *Holistic nursing: A handbook for practice* (5th ed., Rev., pp. 229–238). Boston, MA: Jones and Bartlett Publishers.

Rothgangel, A. S., Braun, S. M., Beuskens, A. J., Seitz, R. J., & Wade, D. T. (2011). The clinical aspects of mirror therapy in rehabilitation: A systematic review of the literature. *International Journal of Rehabilitation Research, 34*(1), 1–13.

Seaward, B. L. (2004). *Managing stress: Principles and strategies for health and well-being* (4th ed., Rev.). Boston, MA: Jones and Bartlett Publishers.

Seers, K. (2006). Pain and older people. In S. J. Redfern & F. M. Ross (Eds.), *Nursing older people* (4th ed., Rev., pp. 457–473). Edinburgh, TX: Churchill Livingstone Elsevier.

Selles, R. W., Schreuders, T. A. R., & Stam, H. J. (2008). Mirror therapy in patients with causalgia (complex regional pain syndrome type II) following peripheral nerve injury: Two cases. *Journal of Rehabilitation Medicine, 40,* 312–314.

So, S., Jiang, Y., & Qin, Y. (2008). Touch therapies for pain relief in adults. *Cochrane Database of Systematic Reviews, 2008*(4), CD006535.

Song, R., Lee, E. O., Lam, P. & Bae, S. C. (2003). Effects of Tai Chi exercise on pain, balance, muscle strength, and perceived difficulties in physical functioning in older women with osteoarthritis: a randomized clinical trial. *Journal of Rheumatology, 30,* 2039–2044.

Stephenson, N., & Dalton, J. A. (2003). Using reflexology for pain management: A review. *Journal of Holistic Nursing, 21,* 179–191.

Stephenson, N., Dalton, J.A., & Carlson, J. (2003). The effect of foot reflexology on pain in patients with metastatic cancer. *Applied Nursing Research, 16,* 284–286.

Stephenson, N. L. N., & Weinrich, S. P. (2000). The effects of foot reflexology on anxiety and pain in patients with breast and lung cancer. *Oncology Nursing Forum, 27,* 57–72.

Sutbeyaz, S., Yavuzer, G., Sezer, N., & Koseoglu, B. F. (2007). Mirror therapy enhances lower-extremity motor recovery and motor functioning after stroke: A randomized controlled trial. *Archives of Physical Medicine and Rehabilitation, 88,* 555–559.

Therapeutic Touch International Association. (2011). *Therapeutic Touch.* Retrieved on September 30, 2011, from http://www.therapeutic-touch.org/channel.php.

Turner, J. A., Mancl, L., & Aaron, L. A. (2006). Short- and long-term efficacy of brief cognitive-behavioral therapy for patients with chronic temporomandibular disorder pain: A randomized controlled trial. *Pain, 121,* 643–657.

Veldhuijzen, D. S., Kenemans, J. L., De Bruin, C. M., Olivier, B., & Volkerts, E. R. (2006). Pain and attention: Attentional disruption or distraction? *The Journal of Pain, 7,* 11–20.

Woods Smith, D., Arnstein, P., Rosa, K. C., & Wells-Federman, C. (2002). Effects of integrating Therapeutic Touch into a cognitive behavioral pain treatment program: Report of a pilot clinical trial. *Journal of Holistic Nursing, 20,* 367–387.

12

The Role of Physical Therapy with Pain and Reconditioning

Reconditioning in this chapter refers to efforts that help older adults experiencing pain regain mobility, activity, and function that were compromised by the pain experience, and thus assume usual and desired activities. The role of physical therapists (PTs) in managing pain and in the reconditioning process of older adults has ancient origins and continues to be a vital therapy today. With normal aging, there is progressive loss of muscle mass. The decrease is from muscle mass being 30% of total body weight at 30 years to being 15% of total body weight at 75 years. With aging, there generally is also loss of isometric contraction force and arthritic changes in the joints. Combined aging changes result in less strength, endurance, and joint stability. These normal aging-related changes are intensified when there is extended inactivity that can occur as a result of hospitalization, illness, or prolonged pain (AHRQ, 2009; Gorevic, 2004; Leveille, 2004; Pagliarulo, 2007).

The effects of disuse have been known for many years. In 1966, Kottke proposed that physical activity can be limited by

- neuromuscular activity restrictions
- physical immobility
- "static positioning in relation to gravity"
- sensory deprivation

Each of these can result from pain experienced by older adults. The resulting effects of inactivity can be devastating physically, emotionally, and socially. With appropriate interventions by PT professionals knowledgeable about the aging process, older adults can recover at least some of the loss, thereby improving function and quality of life (APTA, 2009a; APTA, 2009b; APTA, 2011a; APTA, 2011b; APTA, 2011c).

THE REHABILITATION ROLE OF PHYSICAL THERAPISTS WITH OLDER ADULTS

Rehabilitation involves working with disabled older adults when the goal is to increase independence through recovery of lost physical, psychological, and social skills. PTs have a reconditioning role in rehabilitation of older people that focuses on improving flexibility, strength, and endurance. In addition to managing pain, using cognitive behavioral techniques, PTs can help to relieve anxiety and fear while improving flexibility, range of motion, strength, coordination, endurance, and function. PTs accomplish this through

- evaluation
- diagnosis
- clinical interactions
- functional assessment
- patient/family education
- consultation in hospitals
- consultation in
  - long-term care facilities
  - community practice settings
  - home health agencies

Through these activities PTs who specialize in working with older adults help older adults to be safer and less prone to falls or other accidents (APTA, 2009a; APTA, 2009b; APTA, 2011a; APTA, 2011b; APTA, 2011c; Collins, 2007; Lewis & Bottomley, 2008; NPC, 2006).

Pearl	Good analgesia promotes good recovery/reconditioning.

ROLE OF PHYSICAL THERAPISTS IN OLDER ADULTS' CHRONIC PAIN AND RECONDITIONING

Goal setting is an important first step for the PT working with an older adult who has reconditioning needs. Goals need to be based upon assessment findings and functional abilities. Functional goals need to be reasonable, attainable, and meaningful. The older patient and family need to be involved partners with PTs in identifying needs, expectations, and planning. Involvement of other members of the health care team is also important to support general health, nutrition, and analgesic needs (APTA, 2009b; Collins, 2007).

Reconditioning Exercises

Reconditioning exercises for older adults with chronic pain are used to recover function by increasing the strength of tissues/muscles that became weak with disuse. In one large systematic review of studies that involved older adults living in long-term care, the results indicated that rehabilitative exercise had a positive effect primarily on mobility, with some benefit seen in strength, flexibility, and balance (Forster, Lambley, & Young, 2010).

Some PTs work with patients in chronic pain within a multidisciplinary pain clinic where cognitive behavioral therapy and operant conditioning are included in physical therapy. In general treatment goals for elders living with chronic pain include the following:

- Reduce the impact of pain.
- Improve patient knowledge about the pain syndrome; older adults are often not well informed on need of education about
  - the etiology and meaning of pain
  - differences between acute and chronic pain
  - the distinction between managing and curing pain
  - what can be beneficial for managing pain
  - what can be harmful or can exacerbate pain and what will not do so
  - the ability of the older adult to actively participate in and manage the pain
- Educate the patient about self-management of pain.
- Resolve those impairments that are treatable.
- Improve function through setting goals for function.
- Decrease disability (Wittink, Cohen, & Michael, 2002).

Therapeutic Ergonomics, Gait, and Posture Training

Therapeutic ergonomics, gait, and posture training are important in helping the older adult relieve pain, regain function, and prevent additional pain/injury. Because fatigue can increase pain and the risk of injury, correct body mechanics can assist with conserving energy through proper postural alignment and muscle balance. In addition to recovery from surgery, injury, or stroke, this education can be helpful with older adults who experience low back and neck pain as well as some headache (NPC, 2006).

PHYSICAL THERAPY INTERVENTIONS

Physical therapy interventions for pain management and reconditioning can be divided into active and passive categories, depending on the needs, capabilities, and involvement of the older adult with the treatments. The following interventions are within the scope of practice of licensed PTs (APTA, 2009b).

Passive Therapies

Passive therapies do not require the active participation of the older patient.

Cryotherapy or application of cold is used with acute trauma, surgery, low back pain (LBP), to reduce swelling, to promote analgesia, and to encourage flexibility of tendons. Ice is most effective when used during the first 48 hours for musculoskeletal inflammation. Caution is needed when used with older adults who may have impaired sensation or impaired circulation in the area affected (APTA, 2009b, NPC, 2006; Stanos, Migilevsky, Rader, McLean, & Baum, 2009).

Thermal therapies or heat modalities can help to improve flexibility. Heat can be effective following acute injuries, LBP, surgery, arthritis, or muscle spasm/pain (NPC, 2006).

Thermal therapy used by PTs can be either superficial or deep. Common forms of thermal therapy include the following:

- Hot packs are pouches containing silica gel, which are soaked in water that is maintained at a set temperature. Hot packs can be used for relaxation, but they are not considered part of skilled PT.
- Paraffin treatments use melted paraffin wax with mineral oil heated to a particular temperature. These treatments are intended to relieve pain as well as encourage relaxation and comfort during range of motion exercise.
- Ultrasound and short-wave diathermy are interventions that use deep heat that penetrates somewhat deeper than moist heat to treat constant pain in joints and tissues that are not affected by superficial

heat. Although the mechanism of action is not clear, they are reported to be effective with some chronic pain situations; however, the indications are very specific.

■ Low-level laser therapy is being used to help manage chronic joint pain in some PT practices.

(Bjordal, Couppé, Chow, Tunér, & Ljunggren, 2003; Collins, 2007; Pagliarulo, 2007; Scudds & Scudds, 2005)

Two cautions for thermotherapy with older adults are to

■ avoid damage to fragile skin and underlying tissue
■ avoid thermotherapy directly over transdermal fentanyl patches because it causes the rapid release of medication, resulting in potential overdose

Electrotherapies are to be used with *caution* in older adults. *Any* implanted devices in the body must be identified because electrical signals can interfere with the device. Particular concerns for use of electrotherapies on older patients include the following:

■ Pacemakers
  ■ unless there is cardiac monitoring, use with older patients with pacemakers is contraindicated
  ■ with cardiac monitoring, caution must be given to the placement of electrodes
■ Poor skin sensation in the area to be treated
■ Skin irritation or sensitivity (Scudds & Scudds, 2005)

Common Forms of Electrotherapies

■ *Transcutaneous electrical nerve stimulation (TENS)* is a portable device, designed to reduce pain through surface electrodes, which emit high or low frequency pulsed electrical currents that selectively stimulate particular sensory or motor nerve fibers (Dreeben, 2007; Somers & Clemente, 2006). Although some patients report good relief when using TENS, the limited research has inconsistent findings. A study using rats indicated that TENS is effective for allodynia and complex regional pain syndrome (Somers & Clemente, 2006). A systematic review reported clinically important results when TENS was used in older patients with osteoarthritis (OA) of the knee (Bjordal et al., 2007). TENS is also recommended for back pain in elders (Hadjistavropoulos & Fine, 2006).

■ *Interferential currents (IFC)* is another type of electrotherapy that works through minuscule electrical impulses into tissues surrounding the painful area. Once they intersect subcutaneously, natural endorphins are secreted in response (Dreeben, 2007). One study reported that because IFC is effective in relieving pain with inflammation, it is most appropriately used with acute pain rather than chronic pain (Jorge, Parada, Ferreira, & Tambeli, 2006). In another study, no difference was seen between IFC and TENS, but IFC was more effective than sham IFC in reducing pain intensity (Johnson & Tabasam, 2003).

- *Percutaneous electrical nerve stimulation* combines acupuncture needles with electrotherapy using neuroanatomy and physiology rather than traditional Chinese medicine principles. The authors of a study with community-dwelling older adults reported decreases in disability and the intensity of pain with increases in mood, personal control, and physical activities (Weiner et al., 2003).
- *Ionotophoresis* involves application of medicine, generally to control pain or inflammation, through continuous direct current applied to skin or mucous membrane. Indications are specific (i.e., tendonitis) (APTA, 2009b; Dreeben, 2007).

Pearl	Additional research is needed with electrotherapies, particularly regarding their use with older adults.

Manual Therapies
Passive Therapies

- *Passive range of motion* is movement of a limb through an arc of movement by the PT or a machine without patient involvement. The intent is to promote joint movement, not muscle activity (Pagliarulo, 2007).
- *Manipulation and mobilization techniques* involve skilled, passive, hands on movements by PTs. They can be used to treat muscle, fascia, and joint conditions affecting older people. Movements are done at speeds and amplitudes ranging from small/low (mobilization) to high (manipulation) (APTA, 2010).
- *Massage* is one of the oldest interventions used to alleviate pain and promote function (Pagliarulo, 2007). A Cochrane review reported that massage may be effective in helping individuals with chronic low back pain and that the effect seems to be increased when combined with exercise and education (Furlan, Brosseau, Imamura, & Irvin, 2002).

■ *Other manual therapy techniques* that can be effective in treating pain and dysfunction include craniosacral therapy, muscle energy technique, acupressure, and myofascial release.

Active Therapies

Active therapies do require the active participation of the older patient.

■ *Stretching exercise* that involve low load with prolonged stretches can be done actively by older adults several times daily. Such stretching results in improved length–tension relationship of joints with their surrounding muscles. The literature is inconsistent as to the preferred length of time for stretching (15, 30, or 60 seconds). Benefits of stretching include increased flexibility and improved muscle performance (Feland, Myrer, Schulthies, Fellingham, & Measom, 2001; Lewis & Bottomley, 2008).

■ *Aerobic exercise* is a form of exercise that uses oxygen for energy. It is associated with modest progress in a number of realms, including attention and executive function. Benefits of aerobic exercise include improved cardiac function, decreased fat, and improved response to stress (Pagliarulo, 2007; Smith, Hoetzer, Greiner, Stauffer & DeSouza, 2003; Smith et al., 2001).

■ *Strength training exercises* need to be individualized to meet the needs of the older person. Generally, they are designed to include low weight with increased repetition, which provides for strengthening the muscles with minimal stress on the joints. Benefits include improved muscle strength, increased bone mass, and improved ability to perform activities of daily living (Lewis & Bottomley, 2008; Pagliarulo, 2007).

■ *Progressive resistance exercises* are structured exercises designed to progressively increase the challenge and repetitions. Results of isolated studies have shown improvement even in older adults who received this training after having been discharged from a traditional physical therapy program (Host et al., 2007).

■ *High-intensity weight bearing* exercises have been done successfully with older adults. One study reported applicability for older adults regardless of cognitive function (Littbrand et al., 2006).

Exercise in Water versus on Land

■ *Hydrotherapy or balneotherapy* is exercising in water that has been heated. It is believed that the warmth and buoyancy of the water reduce pain and stress on joints. Because this is an expensive therapy, it is used only in selected situations (Fransen, 2004; Fransen, Nairn, Winstanley, Lam, & Edmonds, 2007).

■ *Aquatic therapy* is exercise that is done within water, either individually or in a group. The buoyancy, hydrostatic pressure, and friction resistance facilitate exercises to improve balance and coordination while easing movement of joints. Aquatic exercise has been effective in improving balance among patients following strokes and increasing muscle strength while reducing LBP in elderly women (Fransen et al., 2007; Han et al., 2011; Lee, Ko, & Cho, 2010; Scudds & Scudds, 2005; Smith et al., 2011).

■ *Tai chi* (discussed in Chapter 11) is an example of the other techniques from which PTs often utilize elements. It has been used in a variety of conditions. In an extensive systematic review, it was found effective in elders who were reconditioning because of low back pain and pain related to osteoarthritis (Klein & Adams, 2004).

Pearl	Although many physical therapy interventions have reported clinical significance, there is a general need for research to substantiate outcomes.

PHYSICAL THERAPISTS AND EDUCATION

An important role of PTs is education. Some particular areas in which PTs educate patients, family members, and caretakers are

■ ways to prevent or lessen impairment
■ ways to avoid or minimize functional limitations
■ safe and easier ways to move and transfer
■ exercises to regain strength and dexterity
■ techniques to regain skills (APTA, 2009b; Collins, 2007)

PHYSICAL THERAPISTS AND ASSISTIVE DEVICES

PTs assess older adults for most appropriate fit of assistive devices. They also teach older adults to appropriately and safely use assistive devices such as crutches, walkers, and canes and adaptive devices such as grab bars to rise from a toilet (APTA, 2009b; Collins 2007).

ROLE OF PHYSICAL THERAPISTS WITH
OLDER ADULTS IN FALLS PREVENTION

As a result of diminution in muscle mass, strength, and joint stability, older people are at increased risk for falling (Gorevic, 2004). Falls and associated injuries among elders are correlated with impaired functioning, admission to long-term care facilities, and increased morbidity and mortality. Falls are reported among one-third of older adults. Preventing falls is an essential public health goal that is expected to reduce serious injuries, emergency department (ED) visits, hospitalizations, and long-term care admissions (American Geriatrics Society, 2010; CDC, 2010; Hausdorff, Rios, Edelberg, 2001). PTs work to realize this goal in a variety of ways.

- *Identification* of patients at high risk for falling is the first role of PTs in falls prevention. One red flag for concern is fear of falling.

  Other risk factors include
  - previous falls
  - OA
  - muscle weakness
  - neurological impairments
  - visual deficits
  - poor balance
  - gait disturbances
  - cognitive changes
  - multiple medications (APTA, 2007; CDC, 2010)

- *Assessment* by a PT for risk of falls involves a variety of tools to test the various risk factors exhibited or likely for the individual older adult (APTA, 2007). One Australian study found that PTs were very accurate in predicting people at risk for falling (Haines, Kuys, Morrison, Clarke, & Bew, 2009).

- *Interventions* to reduce the risk of falls must be based on assessment findings and designed to meet the limitations and needs of each older person. Therapeutic exercise for strengthening, balance, neuromuscular reeducation programs, and vestibular rehabilitation are among the techniques PTs use as interventions to decrease risk of falls.

  Some characteristics of successful plans include
  - simple, low-cost design for continuous participation
  - interventions to minimize pain and instability
  - exercises to increase core and lower body strength
  - improvement in posture

- balance training (e.g., tai chi)
- improving gait (APTA, 2007; CDC, 2010; Hanley, Silke, & Murphy, 2011)

In one meta-analysis, physical therapy was reported to be effective to improve muscle strength and functional performance among older persons (Steib, Schoene, & Pfeifer, 2010). Descending stairs can be a source of falling in older adults. The neuromotor control needed for safe stair descent can be improved through supervised exercises that improve strength and "tension development rate" (Hsu, Wei, Yu, & Chang, 2007).

- *Assistive devices* can be helpful for older adults. They are also associated with increased risk of falling; however, it is not clear whether this occurs because
  - they contribute to falling
  - those who use them are at increased risk
  - there is great need for proper fitting
  - education how to properly use them (Quinlan-Colwell & Taylor, 2006)

When older adults use assistive devices, PTs can assess the appropriateness of the device for

- meeting the needs for assistance
- the physique of the individual older person

PTs can also educate the elder in proper use of the device.

EVALUATION OF LIVING ENVIRONMENTS

In addition to enhancing strength, balance, posture, and gait, PTs can be consulted to evaluate the living environments of older adults to improve safety and reduce the risk of falling through recommendations to improve safety of the environment. Evaluation includes the areas of access to the building as well as the actual structure. Homes and other living areas should be free of hazards, have adequate lighting, and include adaptive devices, such as railings or grab bars as appropriate (APTA, 2007; APTA, 2011c; CDC, 2010, Collins, 2007; Ryburn, Wells, & Foreman, 2009).

GUIDELINES AND RESOURCES

American Geriatric Society www.americangeriatrics.org/products/position papers/Falls.pdf
American Physical Therapy Association http://www.apta.org

Philadelphia Panel Evidence-based Clinical Practice Guidelines on selected
rehabilitation interventions for knee pain. (2001). *Physical Therapy, 81,*
1675–1700
The Arthritis Foundation http://www/arthritis.org

Mr. Parks is an 82-year-old man. He was recently admitted to a
skilled nursing facility after falling and sustaining fractures to his
left hip and left wrist. Until the fall, he had been fairly active in his
yard since his pacemaker was placed 3 years ago. Now he has pain
in his left leg and wrist. It is difficult for him to walk and he can no
longer take care of himself without assistance. He wants to go home.

Questions

1. What options does the facility PT have that may be of help to
   Mr. Parks?
2. What cautions and limitations will the PT need to consider
   when working with Mr. Parks?
3. Does the PT have a role in assessing and modifying Mr. Parks'
   living area?

REFERENCES

Agency for Healthcare Policy and Research (AHRQ). (2009). Choosing nonopi-
oid analgesics for osteoarthritis: Clinician summary guide. *Journal of Pain &
Palliative Care Pharmacotherapy, 23,* 433–437.
American Geriatric Society (2010). Summary of the updated American Geriatrics
Society/British Geriatrics Society clinical practice guideline for prevention of
falls in older adults. *Journal of the American Geriatric Society, 58,* 1–10.
American Physical Therapy Association (APTA). (2007). *Physical fitness and
falls risk reduction based on best available evidence.* Retrieved May 21, 2011,
from http://www.apta.org/uploadedFiles/APTAorg/Practice_and_Patient_
Care/Patient_Care/Physical_Fitness/Members_Only/PocketGuide_Falls
.pdf#search=%22falls%22
American Physical Therapy Association (APTA). (2009a). *Clinical specialization in
physical therapy (HOD P06-06-22-15) updated 12/14/2009.* Retrieved May 21,
2011, from http://www.apta.org/uploadedFiles/APTAorg/About_Us/Policies/

HOD/Specialization/ClinicalSpecialization.pdf#search=%22HOD%20 P06%22

American Physical Therapy Association (APTA). (2009b). *Guidelines: Defining physical therapy in state practice acts (BOD G03-00-16-38) updated 12/14/2009.* Retrieved May 21, 2011, from http://www.apta.org/uploaded Files/APTAorg/About_Us/Policies/BOD/Practice/DefiningPTinState PracticeActs.pdf#search=%22cryotherapy%22

American Physical Therapy Association (APTA). (2010). *Manipulation safety and physical therapist practice.* Retrieved May 21, 2011, from http://www.apta .org/uploadedFiles/APTAorg/Advocacy/State/Issues/Manipulation/ ManipulationSafetyandPTPractice.pdf#search=%22passive%22

American Physical Therapy Association (APTA). (2011a). *Diagnosis by physical therapists (HOD P06-08-06-07) updated 02/03/2011.* Retrieved May 21, 2011, from http://www.apta.org/uploadedFiles/APTAorg/About_Us/Poli cies/HOD/Practice/Diagnosis.pdf#search=%22HOD%20P06%22

American Physical Therapy Association (APTA). (2011b). *Physical therapy as a health profession (HOD P06-99-19-23) updated 02/03/2011.* Retrieved May 21, 2011, from http://www.apta.org/uploadedFiles/APTAorg/About_Us/Policies/HOD/ Practice/HealthProfession.pdf#search=%22HOD%20P06%22

American Physical Therapy Association (APTA). (2011c). *Physical therapy for older adults (HOD P06-06-08-04) updated 02/03/2011.* Retrieved May 17, 2011, from http://www.apta.org/uploadedFiles/APTAorg/About_Us/Policies/HOD/ Practice/OlderAdults.pdf#search=%22HOD%20P06%22

Bjordal, J. M., Couppé, C., Chow, R. T., Tunér, J., & Ljunggren, E. A. (2003). A systematic review of low-level laser therapy with location-specific doses for pain from chronic joint disorders. *Journal of Physiotherapy, 49,* 107–116.

Bjordal, J. M., Johnson, M. I., Lopes-Martins, R. A., Bogen, B., Chow, R., & Ljunggre, A. E. (2007). Short-term efficacy of physical interventions in osteoarthritic knee pain. A systematic review and meta-analysis of randomized placebo-controlled trials. *BMC Musculoskeletal Disorders, 8,* 51. Retrieved May 21, 2011, from http:// www.biomedcentral.com/1471-2474/8/51

Centers for Disease Control and Prevention (CDC). (2010). Falls among older adults: An overview. *Injury Prevention & Control: Home and recreational safety.* Retrieved May 21, 2011, from http://www.cdc.gov/HomeandRecre ationalSafety/Falls/adultfalls.html

Collins, J. (2007). Physical therapy for the older adult. In M. A. Pagliarulo (Ed.), *Introduction to physical therapy* (3rd ed., pp. 337–361). St. Louis, MO: Mosby Elsevier.

Dreeben, O. (2007). *Introduction to physical therapy for physical therapist assistants.* Boston, MA: Jones and Bartlett.

Feland, J. B., Myrer, J. W., Schulthies, S. S., Fellingham, G. W., & Measom, G. W. (2001). The effect of duration of stretching of the hamstring muscle group for increasing range of motion in people aged 65 years or older. *Physical Therapy, 81,* 110–117.

Forster, A., Lambley, R., & Young, J. B. (2010). Is physical rehabilitation for older people in long-term care effective? Findings from a systematic review. *Age and Aging, 39,* 169–175.

Fransen M. (2004). When is physiotherapy appropriate? *Best Practice & Research Clinical Rheumatology, 18,* 477–489.

Fransen, M., Nairn, L., Winstanley, J., Lam, P., & Edmonds, J. (2007). Physical activity for osteoarthritis management: A randomized controlled clinical trial evaluating hydrotherapy or Tai chi classes. *Arthritis & Rheumatism, 57,* 407–414.

Furlan, A. D., Brosseau, L., Imamura, M., & Irvin, E. (2002). Massage for low back pain. *Cochrane Database Systematic Review, 2:CD001929.*

Gorevic, P. D. (2004). Osteoarthritis: A review of musculoskeletal aging and treatment issues in geriatric patients. *Geriatrics, 59*(8), 28–32.

Hadjistavropoulos, T., & Fine, P. G. (2006). Chronic pain in older persons: Prevalence, assessment and management. *Reviews in Clinical Gerontology, 16,* 231–241.

Haines, T., Kuys, S. S., Morrison, G., Clarke, J., & Bew, P. (2009). Cost-effectiveness analysis of screening for risk of in-hospital falls using physiotherapist clinical judgement. *Medical Care, 47,* 448–456.

Han, G., Cho, M., Nam, G., Moon, T., Kim, J., Kim, S., Cho, B. (2011). The effects of muscle strength and visual analog scale pain of aquatic therapy for individuals with low back pain. *Journal of Physical Therapy Science, 23,* 57–60.

Hanley, A., Silke, C., & Murphy, J. (2011). Community-based health efforts for the prevention of falls in the elderly. *Clinical Interventions in Aging, 6,* 19–25.

Hausdorff, J. M., Rios, D. A., & Edleberg, H. K. (2001). Gait variability and fall risk in community-living older adults: A 1 year prospective study. *Archives of Physical Medicine and Rehabilitation, 82,* 1050–1056.

Host, H. H., Sinacore, D. R., Nohnert, K., Steger-May, K., Brown, M., & Binder, E. F. (2007). Training-induced strength and functional adaptations after hip fracture. *Physical Therapy, 87,* 292–303.

Hsu, M. J., Wei, S., Yu, Y., & Chang, Y. (2007). Leg stiffness and electromyography of knee extensors/flexors: Comparison between older and younger adults during stair descent. *Journal of Rehabilitation Research & Development, 44,* 429–436.

Johnson, M. I., & Tabasam, G. (2003). An investigation into the analgesic effects of interferential currents and transcutaneous electrical nerve stimulation on experimentally induced ischemic pain in otherwise pain-free volunteers. *Physical Therapy, 83,* 208–223.

Jorge, S., Parada, C., Ferreira, S. H., & Tambeli, C. H. (2006). Interferential therapy produces antinociception during application in various models of inflammatory pain. *Physical Therapy, 86,* 800–808.

Klein, P. J. & Adams, W. D. (2004). Comprehensive therapeutic benefits of Taiji: a critical review. *American Journal of Physical Medicine and Rehabilitation, 83,* 735–745.

Kottke, F. J. (1966). The effects of limitation of activity upon the human body. *Journal of the American Medical Association, 196,* 825–830.

Lee, D., Ko, T., & Cho, Y. (2010). Effects on static and dynamic balance of task-oriented training for patients in water or on land. *Journal of Physical Therapy Science, 22,* 331–336.

Leveille, S. G. (2004). Musculoskeletal aging. *Current Opinions in Rheumatology, 16,* 114–118.

Lewis, C. B. & Bottomley, J. M. (2008). *Geriatric rehabilitation: A clinical approach* (3rd ed.). Upper Saddle River, NJ: Pearson Prentice Hall.

Littbrand, H., Rosendahl, E., Lindelof, N., Lundin-Olsson, L., Gustafson, Y., & Nyberg, L. (2006). A high-intensity functional weight-bearing exercise program for older people dependent in activities of daily living and living in residential care facilities: Evaluation of the applicability with focus on cognitive function. *Physical Therapy, 86,* 489–498.

National Pharmaceutical Company (NPC). (2006). *Pain: Current understanding of assessment, management, and treatment.* Retrieved May 21, 2011, from www.npcnow.org

Pagliarulo, M. A. (2007). *Introduction to physical therapy,* (3rd ed.). St. Louis, MO: Mosby Elsevier.

Quinlan-Colwell, A., & Taylor, C. (2006). Falls in the elderly: A secondary analysis of the Longitudinal Study of Aging. Unpublished data.

Ryburn, B., Wells, Y., & Foreman, P. (2009). Enabling independence: Restorative approaches to home care provision for frail older adults. *Health and Social Care in the Community, 17,* 225–234.

Scudds, R. J., & Scudds, R. A. (2005). Physical therapy approaches to the management of pain in older adults. In S. J. Gibson & D. K. Weiner(Eds.), *Pain in older persons* (pp. 223–237). Seattle, WA: IASP Press.

Smith, D. T., Hoetzer, G. L., Greiner, J. J., Stauffer, B. L., & DeSouza, C. A. (2003). Effects of ageing and regular aerobic exercise on endothelial fibrinolytic capacity in humans. *The Journal of Physiology, 546,* 289–298.

Smith, P. J., Blumenthal, J. A., Hoffman, B. M., Cooper, H., Strauman, T. A., Welsh-Bohmer, K., Sherwood, A. (2011). Aerobic exercise and neurocognitive performance: A meta-analytic review of randomized controlled trials. *Psychosomatic Medicine, 72,* 239–252.

Somers, D. L., & Clemente, F. R. (2006). Transcutaneous electrical nerve stimulation for the management of neuropathic pain: The effects of frequency and electrode position on prevention of allodynia in a rat model of complex regional pain syndrome type II. *Physical Therapy, 86,* 698–709.

Stanos, S., Migilevsky, M., Rader, L., McLean, J., & Baum, A. (2009). Physical medicine approaches to pain management (). In H. J. Smith (Ed.), *Current therapy in pain* (pp. 527–540). Philadelphia, PA: Saunders Elsevier.

Steib, S., Schoene, D., & Pfeifer, K. (2010). Dose-response relationship of resistance training in older adults: A meta-analysis. *Medicine & Science in Sports & Exercise, 42,* 902–914.

Weiner, D. K., Rudy, T. E., Glick, R. M., Boston, J. R., Lieger, S. J., Morrow, L. A., et al. (2003). Efficacy of percutaneous electrical nerve stimulation for the treatment of chronic low back pain in older adults. *Journal of the American Geriatrics Society, 51,* 599–608.

Wittink, H., Cohen, L. J., & Michael, T. H. (2002). Pain rehabilitation: Physical therapy treatment. In H. Wittink & T. H. Michel (Eds.), *Chronic pain management for physical therapists* (2nd ed., pp. 127–160). Woburn, MA: Elsevier Science.

13

Palliative Care: Techniques to Promote Comfort

PALLIATIVE CARE DEFINITIONS AND CONCEPTS

Palliative care is an interdisciplinary, comprehensive approach that is intended to support and improve the highest quality of life of patients and families. This is accomplished by the prevention and relief of suffering through understanding the individual patient situation, including difficulties associated with life-limiting or life-threatening illness. This is done through early identification and assessment, with respect for patient and family values and preferences, irrespective of prognosis, stage of disease, or therapies being pursued. Physical, psychosocial, and spiritual treatment focus on alleviating pain and other troublesome symptoms (American Academy of Hospice and Palliative Medicine [AAHPM], 2006; Meier, 2002; WHO, 2004).

The National Hospice and Palliative Care Organization (NHPCO, n.d.) describes *palliative care* in relation to hospice care with the focus of hospice on caring for the dying person rather than curing the disease, whereas palliative care utilizes an expansion of the hospice principles to individuals for whom such care is beneficial at an earlier time in their illness. This is illustrated in Figure 13.1, (CAPC, 2009). Palliative care practitioners utilize hospice principles to alleviate pain and suffering with individuals who may still be pursuing medically appropriate curative or life-prolonging interventions (Meier, 2002). It is important to understand that palliative care is for individuals who suffer with symptoms from any chronic illness, which may be cardiac, pulmonary, and cognitive in nature. From this perspective palliative care and hospice can be considered on a continuum of health trajectory where progressively more involved care is required (Figure 13.2).

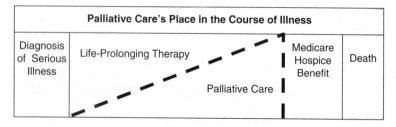

Figure 13.1 ■ Palliative care's place in the course of illness. Adapted and used with permission from the Center to Advance Palliative Care.

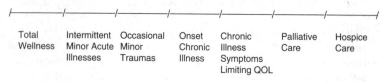

Figure 13.2 ■ Continuum of health care trajectory. *Note:* QOL, quality of life.

Palliative care is both a philosophy and a coordination of care delivery that involves an interdisciplinary approach to manage the frequently complicated symptoms of older adults for whom quality of life is significantly hampered by chronic illness. The goal, whenever possible, is to avoid suffering. It is also to relieve suffering when it does occur while facilitating and supporting optimal quality of life for the older adult and family. This is done by managing physical, psychosocial and spiritual symptoms, distress, suffering, and practical needs (AAHPM, 2006; National Consensus Project For Quality Palliative Care [NCPQPC], 2004). Throughout the illness process, "palliative care affirms life by supporting" goals of the patient and family, including hopes for possible cure, continuation of life, peace, and dignity (AAHPM, 2006). Regardless of the etiology of the illness, effective pain management is a crucial element in promoting patient comfort and relieving suffering (Meier, 2002). *Palliative medicine* is defined as "the study and management of patients with active, progressive, far-advanced disease, for whom the prognosis is limited and the focus of care is on the quality of life" (Doyle, Hanks, Cherny, & Calman, 2005).

Pearl	The focus of palliative care is on symptom management for chronic conditions regardless of whether the older individual is seeking curative or life-prolonging care.

THE IMPORTANCE OF PALLIATIVE CARE AMONG OLDER ADULTS

The percentage of older people in the populations of the United States and Europe has steadily increased and is projected to continue to increase during the next decade. In addition, the distribution and types of diseases causing death have changed, with a greater number of older people dying of chronic nonmalignant illnesses. The relationship between longevity and disability is not clear, but in at least some situations they are interrelated. Situations are complicated when the older person is living with multiple chronic illnesses resulting in cumulative symptoms, pain, and limitations (Andrews, 2001; WHO, 2004).

Living, aging, and dying have changed throughout the past 120 years. Some significant changes can be seen in Table 13.1.

The prevalence of pain during the final years of life has not been captured well. One large (4,703 participants) observational study investigated the occurrence of pain during the last 2 years of life. The researchers reported that 25% of the elderly participants had pain of moderate or greater severity during the last 2 years of their lives. The prevalence continued to increase with age and during the last 4 months of life. Often, there is an inverse relationship between age and analgesic prescriptions with the oldest patients often receiving the least or no pain medicine. This was seen in the noteworthy study by Bernabei and colleagues who assessed analgesic use with 4,003 older adults in nursing homes and found that patients older than 85 received less analgesia than their younger counterparts and in fact they often received no analgesia. Although arthritis is never the cause of death, it was the comorbid illness in 62.2% of that sample and was strongly associated with the pain experienced. The authors recommended that physicians caring for older adults should refer them to providers who specialize in pain or palliative care when pain is an issue (Bernabei et al., 1998; Constantinii, Viterbori, & Flego, 2002; Smith et al., 2010; WHO, 2004).

Table 13.1 ■ *Changes in Living and Dying Over 100 Years*

	1900	*2000*
Health	Illness and disability common	Healthy entering old age
Life expectancy	47	75 (77 for women) (75 for men)
Acute vs. chronic disease	90% acute	90% chronic
Common causes of death	Pneumonia Tuberculosis Diarrhea Enteritis Injuries	Cardiac disease Cancer Stroke Chronic respiratory disease Injuries Diabetes
Duration of illness preceding death	Short (days to weeks)	Often prolonged (months to years)
Location during final days	Home	Hospitals
Primary caregivers	Family	HCPs and paraprofessionals
Payer of financial costs	Family	Medicare and/or Medicaid

Sources: Adapted with permission from Lynn and Adamson (2003); Taylor and Kurent (2003); Taylor, Kurent, Heffner, and Brescia (2003).

Pearl	Although palliative care, palliative nursing, and palliative medicine are specialty areas, all health care providers (HCPs) working with older adults need to actively participate in managing pain and other symptoms that contribute to suffering, regardless of primary diagnosis.

KEY COMPONENTS OF PALLIATIVE CARE

Patient- and Family-Centered Care

An important aspect of palliative care is that it is patient- and family-centered care. There is an appreciation that for older adults in pain to receive optimal understanding and care, family caregivers need to be supported and educated in their caregiving responsibilities.

Adequate Assessment

To adequately address the needs of older people who are living with chronic illness, appropriate and adequate assessment is crucial. Controlling pain is an important component in alleviating suffering, improving comfort, and quality of life. Techniques and tools used to assess pain in older adults are discussed in Chapters 3, 4, and 5. In addition to the usual assessment tools, encouraging older adults or their caregivers to maintain a pain diary can be very useful in managing pain. One systematic review reported that nursing interventions using a pain diary was the most effective pain management strategy for working with patients living with chronic pain, including older adults (Allard, Maunsell, Labbe, & Dorval, 2001). Although there are a number of pain diary formats available, it is often most helpful to use a format that is individualized to the life style and needs of the particular older person as in Figure 13.3. In this way, the activities of the person, the pain intensity/description, the scheduled medications and breakthrough medications can be included in the diary and adjusted as needed.

PHARMACOLOGICAL MANAGEMENT OF SYMPTOMS

For specific information about analgesic medications, the reader is referred to Chapters 7, 8, and 9. No one medication is recommended for use with older adults. Information is provided for the HCP to make the best selection for the older person. Individual selection of appropriate medication needs to be based on several factors.

Example of Individualized Pain Diary

Date/ Time	Scheduled Analgesic	Activity	How long doing activity	Emotion Feeling	Pain description	Pain score	Analgesia and dose

Figure 13.3 ■ Example of individualized pain diary.

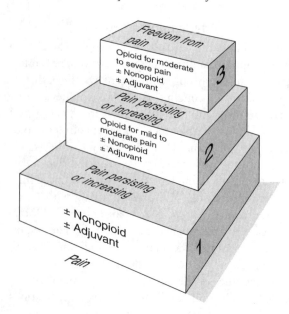

Figure 13.4 ■ WHO ladder. (World Health Organization, 2011)

General principles for using analgesic medications in palliative care follow.

1. Pain intensity is an important first consideration. Although evidence surrounding it has been questioned, in palliative care the pharmacological management of symptoms frequently begins with the concepts of the WHO ladder (Figure 13.4). It is anticipated that by utilizing these guidelines and incorporating the principles of correct medication administration in the correct dose on a scheduled basis, adequate pain management can be achieved in 70% to 90% of patients (Hanks, Cherny, & Fallon, 2005; Lenz, 2003; WHO, 2011).

   From the WHO ladder perspective, analgesia treatment should begin with nonopioids such as acetaminophen or aspirin. If pain is unrelieved or increases, a mild opioid (i.e., tramadol) should be added to the nonopioid, or should replace the nonopioid. If pain continues to be unrelieved or increases, a stronger opioid (i.e., morphine, oxycodone) should be added to, or replace the nonopioid, and replace the mild opioid. On any step of the ladder, adjuvants should be added to help manage symptoms of fear and/or anxiety. The WHO guidelines encourage scheduling the administration of analgesia rather than administering it on a "prn" or "as needed" basis (WHO, 2011).

2. The second factor to consider in the appropriate selection of analgesia is the pharmacokinetics of medications. This includes the duration of action, half-life, and metabolism of the medications. For older patients who have moderate intermittent pain, scheduled doses of a mild opioid and nonopioid may be beneficial. For patients who need continuous analgesia to manage severe pain, a sustained release or long-acting opioid is most appropriate. This can be supplemented with short-acting analgesia for breakthrough pain (BTP). Sustained release or long-acting medications may be preferable with older patients who dislike taking or swallowing medications. Appropriate selection becomes complicated when the older adult has comorbid kidney or liver illness that must be considered in selecting analgesics.

3. The third factor to consider is the most appropriate route of medication. Oral analgesia is always the preferred route. When the oral route is no longer appropriate or possible, opioids can be administered via alternate routes:

   ■ Sustained release or continuous administration can be accomplished
     ■ transdermally (fentanyl)
     ■ subcutaneously (SC) (morphine, hydromorphone)
     ■ epidurally (opioids, local anesthetics, clonidine, baclofen)
     ■ intrathecally (opioids, local anesthetics, clonidine)
   ■ Immediate release for scheduled administration or BTP can be accomplished
     ■ transmucosally (fentanyl)
     ■ sublingually (fentanyl)
     ■ via nasogastric or feeding tubes
     ■ rectally
     ■ via patient controlled analgesia through SC or epidural routes (opioids, local anesthetics) (Hanks et al., 2005; Lenz, 2003; Simpson & Bush, 2004)

In addition, most medications can be prepared for administration via alternate routes by compounding pharmacies (Wowchuk et al., 2009). At such pharmacies, medications can be prepared for topical administration, and hydrocodone that is commercially available only in combination form can be prepared without the acetaminophen or ibuprophen if necessary.

4. The fourth factor to consider is appropriate dosing. As with all older adults, the golden rule is to start low and go slow, remembering that older adults may be more sensitive to the effects of medications. Clearance of medications, including opioids, is slower in older adults, and the receptors in older adults may be more sensitive to medications (Hanks et al., 2005; Lenz, 2003).

When considering the breakthrough medications, general rules are as follows:

- When available, use the short-acting form of the sustained release medication being used.
- Dose should be 10% to 20% of the daily total use (Lenz, 2003).
- Always consider that reduced hepatic and renal clearances may cause medication doses to last longer than usual, thus doses may need to be smaller than usual.

Pearls	Nonopioid medications have ceiling effects or maximum daily doses.
	Opioid medications do not have ceiling effects.

5. The fifth factor to consider is medication side effects. The focus of palliative care is to promote comfort through management of symptoms that cause distress. All medications have potential side effects. It is crucial to avoid medications that have common side effects known to be problematic for older adults and to proactively manage untoward side effects that do develop.

6. The sixth factor to anticipate is that titration in dose or change of medications will be necessary:

- As symptoms change with the course of the disease
- As the older adult may become tolerant to the effects of opioids
- If side effects develop or worsen

7. A final consideration is to identify the degree to which the older adult wants to actively participate in managing pain and other symptoms. Some older adults want to be active participants and control their analgesia, whereas others do not. The older adult receiving palliative care should have as much control over analgesia as he or she desires (Simpson & Bush, 2004).

It is important to note that although methadone can be an important medication for patients receiving palliative care, caution is needed when using it with older adults. The American Geriatrics Society (AGS) recommends that it should not be used as a first-line medication and that use is restricted to HCPs experienced with it and knowledgeable about prescribing it. Side effects of dizziness, light-headedness, and sedation and the long half-life are recognized concerns among older people (AGS, 2009; Shaiova et al., 2008).

Surgical Interventions for Palliative Pain Management

Palliative surgery involves surgical procedures that are performed with the intent of relieving suffering and symptoms, rather than curing or prolonging life, when cure is not the goal. Common palliative surgical interventions to manage pain include

- thoracoscopic splanchnicectomy or celiac plexus blockade to relieve pain resulting from pancreatic cancer
- correction of obstructions caused by tumor

Stereotactic cingulotomy is an extreme procedure in older individuals who are desperate for relief from suffering. It is rarely used to relieve intractable pain that has proven to not be responsive to any other measure.

The decision for any surgical intervention requires careful consideration weighing the risks of increased pain and suffering versus the benefit of relieving pain and suffering. The intensity, extent, and duration of anticipated recovery are important factors to consider. Some procedures are usually not considered to be justified because the anticipated recovery is extensive and long (Johnson, 2004a, 2004b; Ng & Easson, 2004; Simpson & Bush, 2004).

Nonpharmacological Interventions

The reader is referred to Chapter 11 for a detailed discussion of a variety of nonpharmacological modalities. Some interventions that have been effective when used by older adults receiving palliative care include

- distraction
- meditation
- relaxation techniques (breathing, progressive muscle relaxation)
- guided imagery

- music therapy
- massage
- pet therapy
- reflexology
- therapeutic touch
- spiritual support
- hypnosis
- acupuncture
- compassionate touch
- aromatherapy (Aghabati, Mohammadi, & Pour Esmaiel, 2010; Chochinov, 2005; Cooke & Ernst, 2000; Hilliard, 2005; Hodgson & Andersen, 2008; Kayes et al., 2009; Woodruff, 2004).

CAREGIVER ISSUES WITH OLDER ADULTS RECEIVING PALLIATIVE CARE

Palliative care is an ongoing process that can be taxing for family members. Caregiver burden among informal caregivers is now recognized as a significant issue. "Anticipatory grief" is common among caregivers of older adults receiving palliative care. It occurs while the older adult is still alive and the family member/s begin grieving the anticipated loss of the older patient (Albinsson & Strang, 2003; Doyle, 2005; WHO, 2004).

Initial and ongoing assessment of the family of the older adult receiving palliative care is important. A minimum assessment of family members and nonprofessional caregivers should include the following:

- Understanding of the disease process and prognosis
- Knowledge of what is required to provide palliative care
- Willingness to provide care
- Ability to provide care that requires knowing diagnoses of acute and chronic illness
- Ability to learn intricate aspects of care
- Available support people
- Financial ability and limitations

Some of the stress involved with caregiver burden that is experienced by family members can be alleviated through frequent and open communication with the palliative care team. This communication is particularly important when the older adult is receiving palliative care in their home (Cherry, 2005).

WHERE IS PALLIATIVE CARE PROVIDED?

Home Setting

Home palliative care involves members of the palliative team guiding the care of the older adult in their home. The team generally includes nurses, advanced practice nurses, physical therapists, occupational therapists, social workers, dieticians, home health aides, and others who work in coordination with a physician. Through this team approach, multidisciplinary care can be coordinated in a multimodal approach to alleviate symptoms (Milone-Nuzzo & McCorkle, 2006). In some areas, medication kits are prepared for the family to maintain in the home and use when needed for an increase or change in symptoms (Wowchuk et al., 2009).

Community Setting

The Program of All-Inclusive Care of the Elderly (PACE) was begun in 1997 as part of the Balanced Budget Act. It is a capitated benefit that joined together Medicare with Medicaid benefits to provide an innovative, holistic, community-based care program for individuals 55 years and older who require long-term care. Rather than being admitted to a long-term care facility, people in PACE remain at home and generally attend a day health center where their medical and psychosocial needs are addressed and symptoms are managed. This comprehensive care program encourages socialization and exercise while providing nutritious food and medications (CMS, 2010; Lynn & Adamson, 2003; National Pace Association, 2010).

Hospitals

As many as 50% of hospitalized patients who are conscious die while experiencing moderate to severe pain (Desbiens & Wu, 2000). Although many older patients who are hospitalized can benefit from palliative care for symptom management, the availability and focus of palliative care services (PCS) within hospital setting varies greatly. The two most common designs of hospital-based palliative care programs are a consultation service for symptom management and a dedicated hospice unit (Pan et al., 2001). One study looked at the impact of a PCS within a hospital and found that the majority of consultations were for patients diagnosed with cancer, dementia, or HIV. Of the recommendations made by the PCS, 91% to 97% were implemented (Manfredi et al., 2000). In addition to improved patient care, hospital-based palliative care has been correlated with fewer transfers to intensive care units, lower cost, and higher quality of care (Penrod et al., 2006). Although the number of hospital-based palliative care programs have increased in recent years, they tend to be in larger hospitals and clustered in certain geographic areas (Morrison, Maroney-Galin, Kralovec, & Meier, 2005).

Long-Term Care Facilities

Although many older adults spend their final days in long-term care facilities, many of these facilities have turned their focus to rehabilitation. As a result, formal palliative care and hospice programs are not common. Nursing homes rarely have palliative care affiliation.

Older patients, who live in nursing homes and have chronic conditions that could benefit from palliative care, may have a diagnosis that requires particular sensitivity during assessment and treatment. These include

- noncancer diagnosis
- cognitive impairment
- underdiagnosed and undertreated pain

Care in this setting is complicated when the older adult has endorsed "Do not resuscitate" status. Unfortunately, that is often interpreted as do nothing. When that interpretation is extended to treating and managing pain, the older adult may be in constant, unrelieved pain. Although most of the available information is descriptive, long-term care facilities, including nursing homes, seem to be an area where palliative care is needed but rarely included. Both research and palliative care programs are needed in long-term care settings (Hanson et al., 2008; Taylor & Kurent, 2003; Zerzan, Stearns, & Hanson, 2000).

GUIDELINES AND RESOURCES

Clinical Practice Guidelines for Quality Palliative Care. http://www.nationalconsensusproject.org/guideline.pdf

Hospice and Palliative Nurses Association (HPNA). http://www.HPNA.org

National Hospice and Palliative Care Organization. http://www.nhpco.org

Shaiova, L., Berger, A., Blinderman, C. D., Bruera, E., Davis, M. P., Derby, S., & Perlov, E. (2008). Consensus guideline on parenteral methadone use in pain and palliative care. *Palliative and Supportive Care, 6,* 165–176.

Weissman, D.E., Meier, D. E., & Spragens, L. H. (2008). Center to Advance Palliative Care Palliative Care Consultation Service Metrics: Consensus recommendations. *Journal of Palliative Medicine, 11,* 1294–1298.

WHO: Better palliative care for older people. http://www.euro.who.int/en/what-we-do/health-topics/environment-and-health/urban-health/publications/2004/better-palliative-care-for-older-people

Case Study

Ms. Snow is an 83-year-old woman. This is her sixth hospitalization during the last 5 months for breathing difficulties related to chronic obstructive pulmonary disease. While hospitalized, she complains about her chronic neck and shoulder pain that resulted from a motor vehicle accident 15 years ago, during which her husband died. During the last 6 months she has lived in a nursing home but wants to live at home with help from her oldest daughter who is retired. She does not have private or long-term insurance, and her medical care is paid through Medicare and Medicaid.

Questions

1. If a hospital-based PCS is available, how could they be helpful with Ms. Snow?
2. What interventions could be helpful for managing her symptoms?
3. What palliative care needs should be included during discharge planning?
4. What options are available for Ms. Snow?

REFERENCES

Aghabati, N., Mohammadi, E., & Pour Esmaiel, Z. (2010). The effect of therapeutic touch on pain and fatigue of cancer patients undergoing chemotherapy. *Evidence Based Complementary and Alternative Medicine, 7,* 375–381.

Albinsson, L., & Strang, P. (2003). Existential concerns of families of late-stage dementia patients. *Journal of Palliative Medicine, 16,* 225–235.

Allard, P., Maunsell, E., Labbe, J., & Dorval, M. (2001). Educational interventions to improve cancer pain control: A systematic review. *Journal of Palliative Medicine, 4,* 191–203.

American Academy of Hospice And Palliative Medicine (AAHPM). (2006, June). Statement on clinical practice guidelines for quality palliative care. *Clinical Practice Guidelines.* Retrieved from http://www.aahpm.org/Practice/default/quality.html

American Geriatric Society (AGS) (2009). Pharmacological management of persistent pain in older adults. *Journal of the American Geriatrics Society, 57,* 1331–1346.

Andrews, G. R. (2001). Promoting health and function in an ageing population. *British Medical Journal, 322,* 728–729.

Bernabei, R., Gambassi, G., Lapane, K., Landi, F., Gatsonis, C., Dunlop, R., Mor, V. (1998). Management of pain in elderly patients with cancer. *Journal of the American Medical Association, 279,* 1877–1882.

Center to Advance Palliative Care (CAPC). (2008). *America's care of serious illness: A state-by-state report care on access to palliative care in our nation's hospitals.* Retrieved May 27, 2011, from Center to Advance Palliative Care website: http://www.capc.org/reportcard/state-by-state-report-card.pdf

Center to Advance Palliative Care (CAPC). (2009). *The Case for Hospital Palliative Care: Improving Quality Reducing Cost.* Retrieved June 11, 2011, from Center to Advance Palliative Care website: http://www.capc.org/support-from-capc/capc_publications/making-the-case.pdf

Cherry, N. I. (2005). The problem of suffering. In D. Doyle, G. Hanks, N. Cherny, & K. Calman (Eds.), *Oxford textbook of palliative medicine* (3rd ed., pp. 7–14). New York, NY: Oxford University Press.

Chochinov, H. M. (2005). Interventions to enhance the spiritual aspects of dying. *Journal of Palliative Medicine, 8S,* S103–S115.

Center to Advance Palliative Care (CAPC). (N.D.) *The Case for Hospital Palliative Care.* Retrieved June 12, 2011, from http://www.capc.org/support-from-capc/capc_publications/making-the-case.pdf

CMS (Centers For Medicare & Medicaid Services) (2010). *Program of All Inclusive Care for the Elderly (PACE) Overview.* Retrieved May 25, 2011, from https://www.cms.gov/pace

Constantinii, M., Viterbori, P., & Flego, G. (2002). Prevalence of pain in Italian hospitals: Results of a regional cross-sectional survey. *Journal of Pain and Symptom Management, 23,* 221–230.

Cooke, B., & Ernst, E. (2000). Aromatherapy: A systematic review. *British Journal of General Practice, 50,* 493–496.

Desbiens, N. A., & Wu, A. W. (2000). Pain and suffering in seriously ill hospitalized patients. *Journal of the American Geriatrics Society, 48,* S183–S186.

Doyle, D. (2005). Palliative medicine in the home: An overview. In D. Doyle, G. Hanks, N. Cherny, & K. Calman (Eds.), *Oxford textbook of palliative medicine* (3rd ed., pp. 1097–1114). New York, NY: Oxford University Press.

Doyle, D., Hanks, G., Cherny, N. I., & Calman, K. (2005). Introduction. In D. Doyle, G. Hanks, N. Cherny, & K. Calman (Eds.), *Oxford textbook of palliative medicine* (3rd ed., pp. 1–4). Oxford, UK: Oxford University Press.

Hanks, G., Cherny, N. I., & Fallon, M. (2005). Opioid analgesia therapy. In D. Doyle, G. Hanks, N. Cherny, & K. Calman (Eds.), *Oxford textbook of palliative medicine* (3rd ed., pp. 316–341). New York, NY: Oxford University Press.

Hanson, L. J., Eckert, J. K., Dobbs, D., Williams, C. S., Caprio, A. J., Sloane, P. D., Zimmerman, S. (2008). Symptom experience of dying long-term residents. *Journal of the American Geriatrics Society, 56,* 91–98.

Hilliard, R. E. (2005). Music therapy in hospice and palliative care: A review of the empirical data. *Evidence Based Complementary and Alternative Medicine, 2,* 173–178.

Hodgson, N. A., & Andersen, S. (2008). The clinical efficacy of reflexology in nursing home residents with dementia. *The Journal of Alternative and Complementary Medicine, 14,* 269–275.

Johnson, A. G. (2004a). Surgery for the control of symptoms in the abdomen. In G. P. Dunn & A. G. Johnson (Eds.), *Surgical palliative care* (pp. 159–172). New York, NY: Oxford University Press.

Johnson, A. G. (2004b). Neurosurgical palliation. In G. P. Dunn & A. G. Johnson (Eds.), *Surgical palliative care* (pp. 207–226). New York, NY: Oxford University Press.

Kayes, L., McCarty, R., Walkinshaw, C., Congdon, S., Kleinberger, J., Hartman, V., & Standish, L. J. (2009). Use of complementary and alternative medicine (CAM by Washington State hospices). *American Journal of Hospice and Palliative Care, 25,* 463–468.

Lenz, K. L. (2003). The pharmacology of symptom control. In G. J. Taylor & J. E. Kurent (Eds.), *A clinician's guide to palliative care* (pp. 19–46). Malden, MA: Blackwell Publishing.

Lynn, J., & Adamson, D. M. (2003). *Living well at the end of life: Adapting health care to serious chronic illness in old age* (Rand health). Retrieved May 24, 2011, from Living well at the end of life website, RAND Corporation website: http://www.rand.org/content/dam/rand/pubs/white_papers/2005/WP137.pdf

Manfredi, P. L., Morrison, R. S., Morris, J., Goldhirsch, S. L., Carter, J. M., & Meier, D. (2000). Palliative care consultation: How do they impact the care of hospitalized patients. *Journal of pain and symptom management, 20,* 166–173.

Meier, D. E. (2002). United States: Overview of cancer pain and palliative care. *Journal of Pain and Symptom Management, 24,* 265–269.

Milone-Nuzzo, P., & McCorkle, R. (2006). Home care. In B. R. Ferrell & N. Coyle (Eds.), *Textbook of palliative nursing* (2nd ed.), p. 771–785. New York, NY: Oxford University Press.

Morrison, R. S., Maroney-Galin, C., Kralovec, P. D., & Meier, D. E. (2005). The growth of palliative care programs in United States Hospitals. *Journal of Palliative Medicine, 8,* 1127–1134.

National Consensus Project For Quality Palliative Care. (2004). *Clinical practice guidelines for quality palliative care.* Retrieved May 25, 2011, from National Consensus Project For Quality Palliative Care website: http://www.national consensusproject.org/guideline.pdf

National Hospice and Palliative Care Organization (NHPCO). (n.d.). *What is hospice and palliative care.* Retrieved May 22, 2011, from http://www.nhpco. org/i4a/pages/index.cfm?pageid=4648&openpage=4648

National Pace Association. (2010). *Program of All-Inclusive care for the elderly, 2000: Integrated acute and long-term care service delivery and financing.* Retrieved May 24, 2011, from http://www.npaonline.org

Ng, A., & Easson, A. M. (2004). Selection and preparation of patients for surgical palliation. In G. P. Dunn & A. G. Johnson (Eds.), *Surgical palliative care* (pp. 16–32). New York, NY: Oxford University Press.

Pan, C. X., Morrison, R. S., Meier, D. E., Natale, D. K., Goldhirsch, S. L., Kralovec, P., & Cassel, C. K. (2001). How prevalent are hospital-based palliative care programs? Status report and future directions. *Journal of Palliative Medicine, 4,* 315–324.

Penrod, J. D., Deb, P., Luhrs, C., Dellenbaugh, C., Zhu, C. W., Hochman, T., Morrison, R. S. (2006). Cost and utilization outcomes of patients receiving hospital-based palliative care consultation. *Journal of Palliative Medicine, 9,* 855–860.

Shaiova, L. Berger, A., Blinderman, C. D., Bruera, E., Davis, M. P., Derby, S., et al. (2008). Consensus guideline on parenteral methadone use in pain and palliative care. *Palliative and Supportive Care, 6,* 165–176.

Simpson, K. H., & Bush, D. J. (2004). Anaesthesia and perioperative pain management. In G. P. Dunn & A. G. Johnson (Eds.), *Surgical palliative care* (pp. 112–132). New York, NY: Oxford University Press.

Smith, A. K., Cenzer, I. S., Knight, S. J., Puntillo, K. A., Widera, E., Williams, B. A., Covinsky, K. (2010). The epidemiology of pain during the last 2 years of life. *Annals of Internal Medicine, 153,* 563–569.

Taylor, G. J., & Kurent, J. E. (2003). Dying of old age: The frail nursing home patient. In G. J. Taylor & J. E. Kurent (Eds.), *A clinician's guide to palliative care* (pp. 177–185). Malden, MA: Blackwell Publishing.

Taylor, G. J., Kurent, J. E., Heffner, J. E., & Brescia, F. J. (2003). Palliation for chronic illness. In G. J. Taylor & J. E. Kurent (Eds.), *A clinician's guide to palliative care* (pp. 1–18). Malden, MA: Blackwell Publishing.

Woodruff, R. (2004). *Palliative medicine* (4th ed.). New York, NY: Oxford University Press.

World Health Organization [WHO]. (2004). *Better palliative care for older people* (ISBN 92890 1092 4). Copenhagen, Denmark: World Health Organization.

World Health Organization [WHO]. (2011). *WHO's pain ladder.* Retrieved October 30, 2011, from http://www.who.int/cancer/palliative/painladder/en/

World Health Organization [WHO]. (2011). *WHO's pain ladder.* Retrieved May 28, 2011, from http://www.who.int/cancer/palliative/painladder/en/index.html

Wowchuk, S. M., Wilson, E. A., Embleton, L., Garcia, M., Harlos, M., & Chochinov, H. M. (2009). The palliative medication kit: An effective way of extending care in the home of patients nearing death. *Journal of Palliative Medicine, 12,* 797–803.

Zerzan, J., Stearns, S., & Hanson, L. (2000). Access to palliative care and hospice in nursing homes. *Journal of the American Medical Association, 284,* 2489–2494.

14

When Is Hospice the Best Option?

Hospice is a concept of care for individuals who are nearing the end of their lives and who are no longer seeking curative interventions. The focus of the interdisciplinary team members is on supporting the person and his or her family through the final days. The promotion of comfort and alleviating pain are important aspects of care (AAHPM, n.d.; Waldrop & Rinfrette, 2009).

THE EVOLUTION OF HOSPICE CARE

The origins of hospice care are found in ancient Greece and Rome. The concept of modern hospice is credited to Dame Cicely Saunders in England in the 1960s. Shortly after Dame Cicely brought the concept to America, an inpatient hospice was started in 1974 in New Haven, Connecticut. The cost effectiveness of hospice care was sufficiently clear that in 1986 the U.S. government confirmed hospice benefit as a permanent Medicare benefit. In 2001, U.S. hospice and palliative care programs numbered over 3,000 (Bennahum, 2003).

PROFILE OF HOSPICE IN 2011 IN THE UNITED STATES

Hospice care is an interdisciplinary, holistic model of patient- and family-centered care that focuses on relieving suffering through the control of pain, promotion of patient and family autonomy, and supporting the emotional, physical, and spiritual needs of the patient and family during the final period of life when cure is no longer feasible (Bergman et al., 2011; Waldrop & Rinfrette, 2009). One criterion for hospice care is that the health care provider (HCP) anticipates that the older person being considered for hospice care will live 6 months or less. This 6-month time frame is not a prediction but rather an expectation. Although some patients live longer on hospice care, many live far less than 6 months. The core hospice team generally includes the attending physician, hospice physician, registered nurses (assessment, primary, on call), social worker, and home health aide. The team may also include a chaplain, homemaker aide, pharmacist, volunteers, and other consultants, depending upon the needs of the older person (Forman, Kitzes, Anderson, & Sheehan, 2003).

Consultation with physical or occupational therapists can be helpful in the following ways:

- Teaching older adults how to safely move without increasing pain
- Teaching family members how to assist and care for older adult without injuring themselves or the older adult
- Assessing the home for safety improvements adaptive equipment
- Assessing the older adult for assistive devices (Kumar & Jim, 2010).

Hospice care can be provided in specialized hospice facilities, hospitals, long-term care facilities, patient homes, or other settings (Forman et al., 2003). One study reported that older patients in nursing homes receive better pain management when they receive hospice care and services (Miller, Mor, Wu, Gozalo, & Lapane, 2002).

Although some older adults are able to have nursing home costs covered by long-term care insurance or Medicaid and the hospice costs covered by Medicare, other older adults may need to pay the cost of one or the other. Since the financial situations and insurance coverage of older adults vary widely, it is strongly recommended that the older person and the family discuss finances, financial needs, and hospice care costs with the hospice social worker or administrator. Since government coverage, laws, and regulations are ever changing, these are important factors to discuss whenever hospice care is needed. Some hospice organizations have funds to assist with, or cover costs for, those who do not have adequate insurance coverage or finances.

In 2002, approximately 25% of those who died in the United States received hospice care (National Hospice and Palliative Care Organization [NHPCO], 2004). Although hospice care is increasingly more available and utilized, many older adults who are eligible do not select hospice care. Those who do select hospice continue to enroll late in the disease process. Between 2000 and 2007, discharges from hospice increased by 68%. The characteristics of those discharged in 2007 included the following:

- Death was the most common basis for discharge (84.3%)
- Of the 15.6% who did not die
  - The health of some improved
  - Some were transferred to another hospice
  - Some were transferred to an inpatient facility or hospital
- 83.1% were 65 years or older
- 90% were Caucasian
- 55.1% were women (slight increase from 2000)
- Most common admission diagnosis was malignancy
- 66.7% received services from a voluntary nonprofit agency
- 31.2% received services through a proprietary agency
- Only 37% received care for 30 days or more
- Mean length of hospice services was 65 days (varied by age but longest was with those over 75 years)
- Median length of time receiving services was 16 days (Caffrey, Sengupta, Moss, Harris-Kojetin, & Valverde, 2011).

During the past 20 years, the composition of primary hospice diagnoses has changed. Although the majority of patients receiving hospice care in 1992 had a primary diagnosis of cancer (74.7%), in 2007 those with a primary noncancer diagnosis were in the majority (57.2%). Since the average number of diagnoses per patient was 3.3, malignant neoplasm remained the most common diagnosis (46.3%). Other diagnoses (not necessarily the primary diagnosis) included

- cardiac disease (32.3%)
  - essential hypertension (23.5%)
  - congestive heart failure (CHF) (15.4%)
- dementia (21.3%)
- chronic obstructive pulmonary disease and associated conditions (14.8%)
- diabetes mellitus (12.2%)
- cerebrovascular disease (10.9%) (Caffrey et al., 2011)

In 2004, among men with terminal prostate cancer who enrolled in hospice care, 25% did so less than 7 days prior to death (Bergman et al., 2011). It is known that when hospice time is that brief, neither the patient nor the family benefit as fully as possible from the available services and care (Bergman et al., 2011; Miller, Kinzbrunner, Pettit, & Williams, 2003). In one study, family members of older adults who were on hospice for a short time reported a positive benefit, but family members of older adults who had received hospice services for longer than 3 months reported greater benefit and noted that the benefit peaked at around 3 months (Rickerson, Harrold, Kappo, Carroll, & Casarett, 2005).

When admission to hospice occurs during the last days of life, there is not adequate occasion to gain an understanding of the needs, desires, and preferences of the older adult and caregivers (Waldrop & Rinfrette, 2009). These admissions may be related to a very stressful crisis situation (Andershed, 2006). Later referrals to hospice are also associated with the older patient needing to be cared for in an inpatient hospice facility rather than at home or in their usual long-term care facility. This is due to the difficulty in being able to adequately manage pain and other symptoms when caregiving resources have not been developed and supported (Miller et al., 2003).

WHEN IS HOSPICE THE BEST OPTION?

Although many or even most older adults and their families heard or know about hospice prior to becoming ill, being provided information about hospice during the terminal illness is the most important factor that prompts patients and families to consider hospice care. Patients and their families are much more likely to enroll in hospice care when the physician talks with them about the illness being terminal (McGorty & Bornstein, 2003), yet many physicians do not discuss hospice as an option even with older adults who are terminally ill with metastatic lung cancer who have significant symptom management needs (Huskamp et al., 2009).

Factors that influence physicians referring older adults for hospice care include

- a perceived need for help in caregiving with increasing needs
- recent choice to withhold or withdraw life support
- difficulty in managing pain and other symptoms
- patient preference for dying at home
- patient and/or family need for support services
- desire for psychological, social, and emotional support (Casarett, Crowley, & Hirschman, 2004; McGorty & Bornstein, 2003)

Hospice is a good option for older individuals who are living with end-stage dementia or Alzheimer's disease. In addition to multiple system and caretaking needs, the caregiver of an older adult in that situation is often suffering with significant caregiver burden. Among the care needs may be physical pain that is not recognized or treated because of impaired communication (Sanders, Butcher, Swails, & Power, 2009). Hospice nurses are skilled in assessing pain in patients who are not able to communicate pain intensity scores. In one study, not only was pain management better when patients with dementia were cared for by hospice nurses, but they exhibited fewer symptoms of restlessness, agitation, nervousness, and aggression (Bekelman, Black, Shore, Kasper, & Rabins, 2005).

HCP BARRIERS TO TIMELY HOSPICE REFERRAL

One study involving nursing home directors and staff members found that hospice referral was influenced by staff perception of patient status and beliefs about hospice. When staff members perceived that death was likely in the near future and when they perceived hospice as beneficial to the patient and staff, referral to hospice was more likely and more timely.

Barriers to timely referral of appropriate patients to hospice care include the following:

- Ability to make a terminal prognosis
- Lack of knowledge about hospice services and philosophy
- Not recognizing terminal aspect of the older person's illness
- Belief that hospice is only for those who are actively dying
- Belief that hospice does not favorably contribute to the care of the older adult
- Discomfort discussing the terminal aspect of illness with older adults
- Not wanting to lose control over patient care
- Personal preference for curative rather than palliative care
- Personal discomfort with the hospice philosophy
- Belief that the older adult or their family would not want hospice care
- Concern that discussing hospice will cause anxiety for the patient/ family
- Difficulty in predicting death within 180 days
- Considering hospice as alternative rather than complementary care (McGorty & Bornstein, 2003; Welch, Miller, Martin, & Nanda, 2007; Waldrop & Rinfrette, 2009)

COMMUNICATION TO FACILITATE TIMELY HOSPICE REFERRAL

There is considerable data about the characteristics of those who benefit from hospice care and moderate information about barriers to hospice referral and care. There is much less known about how the concept of hospice is presented to those who are likely to benefit from it. It is suggested that since physicians are not knowledgeable about hospice, they may be less likely to discuss hospice with older adults than they are to simply refer them to hospice for the hospice staff to explain the program and benefits (Casarett et al., 2004).

When the discussion of hospice is initiated, it is helpful to be prepared to address patient and family concerns. Most patients and families have at least some hesitation about enrolling with hospice services. The most common reservation is that agreeing to hospice care confirms the diagnosis is terminal. Two other common concerns are whether hospice can provide the services and support needed and whether the services are affordable (Casarett et al., 2004).

Although it is not possible to change the terminal diagnosis, it can be very helpful to provide a safe environment for the older adult and family members to express what they are feeling about the terminality. It also can be helpful to assure the older person and family that the older adult or health care power of attorney

■ is autonomous in making this decision
■ is entitled to have hospice care provided "his/her way"
■ can request a change in services or change in staff as needed
■ can at any point cancel hospice services
■ can at any point have the services reinstated (personal experience of author).

It may not be possible for the hospice team to provide all services that the individual older adult will need (e.g., 24-hour caregivers); however, they generally are able to significantly improve the patient/family situation.

Hospice is a covered Medicare benefit. As such, when the older adult meets the Medicare criteria, there is often no cost to the older adult or the family. Medicare criteria are that the older individual

■ is determined to be terminally ill with a life expectancy of 180 days or less
■ wants hospice care (is no longer interested in pursuing curative treatment)

■ is under the care of a physician who is agreeable to providing medical care/consultation (Dahlin, 2003)

Physicians and nurses need to be educated in the various services provided by hospice, so they will be able to educate the older patient and family about them. In a sample of 99 family survivors of older adults who were cared for by hospice, the survivors identified a number of hospice benefits that they valued but had not known to expect. These included

■ spiritual and emotional support (which many said they did not know they or the older patient needed)

■ 24-hour on-call availability of hospice team members (for questions, care, and emergencies)

■ regular nursing care and visits (provided care, support, education, and reassurance)

■ coordination of care and services (relieving caregiver burden)

■ Time of death arrangements (Casarett et al., 2004).

Earlier referrals to hospice care enable the older patient, caregivers, and family members greater opportunity to benefit from the specialized care. Fifty-three hospice professionals made the following recommendations to facilitate more timely referrals to hospice services:

■ Clear communication by the physician that the prognosis is terminal enables the older patient and family to move from curative goals to palliative goals with more insight.

■ Symptom management needs that are either anticipated or in an early stage.

■ Referral at least 4 weeks prior to anticipated death, but preferably longer (Waldrop & Rinfrette, 2009).

Casarett and Quill (2007) suggest an eight-step approach for effectively discussing hospice with patients for whom it may be appropriate (poor prognosis with limited treatment options). These steps are the following:

■ "Establish the Medical Facts." Communicate with other providers to ensure that all are on the same page and there will not be mixed messages.

■ "Set the Stage." Schedule a specific time and place for a meeting with patient and appropriate family members.

■ "Assess the Patient's Understanding of His or Her Prognosis." Ask the patient and family about their understanding of the disease and prognosis.

■ "Define the Patient's Goals for Care." Allow time to incorporate and process information.

- "Identify Needs for Care." Consider the needs of the patient as well as the needs of the family in providing care.
- "Introduce Hospice." Present it as one way to achieve the patient/family goals and needs for care.
- "Respond to Emotions Elicited and Provide Closure." Discuss and address concerns as well as any negative concepts or experiences about hospice.
- "Recommend Hospice and Refer." Take this step if the patient and family are agreeable to learn more from the hospice team (Casarett & Quill, 2007, pp. 445–447).

In conclusion, it is recommended that primary HCPs, including nurses, educate themselves about hospice services and care, develop comfort with discussing end of life issues with older patients/families, and initiate conversations about hospice when it is first anticipated that the older patient may not live longer than 180 days.

BEREAVEMENT CARE

Bereavement care for family members is often not thought about when older adults and their families consider hospice care. The scope of bereavement services varies widely from hospice to hospice. Some are limited by staff or finances and are only able to send cards and make telephone calls to the family members. Other hospices have significant bereavement departments where home visits are made, groups are coordinated to help with the grief process, and camps are available for surviving children (Demmer, 2003; personal experience of the author). This is a valued aspect of hospice that is much appreciated by those surviving the older adult. Often the hospice patient expresses gratitude for knowing that this bereavement service will be available for their loved ones after they have left.

GUIDELINES AND RESOURCES

American Academy of Hospice and Palliative Medicine. http://www.aahpm.org

Casarett, D. J., & Quill, T. E. (2007). "I'm not ready for hospice": Strategies for timely and effective hospice decisions. *Annals of Internal Medicine, 146,* 443–449.

Clinical Practice Guidelines for Quality Palliative Care. http://www
.nationalconsensusproject.org/guideline.pdf
Hospice and Palliative Nurses Association. https://www.hpna.org
Hospice Association of America. http://www.nahc.org/haa/
National Hospice and Palliative Care Organization. https://www
.nhpco.org

Case Study

Mr. Barnes is an 84-year-old man whose health has slowly but progressively declined over the past 2 years. He has had prostate cancer for 4 years with minor difficulty voiding. He also has CHF and osteoarthritis of both hips and knees. Recently, he has developed back pain. The cardiologist and orthopedist told him that he is not a surgical candidate because his CHF has worsened during the past year. Mr. Barnes now has dyspnea at rest and is now dependent upon supplemental oxygen. He has pitting edema in both lower legs. Treatment with ACE inhibitor (angiotensin converting enzyme inhibitor) and diuretic has been optimized. Mrs. Barnes tells you that he seems to get worse every week. Mr. Barnes tells you that his wife is exhausted from caring for him so much.

Questions

1. Do you think that Mr. Barnes is a candidate for hospice care?
2. On what is your decision based?
3. If Mr. Barnes is a candidate for hospice, how would you begin the conversation with him and his wife?
4. What would you tell the Barnes' about hospice and what hospice services can offer them?

REFERENCES

American Academy of Hospice and Palliative Medicine (AAHPM). (n.d.). *Definition of hospice and palliative care*. Retrieved June 07, 2011, from http://www.aahpm.org/about/default/overview.html#Definition

Andershed, B. (2006). Relatives in end-of-life care-Part 1: A systematic review of the literature the last five years, January 1999–February 2004. *Journal of Clinical Nursing, 15,* 1158–1169.

Bekelman, D. B., Black, B. S., Shore, A. D., Kasper, J. D., & Rabins, P. V. (2005). Hospice care in a cohort of elders with dementia and mild cognitive impairment. *Journal of Pain and Symptom Management, 30,* 208–214.

Bennahum, D. A. (2003). The historical development of hospice and palliative care. In W. B. Forman, J.A. Kitzes, R. P. Anderson, & D. K. Sheehan (Eds.), *Hospice and palliative care concepts and practice* (2nd ed., pp. 1–11). Boston, MA: Jones and Bartlett Publishers.

Bergman, J., Saigal, C. S., Lorenz, K. A., Hanley, J., Miller, D. C., Gore, J. L., & Littwin, M. S. (2011). Hospice use and high-intensity care in men dying of prostate cancer. *Archives of Internal Medicine, 171,* 204–210.

Caffrey, C., Sengupta, M., Moss, A., Harris-Kojetin, L., & Valverde, R. (2011). Home health care and discharged hospice care patients: United States, 2000 and 2007. *National Health Statistics Reports, 38*(April 27, 2011), 1–28. Retrieved from http://www.cdc.gov/nchs/data/nhsr/nhsr038.pdf

Casarett, D. J., Crowley, R. L., & Hirschman, K. B. (2004). How should clinicians describe hospice to patients and families? *Journal of the American Geriatrics Society, 52,* 1923–1928.

Casarett, D. J., & Quill, T. E. (2007). "I'm not ready for hospice": Strategies for timely and effective hospice decisions. *Annals of Internal Medicine, 146,* 443–449.

Dahlin, C. M. (2003). Eligibility and reimbursement for hospice and palliative care. In W. B. Forman, J. A. Kitzes, R. P. Anderson, & D. K. Sheehan (Eds.), *Hospice and palliative care concepts and practice* (2nd ed., pp. 35–45). Boston, MA: Jones and Bartlett Publishers.

Demmer, C. (2003). A national survey of hospice bereavement services. *OMEGA, Journal of Death and Dying, 47,* 327–341.

Forman, W. B., Kitzes, J. A., Anderson, R. P., & Sheehan, D. P. (Eds.). (2003). *Hospice and palliative care concepts and practice* (2nd ed.). Boston, MA: Jones and Bartlett Publishing.

Huskamp, H. A., Keating, N. L., Malin, J. L., Zaslavsky, A. M., weeks, J. C., Earle, C. C., & Ayanian, J. Z. (2009). Discussions with physicians about hospice among patients with metastatic lung cancer. *Archives of Internal Medicine, 169,* 954–962.

Kumar, S. P., & Jim, A. (2010). Physical therapy in palliative care: From symptom control to quality of life: A critical review. *Indian Journal of Palliative Care, 16,* 138–146.

McGorty, E. K., & Bornstein, B. H. (2003). Barriers to physician's decision to discuss hospice: Insights gained from the United States hospice model. *Journal of Evaluation in Clinical Practice, 9,* 363–372.

Miller, S. C., Kinzbrunner, B., Pettit, P., & Williams, J. R. (2003). How does the timing of hospice referral influence hospice care in the last days of life? *Journal of the American Geriatrics Society, 51,* 798–806.

Miller, S. C., Mor, V., Wu, N., Gozalo, P., & Lapane, K. (2002). Does receipt of hospice care in nursing homes improve the management of pain at the end of life. *Journal of the American Geriatrics Society, 50,* 507–515.

National Hospice and Palliative Care Organization (NHPCO). (2004). *National trend summary 2002.* Retrieved from http://www.nhpco.org

Rickerson, E., Harrold, J., Kappo, J., Carroll, J. T., & Casarett, D. (2005). Timing of hospice referral and families' perceptions of services: Are earlier hospice referrals better? *Journal of the American Geriatrics Society, 53,* 819–823.

Sanders, S., Butcher, H. K., Swails, P., & Power, J. (2009). Portraits of caregivers of end-stage dementia patients receiving hospice care. *Death Studies, 33,* 521–556.

Waldrop, D. P., & Rinfrette, E. S. (2009). Making the transition to hospice: Exploring hospice professionals' perspectives. *Death Studies, 33,* 557–580.

Welch, L. C., Miller, S. C., Martin, E. W., & Nanda, A. (2007). Referral and timing of referral to hospice care in nursing homes: The significant role of staff members. *The Gerontologist, 48,* 477–484.

SECTION VI: PAIN CONDITIONS COMMON IN OLDER ADULTS

15

Osteoarthritis and Gout

Arthritis literally means inflammation. More than 100 diseases affecting the joints fall under this broad category. The focus of this chapter will be osteoarthritis (OA) and gout. These disorders frequently affect older adults resulting in physical pain with impaired function and quality of life.

SECTION I ARTHRITIS

Epidemiology of Arthritis

Arthritis, which is common among older adults, is a significant source of disability, impaired quality of life, and increased health care costs (CDC, 2006). It is costly with annual medical costs estimated at $128 billion (CDC, 2011). It is also costly to the aging population from the perspective of disability. Internationally, OA will affect public health through costs related to

- loss of productivity
- increased health services
- increased use of physiotherapy
- pharmaceuticals
- increased surgical interventions (Brooks, 2003)

Prevalence of OA

Between 2003 and 2005, it was estimated that 46.4 million people (21.6%) of the adult population were diagnosed by physicians as having arthritis and rheumatic disorders, and 17.4 million had activity limitations related to arthritis. In 2001, Sharma (2001, 2003) reported that among those older than 50 years, 80% have evidence of OA on X-rays, and among those older than 75 years, 80% have clinical OA. It is predicted that by 2030, that figure will increase to 67 million adults. Women are diagnosed with arthritis slightly more frequently (Table 15.1). Obesity is strongly correlated with arthritis, with 54% higher prevalence of obesity among those diagnosed with arthritis compared with those not diagnosed (CDC, 2006, 2011; Heim, Snijder, Deeg, Seidell, & Visser, 2008; Wright, Riggs, Lisse, & Chen, 2008).

Racial and Ethnic Differences

Recently arthritis has been considered from a racial and ethnic perspective. In one national survey with self-report, no differences were found in how pain interfered with life in general among African American, Hispanic, and non-Hispanic Caucasians (Portenoy, Ugarte, Fuller & Haas, 2004).

Information from the Women's Health Initiative showed that African American, American Indian, and Hispanic women generally had more risk factors (i.e., obesity, diabetes) for developing OA. Those same groups also had fewer protective factors (i.e., physical activity and better finances) (Wright et al., 2008).

In another national survey, African American and Hispanic older adults were 1.8 times more likely than non-Hispanic Caucasians to report joint pain as severe and 1.3 times more likely to report pain that interfered with activity (Bolen et al., 2010). Greater difficulty in coping with arthritic pain was reported by African Americans than Caucasians (Ruehlman, 2005). Arthritic pain was reported as markedly more frequently experienced by American Indians (Yoon &

Table 15.1 ■ *Arthritis Prevalence Comparison per Demographic Characteristic*

Demographics	High Prevalence	Low Prevalence	Lower Prevalence
Gender	Women 40.1%	Men 36.6%	
Race	Black 45.7%	Hispanic 43.8%	White 37.4%
Education	<High School 50.6%	≥High School 36.1%	
Body mass	Obese 46.4%	Lean 34.3%	
Physical activity	Inactive 52.6%	Active 31.3%	

Source: Adapted from information presented in CDC (2006).

Doherty, 2008). Jorge and McDonald (2011) remind us that it is important to provide adequate time and inquire about interference with function as well as the use of complementary modalities when assessing pain in all individuals, and this is particularly important when working with older adults who are Hispanic.

Gender Differences

There are gender differences in musculoskeletal pain, which in general, are more prevalent among older women than among older men (Leveille, Zhang, McMullen, Kelly-Hayes, & Felson, 2005). OA of the hands and knees are reported more frequently in older women. OA of the hips and gout and spondylitis are reported more frequently in older men (American Geriatrics Society [AGS], 2001; Yoon & Doherty, 2008). Research study results are inconsistent when looking at differences in pain perception and coping among postmenopausal women receiving hormone replacement therapy (HRT), postmenopausal women not receiving HRT, and men (France, Keefe, Emery, Affleck, France & Waters, 2004).

Mobility disability is not necessarily related to physical or functional limitations or psychological symptoms. In one study with older women, a direct relationship that predicted disability in walking and stair climbing was found with widespread pain, but not with moderate pain (Leveille, Bean, Ngo, McMullen, & Guralnik, 2007). This suggests that more aggressive management of pain in older women can reduce or even prevent disability.

Risk Factors Associated with OA

There are a number of factors that are known to increase the risk of developing and/or the progression of OA. Modifying those that can be modified is not only preventive but also helps to manage the symptoms. Risk factors for OA include

- genetic predisposition
- aging process
- obesity
- gender
- injury to joints
- joint instability
- inactivity

- reduced muscle strength
- ligament laxity
- physical activity/inactivity
- repetitive movements involving joints
- heavy physical activity
- impaired proprioception (AGS, 2001; America Pain Society [APS], 2003; Brooks, 2003).

Diagnostic Criteria for OA

OA results from progressive tissue response and mechanical changes of the cartilage of joints leading to a failure in the ability to function. Although the weight bearing joints of the spine, hips, knees, ankles, and feet are most commonly affected, joints of the fingers, wrist, and neck can also be affected (AGS, 2001). Diagnosis is generally based on clinical presentation that includes report of stiffness and difficulty moving upon arising in the morning. Often, after sitting or driving the older adult will report a "gel" phenomenon that is a stiffness that improves upon movement. In both cases the stiffness typically resolves in about 30 minutes; however, pain occurs throughout the day as joints are used and bear weight. X-rays may be useful in confirming the diagnosis (APS, 2002; Hochberg, 2001).

Multimodal Management of OA

To date there are no cures for OA (AGS, 2001). Two important goals of pain management among older adults with OA are to improve quality of life and improve function. These goals can be approached through a combination of pharmacological and nonpharmacological interventions.

Education

Education is one extremely important aspect in helping older adults manage the pain associated with arthritis. Education should occur initially upon diagnosis, followed with frequent reinforcement and updates of information.

Important aspects of education include
- OA disease process
- prognosis
- treatment options

- self-management options
- resources

    Education can be offered through

- professional counseling
- formal community-based programs
- publications and brochures (AGS, 2001; Seed, Dunican, & Lynch, 2009).

Exercise

Exercise is an essential component of the multimodal approach to achieving goals of improving function and decreasing pain and disability. Although there may be concern that exercise will increase the pain and symptoms, research indicates that exercise in fact is beneficial for the symptoms of OA.

Exercises should be designed to increase or improve

- strength/reconditioning exercises
- stretching
- mobility
- flexibility
- weight reduction
- balance (to prevent falls) (AGS, 2001; Hernandez-Molina, Reichenbach, Zhang, LaValley, & Felson, 2008; Poitras et al., 2007)

There are a variety of exercises that can be helpful in managing pain associated with arthritis. Regardless of the type selected, it is recommended to refer older patients to physical therapists and exercise trainers who have expertise in working with older adults (Collins, 2007). The following exercise interventions have been shown to be helpful with older adults managing pain and disability related to OA.

- The AGS recommends that all prescriptions for exercise for older adults living with arthritis specify the following:
    - *Intensity*, that is, the effort or exertion to be expended
    - *Volume*, that is, for how long the exercise should be performed
    - *Frequency*, that is, how many times per week the exercise should be done
    - *Progression*, that is, for how and what period of time it should take for the older adult to adapt to the exercise (generally 2 to 3 months) *(AGS, 2001)*
- The *Arthritis Foundation Exercise Program* was specifically designed to increase joint flexibility and range of motion while maintaining

muscle strength. Classes are taught by instructors trained by the organization (Arthritis Foundation, 2011).

■ *Tai chi* is an exercise that comes from China and promotes balance and strength through a series of postures and movements (Chu, 2004). Tai chi has been used with older people living with arthritis with the intent of increasing flexibility, strength, and balance both in their own homes and in residential care settings (Adler, Good, Roberts, & Snyder, 2000; Adler & Roberts, 2006; Choi, Moon, & Song, 2005; Wang, Collet, & Lau, 2004). Tai chi is also discussed in Chapter 11.

■ *S.M.A.R.T.* is an acronym to help older people remember important tips for older adults with arthritis to remember when beginning or continuing a program in physical activity.

  ■ *S*tart low and go slow. Starting with a small amount of exercise that is low in intensity. Then slowly increase the time and intensity allowing time for the body to adjust. This method positions the older adult for greater success.

  ■ *M*odify activity as necessary. It is important to adjust duration and/or intensity as necessary. It may be necessary to change or alter types of exercise.

  ■ *A*ctivities should be joint friendly. Walking, bicycling, water exercises, and dancing are generally good exercises for older adults with arthritis because they do not put stress on joints.

  ■ *R*ecognizing safe places and ways to be active is important. Many older adults with OA feel most comfortable attending classes specially designed for older adults with OA. The Arthritis Foundation Exercise Program and Aquatics Program are offered at local chapters in many communities.

  ■ *T*alking to an health care provider (HCP) who can advise and guide older people in appropriate exercise is also important (CDC, 2010a).

Weight Management

Weight management is an extremely important modifiable factor in the management of arthritis. It is a risk factor being associated with progression of the illness negatively affecting physical function, impaired quality of life, and poor outcomes following joint replacement surgery. Patients should be screened for comorbidities of arthritis and obesity. Among older adults, the prevalence of musculoskeletal pain, including back pain, increased in accordance with increased BMI levels (Andersen, Crespo, Bartlett, Barthon, & Fontaine, 2003). Those with arthritis who have a BMI of 30 or greater should be counseled and referred for appropriate weight management intervention. This is particularly important for women who have osteoarthritis of the knee (OAK) (CDC, 2010b; Messier, Gutekunst, Davis & DeVita, 2005; Wright et al., 2008). A small, recent study in Japan indicated that OAK combined with obesity in postmenopausal women is associated with future coronary heart disease (Michishita, Shono, Kasahara, Katoku, & Tsuruta, 2008).

Complementary Modalities

Complementary modalities are discussed in detail in Chapter 11.

- *Music therapy* has been reported to be highly effective among orthopedic patients to manage postoperative pain (Lukas, 2004). Similar results were reported among 66 community-dwelling elders living with OA who had less pain following 20 minutes of daily music (McCaffrey & Freeman, 2003).
- *Cognitive behavioral (CB) interventions* to support self-efficacy in the areas of reducing weight and being physically active, in conjunction with pain-coping skills, can be an important part of the multimodal approach to managing the pain of arthritis in older adults. It is important to support older adults in believing (self-efficacy) that they can reduce weight and remain physically active (Pells et al., 2008). Some CB interventions that have been effectively used with older people who live with OA are briefly discussed here; the reader is also referred to Chapter 11.
- *Self-management strategies* are more frequently seen as being potentially effective for use by older adults living with OA. Although outcomes of self-management efforts are ambiguous, they do indicate potential benefit, particularly regarding functional improvement. Additional research, with well-designed studies in diverse groups, is needed (Nunez, Keller, & Der Ananian, 2009; Reid et al., 2008).
- *Coping skills training* with older people with OA, and, more recently, including their spouses, was effective. In the groups where the spouse attended the training as well, communication and mutual goal setting skills were included. The benefits were greater among older adults in spouse attended groups (Keefe et al., 2002).

Coping skills can include
- diversional activities
- activity-based skills
- cognitive coping skills, including problem solving
- *Goal setting* is a technique that was successfully used in a small sample of older adults who were living with OA. This simple CB intervention supported the self-efficacy of the participants who generally reported satisfaction with the process and managing their pain. Each participant identified a specific, individualized goal and maintained a record of their progress working toward their goal (Davis & White, 2008).

Assistive Devices

Canes are often used by older people living with OA; however, no identified benefit has been shown and reaction may be impaired by 50% with their use (Seed et al., 2009). If a cane is used, it should be used in the hand contralateral to the affected joint (Pendleton et al., 2000).

Taping of joints and use of *braces* can help to relieve pain. Unloader braces are reported to be superior in managing symptoms than neoprene sleeve braces (Hinman, Crossley, McConnell, & Bennell, 2003; Seed et al., 2009).

Medication Management

- *Acetaminophen* is often the medication that older people use for pain associated with arthritis. It is the recommended first-line medication for older adults with mild to moderate pain due to OA (AGS, 2009; AHPR, 2009; Reuben et al., 2005). Acetaminophen was effective for OA pain in a review with 5,986 participants (Towheed et al., 2006).

  Cautions are that the daily dose from all sources should not to exceed the 4 g limit and that it should be avoided in individuals who are sensitive to the medication, for whom there is concern for liver impairment or risky alcohol consumption (APS, 2003).
- *Nonsteroidal anti-inflammatory drugs (NSAIDs)* are reported to be superior to acetaminophen (Towheed et al., 2006); however, the side effects related to NSAIDs cause these medications either not to be recommended for use or to be used with particular caution with older adults.

The AGS recommends strategies for the use of NSAIDs with older adults:

■ Nonacetylated NSAIDs, such as salsalate, may have less gastro-intestinal (GI) toxicity; however, the studies were small and more data are needed.

■ COX-2-selective inhibitor NSAIDs have fewer GI side effects; however, they do have other NSAID-related side effects.

■ Some protection can be obtained when NSAIDs are administered along with a proton pump inhibitor (AGS, 2009).

If NSAIDs are used to manage pain related to OA in older adults, the choice of the NSAID must be made considering the comorbidities of the individual and the side effects of the NSAID (see Chapter 7). Cost of the medication is an additional factor to consider (if the older person cannot afford the medication, it will not be an effective choice).

■ *COX-2-selective NSAIDs* (celecoxib) were designed to protect against the adverse side effects of NSAIDs; however, the AGS (2009) cautions that COX-2-selective protection from GI bleeding is incomplete, and there are essentially no differences with other NSAID-related side effects or toxicities. Although several professional organizations recommend the COX-2-selective NSAIDs for patients with GI risk factors, they must be used with caution in older patients (Poitras et al., 2007).

■ *Tramadol combined with acetaminophen,* in doses of 37.5 mg trama-dol and 325 mg acetaminophen, proved to be effective in controlling OA-associated pain in 113 older people in one industry sponsored study. With an average daily dose of 4.5 tablets, specific results included

■ reduction in pain intensity scores

■ increase in pain relief scores

■ no serious adverse effects

■ side effects: nausea, vomiting, and dizziness

■ constipation that was 4.3% compared with placebo of 2.3% (Rosenthal, Silverfield, Wu, Jordan, & Kamin, 2004).

■ *Mu opioids* (i.e., morphine, oxycodone, hydromorphone) as treatment of musculoskeletal pain have been the source of debate. Although opioids are now often considered safer in older adults than the side effects associated with NSAIDs and COX-2-selective inhibitors, a very large study (12,840 participants with a mean age of 80) reported increased safety risks necessitating hospitalization for older community-dwelling adults (Solomon et al., 2010). This must be considered with the results of a meta-analysis that showed that opioids had moderate to large effect in reducing pain intensity and small to moderate improvement in function (Zhang et al., 2010). Another meta-analysis of opioid use in older adults who had non-cancer pain showed that opioids were beneficial for short-term use in older adults with chronic pain who did not have comorbidities that contradicted their use. The authors recommended further research to determine long-term safety and effectiveness as well as abuse potential among diverse groups of elders (Papaleontiou et al., 2010).

Professional organizations recommend opioid treatment for older patients with OA when NSAIDs are not indicated or not effective and quality of life is impaired by the pain (AGS, 2009; APS, 2002; Poitras et al., 2007). Decisions must be individualized considering the limitations caused by pain and comorbidities of the person.

Pearl	Rather than using opioids in combination with acetamino-phen, it may be more desirable to schedule acetaminophen around the clock (i.e., 650 mg every 6 hours) and have range orders for opioids (i.e., 5–15 mg oxycodone every 4 hours as needed).

> In this way, the benefit of acetaminophen is achieved without limiting the amount of opioid that can be used.

Topical Analgesic Preparations

Topical NSAIDs, lidocaine, and capsaicin can be good options for older adults. Topical medications differ from transdermal medications in that they act locally, rather than using the skin and subcutaneous tissue as a vehicle for systemic action. Since they avoid any significant systemic absorption and resulting metabolism, they are considered to be generally safe for older adults. They are reported to be at least potentially effective for managing OA-related pain. Additional research is needed to confirm safety and efficacy (AGS, 2009; Biswal, Medhi, & Pandhi, 2006; Seed et al., 2009).

- *Topical NSAIDs* (i.e., diclofenac) solution (Pennsaid) was reported to be as effective as oral diclofenac 50 mg three times per day in patients with OAK (Tugwell, Wells, & Shainhouse, 2004). Diclofenac gel (Voltaren gel) was reported to be statistically and clinically effective in reducing pain reports as well as pain with movement in patients with OAK (Barthel, Haselwood, Longley, Gold, Altman, 2009). Cautions are that topical NSAIDs can cause local skin irritation and there is potential for systemic side effects. GI side effects are a greater risk with older adults who have previously experienced them with systemic NSAIDs (Moody, 2010; Sawynock, 2003).

- *Lidocaine 5% topical patches* provide analgesia rather than nerve blockade. In one 12-week study with 143 older people living with OA that was described as moderate to severe, there was no statistical difference found in pain between those who received 200 mg celecoxib daily and those who received a 5% lidocaine patch (Kivitz et al., 2008).

  Lidocaine 5% topical patches are not approved for use in OA. Although systemic side effects have been rare, the following cautions should be observed:
  - The patch should be placed only on intact skin.
  - Use with caution in patients also receiving class I antiarrhythmic medications (i.e., tocainamide, mexiltene).
  - Calculate total local anesthetic exposure with other agents.
  - Skin reactions have included blisters, bruise, depigmentation, and burning at the site of application (Endo, 2010; Moody, 2010).
- *Capsaicin cream* (0.025% to 0.07%) is derived from the active ingredient in hot chili peppers. Through an involved chemical reaction process, it has antinociceptive properties through desensitization of small diameter afferent nerves. It can be effective in helping to relieve musculoskeletal pain in older adults, either as an adjunct to other medications or as a single therapy. Two cautions are that it generally takes one or even several weeks to realize peak analgesia, and patients can experience a burning sensation of the skin that can be uncomfortable (Mason, Moore, Derry, Edwards, McQuay, 2004; Poitras et al., 2007; Sawynock, 2003; Wang, Hong, Chiu, & Fang, 2001).
- *Nonprescription topical preparations* include counterirritant substances such as capsaicin, that desensitize to painful irritants and products from the salicylate group. Most of these agents do not require a prescription and are intended for only short-term use. The most common products used by older adults to manage the pain of OA include
  - methyl salicylate cream or ointment (i.e., BenGay)
  - menthol cream, gel, ointment, or patch (i.e., Icy hot)
  - camphor with menthol cream (i.e., Tiger balm)
  - tolamine salicylate cream or lotion (i.e., Aspercreme) (Moody, 2010)

Supplements and Food Products

■ *Glucosamine sulfate* is a nonprescription, nutritional supplement that functions as a basic component of joint cartilage that can be used alone or in combination with *chondroitin, which* is another dietary supplement (Seed et al., 2009). Some guidelines recommend glucosamine and chondroitin as part of a multimodal plan for managing the pain of OA in older people (Institute of Clinical Systems Improvement, 2006; Jordan et al., 2003). The analgesic benefit of glucosamine alone and with chondroitin, in older adults with OA, is ambiguous (Clegg et al., 2006). The authors of one meta-analysis concluded that despite flaws in the studies reviewed, some benefit and efficacy is likely (McAlindon, LaValley, Gulin, & Felson, 2000). In a subsequent meta-analysis, the authors concluded that glucosamine sulfate, but not glucosamine hydrochloride, in combination with chondroitin sulfate has a small to moderate effect on the symptoms of OA (Bruyere & Reginster, 2007). A more recent study from Europe reported no benefit of glucosamine and chondroitin over placebo (Wandel et al., 2010).

■ *Flavocoxid (Limbrel)* is not a medication but does require physician supervision and prescription. This Federal Drug Administration-approved product is composed of the natural flavonoids baicalin and batechin derived from plants. It acts through inhibition of arachidonic acid metabolism and antioxidant action.

The report from one study, of 103 older adults, that was supported by the manufacturer of Limbrel, was promising. The researchers reported no difference in analgesia or side effects in flavocoxid compared with naproxen (Levy, Saikovsky, Shmidt, Khokhlov, & Burnett, 2009). A second study reported that flavocoxid could result in lower overall costs compared with that of naproxen (Walton, Schumock, & McLain, 2010). Additional research is needed with larger samples.

■ *Avocado soybean unsaponifiables (ASUs)* are the part of the oils of avocados and soy beans that remain after hydrolysis renders soap. It is hypothesized that these oils may slow down the degradation of cartilage while promoting its repair in OA chondrocytes (Henrotin et al., 2003). One study of middle-aged and older adults reported improvement in analgesia with more than 50% reduction in analgesic medications (Appelbloom, Schuermans, Verbruggen, Henrotin, & Reginster, 2001). A meta-analysis report was that improvements were seen with ASU and that it was twice as effective as placebo (Christensen, Bartels, Astrup, & Bliddal, 2009; Henrotin et al., 2003). More study is needed with this agent. Although no adverse reactions were reported in clinical trials, caution is for possible cross-sensitivity with latex.

■ *S-adenosyl L-methionine (SAMe)* is found naturally in the human body and is also used as a supplement by people living with OA. Among the many functions of SAMe are analgesia and anti-inflammatory actions. It is hypothesized to also promote the growth and repair of articular cartilage (Prestwood, 2005). In some studies, when compared with placebo SAMe was demonstrated to be effective, and when compared with NSAIDs there was no statistical difference (AHRQ, 2002). In others no significant improvement was shown (Soeken, Lee, Bausell, Agelli, & Berman, 2002).

Herbal Remedies

■ *Devil's claw (Harpagophytum procumbens)* was originally used in Southern Africa as a treatment for musculoskeletal problems and has long been used in Europe as a treatment for OA (Gagnier, Chrubasik, & Manheimer, 2004). It was the focus of a number of studies, including four that were double blind, placebo controlled (Brien, Lewith, & McGregor, 2006). In other studies when more than 50 mg per day was used, analgesia was demonstrated (Chrubasik, Roufogalis, & Chrabasik, 2007). Additional research regarding the effectiveness is needed. The most frequent side effect is diarrhea.

■ *Dog rose or rose hip powder (Rosa canina)* extracts have been reported to be effective in improving mobility and alleviating pain in people with OA, with no negative side effects. A study in Denmark of 94 people ranging in age from 48 to 85 reported that data were promising that rose hip is effective for alleviating OA symptoms (Winther, Apel, & Thamsborg, 2005). Rose hip powder was tested in three studies with a total of 287 people living with OA. The results showed a significant but small analgesic effect (Christensen, Bartels, Altman, Astrup, & Bliddal, 2008). Additional research is needed. A caution is that rose hip species differ and may have different activities.

Interventional Options

Intra-articular Injections

■ *Intra-articular corticosteroid (IAC) injections* have had positive analgesic effects for relatively short periods of time (3 to 6 weeks). In one study, despite periodic injections, the analgesic effect was no longer noted after 2 years (Bellamy et al., 2006). IAC may be helpful in older adults with tense effusions in affected joints (Cosby, 2009; Zhang et al., 2010).

■ *Intra-articular hyaluronic acid (IAHA) injections* have also been reported for analgesia for relatively short periods and diminished over time. IAHA has been more effective than *IAC* in maintaining analgesia over 12 weeks. There are no significant safety concerns for IAHA; however, the following needs to be considered:

  ■ It is recommended for older adults who are highly functioning with significant pain or limitation.
  ■ When high molecular weight hylan was used for injection, subsequent flares in pain were more frequent (consider avoiding this product).
  ■ Use with caution in older patients who are morbidly obese (Cosby, 2009; Zhang et al., 2010).

Acupuncture

Acupuncture has been reported to be effective in relieving pain, improving sleep, and improving quality of life in older adults with OAK, in small studies and case reports (Huang, Bliwise, Carnevale, & Kunter, 2010; Bareta, Berman, Hadhazy, Lao, & Singh, 2001). One meta-analysis of acupuncture use with OAK found great variety in results, but both acupuncture and sham acupuncture were more effective than no intervention (Manheimer, Linde, Lao, Bouter, Berman, 2007). Further investigation is needed; however, the safety profile has been good for acupuncture in older adults (see Chapter 11).

Surgical Interventions

These are recommended for older adults for whom medical management of OA has not been effective. Consideration must be given to comorbidities and whether the older patient is an appropriate surgical candidate. Referral to an orthopedic surgeon is necessary. The most common surgical interventions recommended for older patients with arthritis are total knee or hip arthroplasty (replacements). For less active patients, unicompartmental knee replacements may be appropriate (APS, 2002; Poitras et al., 2007; Porcheret, Jordan, & Croft, 2006).

Although additional research is needed, a recent study indicates that prehabilitation, a formal exercise program prior to surgical intervention, improves strength and may facilitate postoperative recovery (Swank et al., 2011). It is imperative that postoperative pain management is appropriate for older adults. When a group of orthopedic patients older than 50 years were treated with a protocol that included scheduled, as needed, and pre-emptive analgesia, they did well postoperatively and generally reported mild postoperative pain (Morrison, Flanagan, Fischberg, Cintron, & Siu, 2009).

SECTION II GOUT

Gout is a chronic, episodic, metabolic disorder that is an inflammatory arthritis resulting from phagocytosis, within the affected joint, of the monosodium urate monohydrate crystals of uric acid.

Gout is considered from four phases:

- Asymptomatic tissue deposition
  - Hyperuricemia and crystals are present in tissues
  - No overt symptoms
- Acute flares
  - Acute inflammation caused by urate crystals
  - Pain ranges from mild to excruciating
  - Initial flares generally occur in lower extremities particularly the great toe (podagra)
  - Multiple joints may be affected in older people
  - May last days or even weeks
- Intercritical segments
  - After the acute flare subsides
  - May have a stage when gout is clinically inactive
  - Deposition of the urate crystals continues
  - May last for long periods of time
- Chronic gout
  - Presents increased risk of kidney stones (CDC, 2010a; Chen & Schumacher, 2006; Lawrence et al., 2008)

Epidemiology and Prevalence

In 2008, the estimated prevalence of self-reported gout among adults in the United States was approximately 3 million, which was a marked increase from the 1995 estimate of 2.1 million. Prevalence increases with age in both genders, but it is more common in men in all age groups. Among men it is the most frequent type of inflammatory arthritis and almost twice as common among African American men as Caucasian men (CDC, 2010a; Lawrence et al., 2008).

Risk factors include obesity, hypertension, alcohol consumption (especially beer and whiskey), diuretics, and heavy consumption of meat and seafood (Eliopoulos, 2001).

Diagnostic Criteria

Generally there is an elevated serum concentration of uric acid. In fact the diagnostic gold standard is aspiration and analysis of urate crystals.

Clinically, acute gout is generally seen as a red, hot, and swollen joint. Radiographic findings in the acute phase show asymmetric swelling. In chronic cases there can be periarticular erosions and overhanging edges (Eggebeen, 2007; Lawrence et al., 2008).

Multimodal Management

Multimodal management is always aimed toward alleviating the pain during a flare and to prevent additional flares, kidney stones, and tophi development (CDC, 2010a).

- *Education* is primarily designed to teach the older person with gout to decrease urate. Avoiding high purine foods and alcohol are important strategies in preventing gout flares.

Some education measures to accomplish this include the following:

- Make sure *Diet* is low purine (avoid anchovies, bacon, brain, herring, legumes, liver, kidney, mackerel, sardines, turkey, and veal).
- *Reduce weight* if overweight or obese.
- *Avoid or reduce* alcohol consumption, especially beer.
- Avoid thiazide diuretics that can increase uric acid levels.
- Risk factors should be reduced or eliminated, including
  - obesity
  - smoking
  - hyperlipidemia (consider fenofibrate that has safer uricosuric effects)
  - hypertension (consider lasartan that has safer uricosuric effects)
  - hyperglycemia (Eliopoulos, 2001; Zhang et al., 2006).
- *Exercise* should be encouraged during nonacute phases to manage weight and improve general function.

- *Complementary interventions,* as discussed in the previous section, may be helpful in managing the pain during an acute flare. (see Chapter 11 for a more detailed account of complementary interventions).
- *Assistive devices,* such as a cane, crutches, or wheel chair, may be necessary during an acute flare of gout in the lower extremities.
- *Supplements and herbs* such as folic acid, vitamin E, and eicosapentaenoic acid may be helpful. Yucca and devil's claw have been reported as helpful in reducing symptoms (Eliopoulos, 2001).
- *Medication management* of gout-associated pain is focused on relieving the cause of the pain—inflammation due to the urate crystals.
  Medications during an acute flare include the following:
- An oral NSAID is the primary medication.
  - May need gastroprotective medication (see Chapter 7 for cautions in older adults)
- Corticosteroids are an option, depending upon comorbidities and risk of osteoporosis.
  - Particular cautions include
    - avoid in older adults with septic joints
    - use with caution with diabetes
- Colchicine or phenylbutazone are used in acute flares.
- Colchicine is effective as second-line therapy to NSAID.
  - Usual dosage is 0.6 mg BID (2 x per day) or TID (3 x per day)
    - dose should be reduced in older adults
    - avoid IV administration
  - Most effective when used during the initial 24 hours of an acute attack
  - Side effects include nausea, vomiting, diarrhea
  - Cautions include
    - can lead to suppression of bone marrow
    - avoid in older adults with severe renal or liver problems
    - can cause neuromyopathy
    - side effects occur with higher doses

Medications used for long-term medication management are intended to lower the urate levels. These include colchicine, allopurinol, probenecid, and indomethacin (Eggebeen, 2007; Eliopoulos, 2001; Zhang et al., 2006).

- *Interventional option:* Intra-articular aspiration with injection of a long-acting steroid is considered safe and effective treatment in an acute flare (Zhang et al., 2006).

GUIDELINES AND RESOURCES

Adler, R., & Hochberg, M. C. (2003). Suggested guidelines for evaluation and treatment of glucocorticoid-induced osteoporosis for the Department of Veterans Affairs. *Archives of Internal Medicine, 163,* 2619–2624.

Agency for Healthcare Policy and Research (AHPR). (2009). Governmental report: Choosing nonopioid analgesics for osteoarthritis: Clinician summary guide. *Journal of Pain & Palliative Care Pharmacotherapy, 23,* 433–457.

American College or Rheumatology. www.rheumatology.org

American Geriatrics Society. (2001). Exercise prescription for older adults with osteoarthritis pain: Consensus practice recommendations. *Journal of the American Geriatrics Society, 49*(6), 808–823.

American Geriatrics Society (AGS). (2009). Pharmacological management of persistent pain in older persons: American Geriatrics Society Panel of the Pharmacological Management of Persistent Pain in Older Adults. *Journal of the American Geriatrics Society, 57,* 1331–1346.

Arthritis Foundation. http://www.arthritis.org

Centers for Disease Control. www.cdc.gov/arthritis/data

Jordan, K. M., Arden, N. K., Doherty, M., Bannwarth, B., Bijlsma, J. W., Dieppe, P., Dougados M. (2003). EULAR Recommendations 2003: An evidence based approach to the management of knee osteoarthritis: Report of a task force of the Standing Committee for International Clinical Studies Including Therapeutic Trials (ESCISIT). *Annals of Rheumatoid Disease, 62,* 1145–11155.

National Center for Complementary and Alternative Medicine. http://www.nccam.nih.gov

National Institute on Aging. http://www.nia.nih.gov/

National Institute of Arthritis and Musculoskeletal and Skin Diseases. www.niams.nih.gov

The Arthritis Society of Canada. http://www.arthritis.ca

Case Study

Mr. and Mrs. Murphy are African Americans in their mid-70s. They came to clinic today to find out what they can do about the problems they are having with their hands and that Mrs. Murphy is having with her knees. They both take oral medications for hypertension, cholesterol elevations, and diabetes. When Mr. Murphy mentions that his wife is significantly overweight and "that is not helping her knees," Mrs. Murphy tells him that at least she does not eat all those hot dogs that he eats all the time with all the beer that he drinks.

Questions

1. What assessments and evaluations are need for Mr. and Mrs. Murphy?
2. What are the most likely diagnoses for them?
3. What risk factors do they have that contribute to those diagnoses?
4. What education should you prepare for them?
5. What factors are likely to complicate treatment?
6. What medications are the best options for each of them?
7. What education do they need about the medications?
8. What nonpharmacological interventions may be helpful to them?

REFERENCES

Adler, P., Good, M., Roberts, B., & Snyder, S. (2000). The effects of tai chi on older adults with chronic arthritis pain. *Journal of Nursing Scholarship, 32,* 377.

Adler, P., & Roberts, B. (2006). The use of tai chi to improve health in older adults. *Orthopaedic Nursing, 25,* 122–126.

Agency for Healthcare Policy and Research (AHPR). (2009). Governmental report: Choosing nonopioid analgesics for osteoarthritis: Clinician summary guide. *Journal of Pain & Palliative Care Pharmacotherapy, 23,* 433–457.

Agency for Healthcare Research and Quality (AHRQ). (2002). S-adenosyl L-methionine for treatment of depression, osteoarthritis, and liver disease. *Evidence Report/Technology Assessment, 64.* Retrieved May 08, 2011, from http://archive.ahrq.gov/clinic/epcsums/samesum.pdf

American Geriatrics Society (AGS). (2001). Exercise prescription for older adults with osteoarthritis pain: Consensus practice recommendations. *Journal of the American Geriatrics Society, 6,* 808–823.

American Geriatrics Society (AGS). (2009). Pharmacological management of persistent pain in older persons: American Geriatrics Society Panel of the

Pharmacological Management of Persistent Pain in Older Adults. *Journal of the American Geriatrics Society, 57,* 1331–1346.

American Pain Society (APS). (2002). *Pain in osteoarthritis, rheumatoid arthritis and juvenile chronic arthritis.* Glenview, IL: American Pain Society.

American Pain Society (APS). (2003). *Principles of analgesic use in the treatment of acute pain and cancer pain* (5th ed.). Glenview, IL: American Pain Society.

Andersen, R. E., Crespo, C. J., Bartlett, S. J., Barthon, J. M., & Fontaine, K. R. (2003). Relationship between body weight gain and significant knee, hip, and back pain in older Americans. *Obesity a Research Journal, 11,* 1159–1162.

Appelbloom, T., Schuermans, J., Verbruggen, G., Henrotin, G., & Reginster, J. Y. (2001). Symptoms modifying effect of avocado/soybean unsaponifiables (ASU) in knee osteoarthritis. *Scandinavian Journal of Rheumatology, 30,* 242–247.

Arthritis Foundation. (2011). *Arthritis Foundation Exercise Program.* Arthritis Foundation. Retrieved May 06, 2011, from http://www.arthritis.org/af-exercise-program.php

Bareta, J., Berman, B. M., Hadhazy, V., Lao, Singh, B. B. (2001). Clinical decisions in the use of acupuncture as an adjunctive therapy for osteoarthritis of the knee. *Alternative Therapies in Health and Medicine, 7(4),* 58–65.

Barthel, H. R., Haselwood, D., Longley, S., Gold, M. S., & Altman, R. D. (2009). Randomized controlled trial of diclofenac sodium gel in knee osteoarthritis. *Seminars in Arthritis and Rheumatism, 39,* 203–212.

Bellamy, N., Campbell, J., Robinson, V., Gee, T., Bourne, R., & Wells, G. (2006). Intraarticular corticosteroid for treatment of osteoarthritis of the knee. *Cochrane Database Systematic Review, CD005328.*

Biswal, S., Medhi, B., & Pandhi, P. (2006). Long term efficacy of topical nonsteroidal anti-inflammatory drugs in knee osteoarthritis: Metaanalysis of randomized placebo controlled clinical trials. *Journal of Rheumatology, 33,* 1841–1844.

Bolen, J., Schieb, L., Hootman, J., Helmick, C., Theis, K., Murphy, L., & Langmaid, G. (2010). Differences in the prevalence and impact of arthritis among racial/ethnic groups in the United States, National Health Interview Survey, 2002, 2003, and 2006. *Preventing Chronic Disease Public Health Research, Practice, and Policy, 7(3),* 1–5.

Brien, S., Lewith, G.T., & McGregor, G. (2006). Devil's claw (*Harpagophytum procumbens*) as a treatment for osteoarthritis: A review of efficacy and safety. *Journal of Alternative and Complementary Medicine, 12,* 981–993.

Brooks, P. (2003). Inflammation as an important feature of osteoarthritis. *Bulleting of the World Health Organization, 81,* 689–690.

Bruyere, O., & Reginster, J. Y. (2007). Glucosamine and chondroitin sulfate as therapeutic agents for knee and hip osteoarthritis. *Drugs Aging, 24,* 573–580.

Centers for Communicable Disease (CDC). (2006). *Prevalence of doctor diagnosed arthritis and arthritis attributable activity limitation—United States*

2003–2005. Retrieved April 27, 2011, http://www.cdc.gov/mmwr/preview/mmwrhtml/mm5540a2.htm

Centers for Communicable Disease (CDC). (2010a). *Gout*. Retrieved May 07, 2011, http://www.cdc.gov/arthritis/basics/gout.htm

Centers for Communicable Disease (CDC). (2010b). *Physical activity and arthritis*. Retrieved May 07, 2011, http://www.cdc.gov/arthritis/pa_overview.htm

Centers for Communicable Disease (CDC). (2011). *Cost Statistics*. Retrieved May 11, 2011, http://www.cdc.gov/arthritis/data_statistics/cost.htm

Chen, L. X. & Schumacher, H. R. (2006). Gout: Can we create an evidence based systematic approach to diagnosis and management? *Best Practice & Research Clinical Rheumatology, 20,* 673–684.

Choi, J. H., Moon, J. S., & Song, R. (2005). Effects of Sun-style Tai Chi exercise on physical fitness and fall prevention in fall-prone older adults. *Journal of Advanced Nursing, 51,* 150–157.

Christensen, R., Bartels, E. M., Altman, R. D., Astrup, A., & Bliddal, H. (2008). Does the hip powder of *Rosa canina* (rosehip) reduce pain in osteoarthritis patients? A meta-analysis of randomized controlled trials. *Osteoarthritis Cartilage, 16,* 965–972.

Christensen, R., Bartels, E. M., Astrup, A., & Bliddal, H. (2009). Symptomatic efficacy of avocado-soybean unsaponifiables (ASU) in osteoarthritis (OA) patients: A meta-analysis of randomized controlled trials. *Osteoarthritis Cartilage, 16,* 399–408.

Chrubasik, J. E., Roufogalis, B. D., & Chrubasik, S. (2007). Evidence of effectiveness of herbal anti-inflammatory drugs in the treatment of painful osteoarthritis and chronic low back pain. *Phytotherapy Research, 21,* 675–683.

Chu, D. A. (2004). Tai chi, Qi gong and Reiki. *Physical Medicine and Rehabilitation Clinics of North America, 15,* 773–781.

Clegg, D. O., Reda, D. J., Harris, C. L., Klein, M. A., O'Dell, J. R., Hooper, M. M., Williams H. J. (2006). Glucosamine, chondroitin sulfate, and the two in combination for painful knew osteoarthritis. *The New England Journal of Medicine, 354,* 795–808.

Collins, J. E. (2007). Physical therapy for the older adult. In M. A. Pagliarulo (Ed.), *Introduction to physical therapy* (3rd ed., pp. 337–361). St. Louis, MO: Mosby Elsevier.

Cosby, J. (2009). Osteoarthritis: Managing without surgery. *Journal of Family Practice, 58,* 354–361.

Davis, G. C., & White, T. I. (2008). A goal attainment pain management program for older adults with arthritis. *Pain Management Nursing, 9,* 171–179.

Eggebeen, A. T. (2007). Gout: An update. *American Family Physician, 76,* 801–808.

Eliopoulos, C. (2001). Gerontological nursing. Philadelphia, PA: Lippincott.

Endo. (2010). *Lidoderm (package insert)*. Chadds Ford, PA: Endo Pharmaceuticals.

France, C. R., Keefe, F. J., Emery, C. F., Affleck, G., France, J. L., & Waters, S. (2004). Laboratory pain perception and clinical pain in post-menopausal women and age-matched men with osteoarthritis: Relationship to pain coping and hormonal status. *Pain, 112,* 274–281.

Gagnier, J. J., Chrubasik, S., Manheimer, E. (2004). Harpagophytum procumbens for osteoarthritis and low back pain: a systematic review. *BMC Complementary and Alternative Medicine, 4,* 4–13.

Heim, N., Snijder, M. B., Deeg, D. J., Seidell, J. C., & Visser, M. (2008). Obesity in older adults is associated with an increased prevalence and incidence of pain. *Obesity a Research Journal, 16,* 2510–2517.

Hernandez-Molina, G., Reichenbach, S., Zhang, B., LaValley, M., & Felson, D. T. (2008). Effect of therapeutic exercise for hip osteoarthritis pain: Results of a meta-analysis. *Arthritis & Rheumatism, 59,* 1221–1228.

Henrotin, Y. E., Sanchez, C., Deberg, M. A., Piccardi, N., Guillou, B., Msika, P., & Reginster, J. Y. (2003). Avocado/soybean unsaponifiables increase aggrecan synthesis and reduce catabolic and proinflammatory mediator production by human osteoarthritic chondrocytes. *Journal of Rheumatology, 30,* 1825–1834.

Hinman, R. S., Crossley, K. M., McConnell, J., & Bennell, K. L. (2003). Efficacy of knee tape in the management of osteoarthritis of the knee: Blinded randomized controlled trial. *British Medical Journal, 327,* 135.

Hochberg, M. C. (2011). Clinical features and diagnosis of osteoarthritis. *Menopause Management, 10,* 12–14.

Huang, W., Bliwise, D. L., Carnevale, C. V., & Kunter, N. G. (2010). Acupuncture for pain and sleep in knee osteoarthritis. *Journal of the American Geriatrics Society, 58,* 1218–1220.

Institute for Clinical Systems Improvement. (2006). *Diagnosis and treatment of degenerative joint disease of the knee.* Retrieved May 04, 2011, from http://www.icsi.org/guidelines and more/guidleines_order__protocols/musculo-skeletal/degenerative_joint_disease/degenerartive_joint_disease_of_the_kne_adult_diagnosis_and_treatment_of_2.htmle

Jordan, K. M. Arden, N. K., Doherty, M., Bannwarth, B., Bijlsma, J. W., Dieppe, P., Dougados, M. (2003). EULAR Recommendations 2003: An evidence based approach to the management of knee osteoarthritis: Report of a task force of the Standing Committee for International Clinical Studies Including Therapeutic Trials (ESCISIT). *Annals of Rheumatoid Disease, 62,* 1145–11155.

Jorge, J., & McDonald, D. D. (2011). Hispanic older adults' osteoarthritis pain communication. *Pain Management Nursing,12,* 173–179.

Keefe, F. J., Smith, S. J., Buffington, A. L., Gibson, J., Sudts, J. L., & Caldwell, D. S. (2002). Recent advances and future directions in the biopsychosocial assessment and treatment of arthritis. *Journal of Consulting and Clinical Psychology, 7,* 640–655.

Kivitz, A., Fairfax, M., Sheldon, E. A., Xiang, Q., Jones, B. A., Gammaitoni, A. R., & Gould, E. M. (2008). Comparison of the effectiveness and tolerability of lidocaine patch 5% versus celecoxib for osteoarthritis-related knee pain: Post hoc analysis of a 12-week, prospective, randomized, active-controlled, open-label, parallel-group trial in adults. *Clinical Therapeutics, 30,* 2366–2377.

Lawrence, R. C., Felson, D. T., Helmick, C. G., Arnold, L. M., Choi, H., Deyo, R. A., Wolfe, F. (2008). Estimates of the prevalence of arthritis and other rheumatic conditions in the United States. *Arthritis & Rheumatism, 58,* 26–35.

Leveille, S. G., Bean, J., Ngo, L., McMullen, W., & Guralnik J.M. (2007). The pathway from musculoskeletal pain to mobility difficulty in older disabled women. *Pain, 128,* 69–77.

Leveille, S. G., Zhang, Y., McMullen, W., Kelly-Hayes, M., & Felson, D. T. (2005). Sex differences in musculoskeletal pain in older adults. *Pain, 116,* 332–338.

Levy, R. M., Saikovsky, R., Schmidt, E., Khokhlov, A., & Burnett, B. P. (2009). Flavocoxid is as effective as naproxen for managing the signs and symptoms of osteoarthritis of the knee in humans: a short term randomized double-blind pilot study. *Nutrition Research, 29,* 298–304.

Lukas, L. K. (2004). Orthopedic outpatients' perception of perioperative music listening as therapy. *The Journal of Theory Construction and Testing, 8,* 7–12.

Manheimer, E., Linde, K., Lao, L., Bouter, L. M., & Berman, B. M. (2007). Meta-analysis: Acupuncture for osteoarthritis of the knee. *Annals of Internal Medicine, 146,* 868–877.

Mason, L., Moore, R. A., Derry, S., Edwards, J. E., & McQuay, H. J. (2004). Systematic review of topical capsaicin for the treatment of chronic pain. *British Medical Journal, 328,* 991.

McAlindon, T. E., LaValley, M. P., Gulin, J. P., & Felson, D. T. (2000). Glucosamine and chondroitin for treatment of osteoarthritis: A systematic quality assessment and meta-analysis. *Journal of the American Medical Association, 283,* 1469–1475.

McCaffrey, R., & Freeman, E. (2003). Effect of music on chronic osteoarthritis pain in older people. *Journal of Advanced Nursing, 44,* 517–524.

Messier, S. P., Gutekunst, D. L., Davis, C., & DeVita, P. (2005). Weight loss reduces knee-joint loads in overweight and obese older adults with knee osteoarthritis. *Arthritis and Rheumatology, 52,* 2026–2032.

Michishita, R., Shono, N., Kasahara, T., Katoku, M., & Tsuruta, T. (2008). The possible influence of osteoarthritis of the knee on the accumulation of coronary risk factors in postmenopausal obese women. *Obesity Research and Clinical Practice, 2,* 29–34.

Moody, M. L. (2010). Topical medications in the treatment of pain. *Pain Medicine News, 8,* 15–21.

Morrison, R. S., Flanagan, S., Fischberg, D., Cintron, A., & Siu, A. L. (2009). A novel interdisciplinary analgesic program reduces pain and improves function in older adults after orthopedic surgery. *Journal of the American Geriatrics Society, 57,* 1–10.

Nunez, D. E., Keller, C., & Der Ananian, C. (2009). A review of the efficacy of the self-management model on health outcomes in community-residing older adults with arthritis. *Worldviews on Evidence-Based Nursing, 6,* 130–148.

Papaleontiou, M., Henderson, C. R., Turner, B., Moore, A. A., Olkhouskaya, Y., Amanfo, L., & Reid, M. C. (2010). Outcomes associated with opioid use in the treatment of noncancer pain in older adults: A systematic review and meta-analysis. *Journal of the American Geriatrics Society, 58,* 1353–1369.

Pells, J. J., Shelby, R. A., Keefe, F. J., Dixon, K. E., Blumenthal, J. A., LaCaille, L., Kraus, V. B. (2008). Arthritis self-efficacy and self-efficacy for resisting eating: Relationships to pain, disability, and eating behavior in overweight and obese individuals with osteoarthritic knee pain. *Pain, 136,* 340–347.

Pendleton, A., Arden, N., Dougados, M., Doherty, M., Bannwarth, B., Bijlsma, J. W., Zimmerman-Gorska, I. (2000). EULAR recommendations for the management of knee osteoarthritis: Report of a task force of the Standing Committee for International Clinical Studies Including Therapeutic Trials (ESCISIT). *Annals of Rheumatic Diseases, 59,* 936–944.

Poitras, S., Avouac, J., Rossignol, M., Avouac, B., Cedraschi, C., Nordin, M., Hilliquin, P. (2007). A critical appraisal of guidelines for the management of knee osteoarthritis using appraisal guidelines research and evaluation criteria. *Arthritis Research & Therapy, 9,* 1–12.

Porcheret, M., Jordan, K., & Croft, P. (2006). Treatment of knee pain in older adults in primary care: Development of an evidence-based model of care. *Rheumatology, 46,* 638–648.

Portenoy, R., Ugarte, C., Fuller, I., & Haas, G. (2004). Population-based survey of pain in the United States: Differences among White, African American, and Hispanic subjects, *The Journal of Pain, 5,* 317–328.

Prestwood, K. (2005). Complementary and alternative medicine for the treatment of pain in older adults. In: S. Gibson & D. Weiner (Eds.), *Pain in older persons* (pp. 285–307). Seattle, WA: IASP Press.

Reid, M. C., Papaleontiou, M., Ong, A., Breckman, R., Wethington, E., & Pillemer, K. (2008). Self-management strategies to reduce pain and improve function among older adults in community settings: A review of the evidence. *Pain Medicine, 9,* 409–424.

Reuben, D. B., Herr, K. A., Pacala, J. T., Pollock, B. G., Potter, J. F., & Semla, T. P. (2005). *Geriatrics at your fingertips* (7th ed.). New York, NY: The American Geriatrics Society.

Rosenthal, N. R., Silverfield, J. C., Wu, S. C., Jordan, D., & Kamin, M. (2004). Tramadol/acetaminophen combination tablets for the treatment of pain associated with osteoarthritis flare in an elderly patient population. *Journal of the American Geriatrics Society, 52,* 374–380.

Ruehlman, L. S. (2005). Comparing the experiential and psychosocial dimensions of chronic pain in African Americans and Caucasians: Findings from a National Community Sample, *Pain Medicine, 6* (1), 49–61.

Sawynock, J. (2003). Topical and peripherally acting analgesics. *Pharmacological Reviews, 55,* 1–20.

Seed, S. M., Dunican, K. C., & Lynch, A. M. (2009). Osteoarthritis: A review of treatment options. *Geriatrics, 64,* 20–28.

Sharma, L. (2001). Epidemiology of osteoarthritis. In R. W. Moskowitz, O. S. Howell, R. D. Altman, J. A. Buckwalter, & V. M. Goldberg (Eds.), *Osteoarthritis: Diagnosis and medical/surgical management* (3rd ed., pp. 3–17). Philadelphia, PA: W. B. Saunders.

Sharma, L. (2003). Examination of exercise effects on knee osteoarthritis outcomes: Why should the local mechanical environment be considered? *Arthritis Care & Research, 49,* 255–260.

Soeken, K. L., Lee, W. L., Bausell, R. B., Agelli, M., & Berman, B. M. (2002). Safety and efficacy of S-adenosylmethionine (SAMe) for osteoarthritis. *Journal of Family Practice, 51,* 425–430.

Solomon, D. H., Rassen, J. A., Glynn, R. J., Lee, J., Levin, R., & Schneeweiss, S. (2010). The comparative safety of analgesics in older adults with arthritis. *Archives of Internal Medicine, 22,* 1968–1976.

Swank, A. M., Kachelman, J. B., Bibeau, W., Quesada, P. M., Nyland, J., Malkani, A., & Topp, R. V. (2011). Prehabilitation before total knee arthroplasty increases strength and function in older adults with severe osteoarthritis. *The Journal of Strength and Conditioning Research, 25,* 318–325.

Towheed, T. E., Maxwell, L., Judd, M. G., Catton, M., Hochberg, M C., & Wells, G. (2006). Acetaminophen for osteoarthritis. *Cochrane Database Systematic Review, 1,* CD004257.

Tugwell, P. S., Wells, G. A., & Shainhouse, G. Z., (2004). Equivalence study of topical diclofenac solution (Pennsaid) compared with oral diclofenac in symptomatic treatment of osteoarthritis of the knee: A randomized control trial. *Journal of Rheumatology, 31,* 2002–2012.

Walton, S. M., Schumock, G. T., & McLain, D. A. (2010). Cost analysis of flavocoxid compared to naproxen in subjects with osteoarthritis of the knee - a subset analysis. *Advances in Therapy, 27,* 953–962.

Wandel., S., Juni, P., Tendal, B., Nuesch, E., Villiger, P. M., Welton, N. J., Trelle, S. (2010). Effects of glucosamine, chondroitin, or placebo in patients with osteoarthritis of hip or knee: Network meta-analysis. *British Medical Journal, 341,* c4675.

Wang, C., Collet, J. P., & Lau, J. (2004). The effect of Tai chi on health outcomes in patients with chronic conditions: A systematic review. *Archives of Internal Medicine, 164,* 493–501.

Wang, Y. Y., Hong, C. T., Chiu, W. T., & Fang, J. Y. (2001). In vitro and in vivo evaluations of topically applied capsaicin and noninvamide from hydrogels. *International Journal of Pharmaceutics, 224,* 89–104.

Winther, K., Apel, K., & Thamsborg, G. (2005). A powder made from seeds and shells of a rose-hip subspecies (*Rosa canina)* reduces symptoms of knee and hip osteoarthritis: A randomized, double-blind, placebo-controlled clinical trial. *Scandinavian Journal of Rheumatology, 34,* 302–308.

Wright, N. C., Riggs, G. K., Lisse, J. R., & Chen, Z. (2008). Self-reported osteoarthritis, ethnicity, body mass index, and other associated risk factors in postmenopausal women-results from the Women's Health Initiative. *Journal of the American Geriatrics Society, 56,* 1736–1743.

Yoon, E. & Doherty, J. B. (2008). Arthritis pain. *Journal of Gerontological Social Work, 50*(Supp#1), 79–103.

Zhang, W., Nuki, G., Moskowitz, R. W., Abramson, S., Altman, R. D., Arden, N. K., Tugwell, L. P. (2010). OARSI recommendations for the management of hip and knee osteoarthritis Part III: Changes in evidence following systematic cumulative update of research published through January 2009. *Osteoarthritis and Cartilage, 18,* 476–499.

Zhang, W., Doherty, M., Bardin, T., Pascual, E., Barskova, V., Conoghan, P., Zimmerman-Gorska, I. (2006). EULAR evidence based recommendations for gout. Part II: Management. Report of a task force of the EULAR Standing Committee for International Clinical Studies Including Therapeutics (ESCISIT). *Annals of Rheumatic Diseases, 65,* 1312–1324.

16

Chronic Back Pain and Osteoporosis

The human skeleton, particularly the back, is the location of pain in many older adults. The focus of this chapter will be chronic back pain and osteoporosis.

LOW BACK PAIN

Epidemiology and Prevalence

It is estimated that low back pain (LBP) is experienced on a regular basis by 51% of people and at some point in time by 84% (McBeth & Jones, 2007). In the United States, pathology of the back and neck is the second leading cause of disability, with more than 15 million physician visits each year due to chronic low back pain (CLBP) (Strine & Hootman, 2007). It is reported that women experience back pain more frequently than men (International Association for the Study of Pain, 2007; Tousignant-Laflamme, Rainville, & Marchand, 2005).

One in three community-dwelling older people live with CLBP (Weiner, Sakamoto, Perrara, & Breuer, 2006). Although Medicare patient coverage increased 131.7% between 1991 and 2002, the increase in Medicare patients with LBP increased 310% and associated Medicare costs increased by 387% (Weiner, Kim, Bonino, & Wang, 2006).

Recurrence is significant with the worldwide recurrence rate after initial injury estimated as 40% to 70% (Ghaffari, Alipour, Farshad, Yensen, & Vingard, 2005). Failed back surgery syndrome is estimated to occur 5% to 40% of the time (Weiner, Sakamoto, et al., 2006). In Canada, it was found that 20% of back pain recurs within 6 months and recurs more with aging (Cassidy, Cote, Carroll, & Kristman, 2005).

Although CLBP "is one of the most common, poorly understood, and potentially disabling chronic pain conditions from which older adults suffer," (Rudy, Weiner, & Lieber, 2007) it is difficult to determine the full impact. That is complicated by comorbid conditions. In their study with 320 community-dwelling older adults, Rudy et al. (2007) found significant biomedical, psychosocial, and functional differences between those with and those without CLBP. Depression, measured by the Geriatric Depression Scale, was marked among those with CLBP.

Diagnostic Criteria

Specific pathoanatomical diagnosis is most often vague. Complicating this is that imaging findings often are not well correlated with symptoms, and similar results are seen in people with and without symptoms. Many of the biomechanical and soft tissue pathologies frequently seen in older adults can be diagnosed through physical examination (Bruer, Pappagallo, Ongesng, Akhtar, & Goldfarb, 2008; Weiner, Sakamoto, et al., 2006).

Multimodal Management

Education is a basic and crucial component in the treatment of LBP. Patients must understand the pathology and that they need to be active participants in the recovery or management process. Education should focus on a healthy lifestyle, attaining and maintaining a healthy weight, and exercise (Patel & Ogle, 2000).

The authors of a systematic review of excercise reported that specific exercises were not successful in treating acute episodes of LBP; however, exercise can be beneficial for people living with chronic low back pain (PLWCLBP) to assume their usual daily activities (van Tulder, Malmivaara, Esmail & Koes, 2000). In a review of 51 RCTs of exercise among PLWCLBP, exercise was found to be a positive intervention (Liddle, Baxter, & Gracey, 2004). This is consistent with staying active being a primary recommendation in the Clinical guidelines from the American College of Physicians/American Pain Society Low Back Pain Guidelines Panel (ACP/APS-LBPGP) (Chou et al., 2007).

Weiner et al. (2008) recently reported a RCT involving 200 older community dwellers comparing percutaneous electrical nerve stimulation with and without general conditioning aerobic exercise (GCAE). They found that although the addition of GCAE seemed to be beneficial in reducing fear, it did not contribute to reducing pain or increasing function.

Physical therapy referral can be very beneficial during acute phases of back pain. Helpful interventions include heat through hydrocolloid packs and ultrasound as well as massage. Evidence does not support traction or transcutaneous electrical nerve stimulation with acute instances of back pain (Patel & Ogle, 2000).

Weight management is an important component of managing musculoskeletal pain. Older adults who are overweight not only experience more pain but are also at greater risk for developing new pain (Heim, Snijder, Deeg, Seidell, & Visser, 2008). Among older adults, the prevalence of musculoskeletal pain, including back pain, increased in accordance with increased BMI levels (Andersen, Crespo, Bartlett, Barthon, & Fontaine, 2003). Encouraging overweight older adults to reduce weight may include referral to a nutritionist or a reputable weight loss program.

Cognitive Behavioral Therapy

The ACP/APS-LBPGP also classifies cognitive behavioral therapy and progressive muscle relaxation as effective interventions for CLBP (Chou et al., 2007). A recent Norwegian systematic review of RCT involving back schools, fear-avoidance training, and brief education found what appeared to be no difference between fear-avoidance training and back fusion surgery (Brox, Storheim, Grotle, Tveito, & Indahl, 2008). Although group therapy for PLWCLBP could be a viable intervention (Keefe, Beaupre, & Gil, 1996), a search of CINAHL, EBSCO, and psycINFO was sparse. A Finnish study supported earlier findings that patient characteristics affected participation and outcomes (Talo, Forssell, Heikkonen, & Puukka, 2001). These are interventions that need further investigation.

Complementary Interventions

CLBP is one of the most common reasons people utilize complementary modalities (Williams et al., 2005).

■ *Meditation* has been studied from several perspectives. One study reported that an 8-week mindfulness meditation program was "feasible among community-dwelling older adults with CLBP" (Morone, Greco, & Weiner, 2008, p. 318). The Carson et al. (2005b) pilot study found that Loving Kindness Meditation (LKM) may be helpful for individuals living with CLBP. This was consistent with an earlier study that found forgiveness related to both anger and pain from a sensory dimension view (Carson et al., 2005a). Through an integrative review of experimental and nonexperimental studies using meditation as an intervention for chronic pain, Tiexeira (2008) concluded that it has potential benefit. Clearly the role of meditation in managing CLBP warrants additional study.

■ *Viniyoga style yoga* for CLBP was recommended by the ACP/APS-LBPGP (Chou et al., 2007). In a small study that warrants replication, *Iyengar yoga* was a statistically more effective therapy than an educational control condition to assist PLWCLBP to reduce analgesia medication (Williams et al., 2005).

Straube, Moore, Derry, & McQuay (2008) concluded in a recent systemic review of 22 studies that investigated vitamin D levels, or benefit for CLBP, that there is no current evidence to support such a link and that additional research is needed.

Paramore (1997) reported that the vast majority, 17.6 million Americans, who utilized complementary modalities did so for chiropractic services. The second largest group was the 8 million who obtained therapeutic massages. In Great Britain, Ernst (1999) compared spinal manipulation with massage, finding mixed results that require further investigation.

The ACP/APS-LBPGP classifies *acupuncture* as a moderately effective intervention for CLBP (Chou et al., 2007). Evaluation of acupuncture study reports noted that acupuncture is more effective than placebo, but long-term effectiveness is not clearly ascertained (Chou & Huffman, 2007). A review of 17 studies involving nearly 5,000 subjects revealed that although more high-quality studies are needed, the real benefit seems to be when acupuncture is integrated with other therapies (Ammendolia, Furlan, Imamura, Irvin, & Van Tulder, 2008). Interestingly in one study using sham acupuncture, the sham version was found to be more effective than standard multimodal analgesia (Haake, et al., 2007; Shih, Costi, & Teixeira, 2008).

Herbal Preparations

Herbal preparations have not been studied as frequently in PLW CLBP as those with osteoarthritis (OA). The ACP/APS-LBPGP noted that although herbal treatments (i.e., devil's claw, willow bark, and capsicum) seem safe as treatment for acute episodes of CLBP, the associated benefits range are small to moderate (Chou et al., 2007). Results of a German double-blind RCT with 320 participants that compared capsicum plaster with a placebo were highly statistically significant ($p < 0.001$) for relieving pain with capsicum (Frericka, Keitelb, Kuhna, & Schmidta, 2003).

Medication Management

Acetaminophen and nonsteroidal anti-inflammatory drugs (NSAIDs) are the primary pharmacological methods recommended to manage CLBP (Chou et al., 2007). One systematic review of 51 studies involving 6,057 participants did not find sufficient support to confirm that NSAIDs are effective for CLBP (van Tulder, Scholten, Koes, & Deyo, 2000). This is a concern since gastrointestinal toxicity is a major adverse event related to their use (Cowan, 2002). Skeletal muscle relaxants, tricyclic antidepressants, benzodiazepines, and neuropathic agents are also prescribed to treat CLBP (Chou et al., 2007).

Back pain is the primary condition for which opioids are prescribed, accounting for 20% to 29% of opioid prescriptions (Kelly, Cook, Kaufman, & Anderson, 2008) with one household survey reporting opioids being used in 11% to 13% of the US population (Luo, Pietrobon, & Hey, 2004). The Trends and Risks of Opioid Use for Pain (TROUP) study assessed opioid use for noncancer pain, including back pain, over a 6-year period from 2000 to 2005 (Sullivan et al., 2008). TROUP found that even though there was no increase noted in noncancer pain diagnosis, all opioid prescriptions increased, with those for short-acting opioids increasing most rapidly. In a 2007 meta-analysis of opioid use for PLWCLBP, it was concluded that although opioids are effective in acute back pain, their efficacy with duration longer than 16 weeks is not clear (Martell et al., 2007). The American Pain Society (2002) does consider opioids an option for noncancer pain when other treatments have not been effective.

Injections

The various injections and interventional options used to treat CLB are discussed in detail in Chapter 10. The prospective multicenter (RCT) PROCESS study that compared spinal cord stimulation (SCS) with conventional medical treatment in patients with failed back surgery found that SCS resulted in better quality of life than medical management alone, in certain patients with neuropathic pain (Kumar et al., 2007).

Surgical Intervention

Surgery is an intervention for CLBP that has varied results. In 2007, Soegaard, Bunger, Christiansen, and Christiansen reported benefit of lumbar fusion in 675 patients. They found that when the net benefit was assessed 2 years postoperatively, the benefit of surgery was highly significant from a functional standpoint that assessed daily work and social functioning. Severity of preoperative disability and preoperative emotional distress was positively correlated with greater benefit postoperatively, whereas cigarette smoking and previous surgery plus degeneration were negatively correlated.

The difference between surgical intervention and medical management in the Spine Patient Outcomes Research Trial observational study was not statistically significant, and the differences narrowed further over time (Weinstein et al., 2007). One study from the Netherlands found poor surgical outcomes were correlated with higher levels of pain, disability, fear of pain, and passive interventions preoperatively (den Boer, Oostendorp, Beems, Munneke, & Evers, 2006). In a randomized study (RCT) of 60 PLWCLBP who had previous surgery, there was no difference in function between those who had repeat surgery and those who had cognitive and exercise interventions (Brox et al., 2008).

OSTEOPOROSIS WITH RESULTING FRACTURES

Osteoporosis is a metabolic disease that involves breakdown of the skeleton as a result of bone loss due to demineralization and deficient filling of resorptive cavities. The result is an increased risk of fracture. It is distinguished by

- low bone mass,
- microarchitectural deterioration of bone tissue,

- increased fragility of bones, and
- increased risk of fractures after even minor trauma (Akesson, 2003; Eliopoulos, 2005).

Epidemiology and Prevalence

Although the prevalence of osteoporosis in the United States has declined over the last two decades, it remains a significant health care concern. In 2006, a national survey reported 10% (4.5 million) women and 2% (0.8 million) men older than 50 years have osteoporosis as diagnosed by bone mineral density (BMD) of the femur (Looker, Melton, Harris, Borrud, & Shepherd, 2010). These figures are expected to increase as the population ages (Ettinger, 2003).

Osteoporosis generally is asymptomatic; however, it can cause back pain and pain occurs in response to resulting fractures. Common sites for fractures related to osteoporosis are spine, hip, forearm, and proximal humerus. Although not specifically listed as a common site in the literature, clinically, rib fractures are often seen among older women with osteoporosis. It is estimated that in developing countries, older women have a 40% probability of sustaining an osteoporotic fracture and more than 20% chance of a hip fracture (Chan, Anderson, & Lau, 2003; World Health Organization [WHO], 2004).

Diagnostic Criteria

Diagnosis is made when BMD is 2.5 standard deviations below the average BMD for healthy young adults. Dual X-ray absorptiometry is the most widely validated method of measuring BMD (WHO, 2004).

The WHO developed the FRAX® or *WHO Fracture Risk Assessment Tool* to assess the risk of fracture in older adults. The FRAX® algorithm provides a 10-year probability of sustaining a significant fracture specific to nationality, race, and gender and is available for interactive use through the web site http://www.shef.ac.uk/FRAX/index.jsp

Although not all people with osteoporosis sustain fractures, the risk of fracture is increased with osteoporosis (Ettinger, 2003). Risk factors for developing osteoporosis and fractures include any disease or behavior that results in inadequate calcium intake, excessive calcium loss, or poor calcium absorption. Specific factors include the following:

- Female sex, particularly women who are
  - small frame and thin,
  - Caucasian with European ancestry,
  - Asian,
  - estrogen deficient—early menopause,
  - aging (women over 65),
  - genetically predisposed (family history),
  - cigarette smokers,
  - high alcohol users (≥3 drinks/day), and
  - sedentary.
- Prolonged use of certain medications, such as
  - corticosteroid (increases male risk),
  - thyroid hormone replacement,
  - anticonvulsants,
- Certain disease processes, including
  - cushing syndrome due to excessive glucocorticosteroid production by the adrenal gland,
  - hyperthyroidism,
  - malabsorption disorders, and
  - reduced estrogen and androgen (American College of Rheumatology [ACR], 2010; Adler & Hochberg, 2003; Eliopoulos, 2005).

Pearl | Although the potential for sustaining fracture is high when osteoporosis is present, the absence of osteoporosis does not eliminate the potential for fracture (WHO, 2004).

Multimodal Management of Osteoporosis and Fractures

Prevention and early intervention to stop progression of bone loss are the most desirable and effective interventions. They include identifying those at risk, education, promoting good nutrition, exercise, and pharmacological treatment (Akesson, 2003).

- *Education* is a crucial component of treatment and should address the following:
  - Diet rich in protein and calcium
  - Supplemental calcium (1,200 mg)
  - Vitamin D (20 mcg or 800 IU)
    - Also effective with improving muscle strength that is important in preventing falls with resulting fractures

- Soy food products to help reduce fractures
- Maintaining an ideal weight
- Avoiding activities that could result in fractures (Akesson, 2003; Eliopoulos, 2005; McLaren, 2006; Zhang et al., 2003).
- *Exercise* goals are to remain active; maintain function; prevent further skeletal decline; improve muscle strength, coordination, flexibility, and balance; and prevent falls. Exercises that are beneficial include the following:
  - Range of motion exercises
  - Aerobics
  - Walking
  - Weight-bearing exercises
  - Resistance training

Tai chi is particularly beneficial since there is little pressure exerted on bones and joints while relaxing muscles and strengthening bones (Bonaiuti et al., 2002; Chan et al., 2003; Choi, Moon, & Song, 2005; Hardy, 2009; McLaren, 2006).

- *Assistive devices* can include
  - braces that can be supportive and help lessen associated spasms
  - bed boards (Eliopoulos, 2001).
- *Physical therapy* has two roles regarding osteoporosis. The first is a preventive role through programs aimed to improve and maintain flexibility, strength, activity, and weight-bearing.

The second role is in rehabilitation following fractures, especially hip fractures. In the acute phase, PTs work with the older adults in transferring, walking, and using assistive devices safely and appropriately. During the rehabilitation phase, PTs work with the older person to reclaim skills that enable functioning and usual living activities (Collins, 2007).

- *Medication management* of osteoporosis can be considered from two perspectives: (a) prevention of further deterioration and fracture and (b) managing pain associated with fractures.
  1. Medications to prevent further deterioration and fractures are as follows:
     - Antiresorptive medications
     - Calcitonin
     - Nitrogen and non-nitrogen containing bisphosphonates
     - Strontium ranelate
     - Selective estrogen receptor modulators
     - *Hormone therapy* with estrogen, testosterone, parathyroid hormone, androgens, and tibolone (a synthetic steroid). Since

estrogen therapy is associated with increased risk of cardiovascular disease and breast cancer, it is not considered a first-line therapy.

- Anobolic agents to offset bone loss
- Growth factors
- Cathepsin K (an osteoclast protease that works on bone collagen)
- Cytokines (ACR, 2010; Adler & Hochberg, 2003; Akesson, 2003; Ettinger, 2003; Zhang et al., 2003).

It is recommended that all older adults who must be treated with glucocorticoids also be treated with calcium (1 g/day) and vitamin D (400 to 800 IU/ day). If moderate doses of glucocorticoids are necessary, considering the addition of bisphosphonate is recommended (Adler & Hochberg, 2003).

2. Medications can be used to manage pain associated with osteoporosis and subsequent fractures. The goal is to improve comfort and to facilitate exercise and function.

Multimodal analgesia is discussed in detail in Chapter 7.

As with the pain associated with OA, management of the spinal pain that can accompany osteoporosis starts with acetaminophen. If that is not effective, NSAIDs or COX-2-selective NSAIDs can be added. If pain persists or increases, opioids can be added to the regimen.

Pain related to fractures among cognitively intact community-dwelling older adults is often under treated. This inadequacy of analgesia increases among older adults with cognitive impairment (Morrison & Siu, 2000). Adequate analgesia is an imperative for older adults who have sustained fractures to provide comfort, promote recovery, promote optimal function, and help to prevent the development of chronic pain (Herrick et al., 2004).

The pain associated with fractures related to osteoporosis may be moderate to severe requiring treatment with an opioid (Herr & Titler, 2009). Selection of the opioid and appropriate dosing will depend upon several factors:

- Pain assessment (see details in Chapters 3, 4, and 5)
- Pain intensity and interference with function
- History of analgesic use
- Comorbidities that may limit or contraindicate particular medications (see Chapter 7)
- Response to previous analgesic medications.

Complementary or nonpharmacological interventions are discussed in more detail in Chapter 11. Therapeutic touch can be beneficial in helping to manage the pain as well as promote healing (Gregory & Verdouw, 2005). Other complementary interventions that are appropriate to use with this group of older adults include the following:

- Positioning/repositioning
- Ice or heat with cautions for frail skin
- Distraction with guided imagery, puzzles, and card games
- Relaxation and breathing (Eliopoulos, 2005; Titler et al., 2003).

Pearls

The best interventions for osteoporosis are those designed to prevent the disorder and subsequent fractures.

When providing care for older adults with osteoporosis, care must be taken to avoid fractures.

GUIDELINES AND RESOURCES

American College of Rheumatology. www.rheumatology.org
Centers for Disease Control and Prevention. www.cdc.gov/arthritis/data
National Center for Complementary and Alternative Medicine. http://www.nccam.nih.gov
National Institute of Arthritis and Musculoskeletal and Skin Diseases. www.niams.nih.gov
National Institute on Aging. http://www.nia.nih.gov/

Case Study

Ms. Brown is admitted to the hospital with a diagnosis of "intractable pain." When approached, she continually moans "oh my," "oh, my." Initially it is difficult to assess her pain because she does not interact well. Her husband tells you that she has osteoporosis and CLBP. When she cries "oh my" she holds onto her lower stomach. She also cries louder when her left foot is touched. Her husband tells you that she had been taking sustained release oxycodone, but last week the pain management physician changed her to methadone 10 mg every 12 hours.

1. What additional assessments are needed to adequately address the pain Ms. Brown is having?
2. What are the first interventions that should be done for Ms. Brown?
3. What other providers need to be included in Ms. Brown's care?
4. What are the most appropriate analgesic medications to be prescribed for Ms. Brown?
5. What complementary interventions could be helpful for Ms. Brown?

REFERENCES

Adler, R., & Hochberg, M. C. (2003). Suggested guidelines for evaluation and treatment of glucocorticoid-induced osteoporosis for the Department of Veterans Affairs. *Archives of Internal Medicine, 163,* 2619–2624.

Akesson, K. (2003). New approaches to pharmacological treatment of osteoporosis. *Bulletin of the World Health Organization, 81,* 657–664.

American College of Rheumatology (2010). *American College of Rheumatology 2010 recommendations for the prevention and treatment of glucocorticoid-induced osteoporosis: Clinician's guide.* Retrieved May 05, 2011, from www.rheumatology.org

American Geriatrics Society (2009). Pharmacological management of persistent pain in older persons: American Geriatrics Society Panel of the Pharmacological Management of Persistent Pain in Older Adults. *Journal of the American Geriatrics Society, 57,* 1331–1346.

American Pain Society. (2002). *Guideline for the management of pain in osteoarthritis, RA, and juvenile chronic arthritis.* Glenview, IL: Author.

Ammendolia, C., Furlan, A. D., Imamura, M., Irvin, E., & Van Tulder, M. (2008). Evidence-informed management of chronic low back pain with needle acupuncture. *The Spine Journal, 8,* 160–172.

Andersen, R. E., Crespo, C. J., Bartlett, S. J., Barthon, J. M., & Fontaine, K. R. (2003). Relationship between body weight gain and significant knee, hip, and back pain in older Americans. *Obesity A Research Journal, 11,* 1159–1162.

Bonaiuti, D., Shea, B., Iovine, R., Negrini, S., Welch, V., & Kemper, H. H. (2002). Exercise for preventing and treating osteoporosis in post menopausal women. *Cochrane Database of Systematic Reviews 2002, 3.*

Brox, J., Storheim, K., Grotle, M., Tveito, T., & Indahl, A. (2008). Evidence-informed management of chronic low back pain with back schools, brief education and fear. *The Spine Journal, 8,* 948–958.

Bruer, B., Pappagallo, M., Ongesng, F., Akhtar, H., & Goldfarb, R. (2008). What is the relationship of low back pain to signs of abnormal skeletal metabolism detected by bone scans. *Pain Medicine, 9,* 222–226.

Carson, J. W., Keefe, F. J., Goli, V., Fras, A. M., Lynch, T. R., Thorp, S. R., & Buechler, J. L. (2005a). Forgiveness and chronic low back pain: A preliminary study examining the relationship of forgiveness to pain, anger, and psychological distress. *Journal of Pain, 6,* 84–91.

Carson, J. W., Keefe, F. J., Lynch, T. R., Carson, K. L., Goli, V., Fras, A. M., & Thorp, S. R. (2005b). Loving-kindness meditation for chronic low back pain: Results from a pilot trial. *Journal of Holistic Nursing, 23,* 287–304.

Cassidy, J. D., Cote, P., Carroll, L. J., & Kristman, V. (2005). Incidence and course of low back pain episodes in the general population. *Spine, 30,* 2817–2823.

Chan, K. M., Anderson, M., & Lau, E. M. (2003). Exercise interventions: Defusing the world's osteoporosis time bomb. *Bulletin of the World Health Organization, 81,* 827–830.

Choi, J. H., Moon, J. S., & Song, R. (2005). Effects of sun-style tai chi exercise on physical fitness and fall prevention in fall-prone older adults. *Journal of Advanced Nursing, 51,* 150–157.

Chou, C., & Huffman, L. H. (2007). Nonpharmacologic therapies for acute and chronic low back pain: A review of the evidence for an American Pain Society/American College of Physicians clinical practice guideline. *Annals of Internal Medicine, 147,* 493–505, W121–W141.

Chou, R., Qaseem, A., Snow, V., Casey, D., Cross, T., & Shekelle, P. (2007). Diagnosis and treatment of low back pain: A joint clinical practice guideline from the American College of Physicians and the American Pain Society. *Annals of Internal Medicine, 147,* 478–491.

Collins, J. E. (2007). Physical therapy for the older adult. In M. A. Pagliarulo (Ed.), *Introduction to physical therapy* (3rd ed., pp. 337–361). St. Louis, MO: Mosby Elsevier.

Cowan, D. (2002). Chronic non-cancer pain in older people: Current evidence for prescribing. *British Journal of Community Nursing, 7,* 420–425.

Eliopoulos, C. (2005). *Gerontological nursing.* (6th ed.) Philadelphia, PA: Lippincott, Williams & Wilkins.

Ernst, E. (1999). Massage therapy for low back pain: A systematic review. *Journal of Pain and Symptom Management, 17,* 65–69.

Ettinger, M. P. (2003). Aging bone and osteoporosis. *Archives of Internal Medicine, 163,* 2237–2244.

Frericka, H., Keitelb, W., Kuhna, U., & Schmidta, S. (2003). Topical treatment of chronic low back pain with a capsicum plaster. *Pain, 106,* 59–64.

Ghaffari, M., Alipour, A., Farshad, A. A., Yensen, I., & Vingard, E. (2005). Incidence and recurrence of disabling low back pain and neck-shoulder pain. *Spine, 31,* 2500–2506.

Gregory, S. & Verdouw, K. (2005). Therapeutic touch: Its application for residents in aged care. *Australian Nursing Journal, 12*(7), 1–3.

Haake, M., Müller, H. H., Schade-Brittinger, C., Bassler, H. D., Helmut, C., Basler, H. D., Maier, C. (2007). German acupuncture trials (GERAC) for chronic low back pain: Randomized, multi-center, blinded, parallel-group trial with 3 groups. *Archives of Internal Medicine, 167,* 1892–1898.

Hardy, S. (2009). Preventing disability through exercise investigating older adults' influences and motivations to engage in physical activity. *Journal of Health Psychology, 14,* 1036–1046.

Heim Heim, N., Snijder, M. B., Deeg, D. J., Seidell, J. C., & Visser, M. (2008). Obesity in older adults is associated with an increased prevalence and incidence of pain. *Obesity A Research Journal, 16,* 2510–2517.

Herr, K., & Titler, M. (2009). Acute pain assessment and pharmacological management practices for the older adult with a hip fracture: Review of ED trends. *Journal of Emergency Nursing, 35,* 312–320.

Herrick, C., Steger-May, K., Sinacore, D. R., Brown, M., Schechtman, K. B., & Binder, E. F. (2004). Persistent pain in frail older adults after hip fracture repair. *Journal of IASP.*

International Association for the Study of Pain. (2007, September). *Global year against pain in women: Real women, real pain.* Retrieved March 15, 2008, from International Association for the Study of Pain website: http://www .iasp-pain.org

Jorge, J., & McDonald, D. D. (in press). Hispanic older adults' osteoarthritis pain communication. *Pain Management Nursing.*

Keefe, F. J., Beaupre, P. M., & Gil, K. M. (1996). Group therapy for patients with chronic pain. In R. J. Gatchel & D. Turk (Eds.), *Psychological approaches to pain management: A practitioner's handbook* (pp. 259–281). New York, NY: Guilford Press.

Kelly, J. P., Cook, S. F., Kaufman, D. W., & Anderson, T. (2008). Prevalence and characteristics of opioid use in the US adult population. *Pain, 138,* 507–513.

Kumar, K., Taylor, R. S., Jacques, L., Eldabe, S., Meglio, M., & Molet, J. (2007). Spinal cord stimulation versus conventional medical management for neuropathic pain: A multicentre randomised control trial in patients with failed back surgery syndrome. *Pain, 132,* 179–188.

Liddle, S. D., Baxter, G. D., & Gracey, J. H. (2004). Exercise and chronic low back pain: What works? *Pain, 107,* 176–190.

Looker, A. C., Melton, L. J., Harris, T. B., Borrud, L. G., & Shepherd, J. A. (2010). Prevalence and trends in low femur bone density among older US adults: NHANES 2005–2006 compared with NHANES III. *Journal of Bone and Mineral Research, 25,* 64–71.

Luo, X., Pietrobon, R., & Hey, L. (2004). Patterns and trends in opioid use among individuals with back pain in the United States. *Spine, 29,* 884–890.

Martell, B. A., O'Connor, P. G., Kerns, R. D., Becker, W. C., Morales, K. H., & Kosten, T. R. (2007). Systematic review: Opioid treatment for chronic back pain: Prevalence, efficacy, and association with addiction. *Annals of Internal Medicine, 146,* 116–127.

McBeth, J., & Jones, K. (2007). Epidemiology of chronic musculoskeletal pain. *Best Practice & Research Clinical Rheumatology, 21,* 403–425.

McLaren, S. M. (2006). Eating and drinking. In S. J. Redfern & F. M. Ross (Eds.), *Nursing older people* (pp. 279–314). Edinburgh, UK: Churchill Livingstone Elsevier.

Morone, N. E., Greco, C. M., & Weiner, D. K. (2008). Mindfulness meditation for the treatment of chronic low back pain in older adults: A randomized controlled pilot study. *Pain, 134,* 310–319.

Paramore, L. C. (1997). Use of alternative therapies: Estimates from the 1994 Robert Wood Johnson Foundation National Access to Care Survey. *Journal of Pain Symptom Management, 13,* 83–89.

Patel, A. T. & Ogle, A. A. (2000). Diagnosis and management of acute low back pain. *American Family Physician, 61,* 1779–1786, 1789–1790.

Rudy, T. E., Weiner, D. K., & Lieber, S. J. (2007). The impact of chronic low back pain on older adults: A comparative study of patients and controls. *Pain, 131,* 293–301.

Shih, M. L., Costi, J. M., & Teixeira, J. E. (2008). Sham acupuncture is not a placebo. *Archives of Internal Medicine, 168,* 1011.

Soegaard, R., Bunger, C. E., Christiansen, T., & Christiansen, F. B. (2007). Determinants of cost-effectiveness in lumbar spinal fusion using the net benefit framework: A 2-year follow-up study among 695 patients. *European Spine Journal, 16,* 1822–1831.

Straube , S., Moore, R. A., Derry, S., & McQuay, H. J. (2008). Vitamin D and chronic pain. *Pain, 141,* 10–13.

Strine, T. W., & Hootman, J. M. (2007). US national prevalence and correlates of low back and neck pain among adults. *Arthritis & Rheumatism, 57,* 656–665.

Sullivan, M. D., Edlund, M. J., Fan, M. Y., Devries, A., Braden, J. B., & Martin, B. C. (2008). Trends in use of opioids for non-cancer pain conditions 2000–2005 in commercial and medicaid insurance plans: The TROUP study. *Pain, 138,* 440–449.

Talo, S. J., Forssell, H., Heikkonen , S., & Puukka, P. (2001). Integrative group therapy outcome related to psychosocial characteristics in patients with chronic pain. *International Journal of Rehabilitation Research, 24,* 25–33.

Tiexeira, M. E. (2008). Meditation as an intervention for chronic pain: An integrative review. *Holistic Nursing Practice, 22,* 225–234.

Titler, M. G., Herr, K., Schilling, M. L., Marsh, J. L., Xie, X, Ardery, G., Everett, L. Q. (2003). Acute pain treatment for older adults hospitalized with hip fracture: Current nursing practices and perceived barriers. *Applied Nursing Research, 16,* 211–227.

Tousignant-Laflamme, Y., Rainville, P., & Marchand, S. (2005). Establishing a link between heart rate and pain in healthy subjects: A gender effect. *The Journal of Pain, 6,* 341–347.

van Tulder, M., Malmivaara, A., Esmail, R., & Koes, B. (2000). Exercise therapy for low back pain: A systematic review with the framework of the Cochrane Collaboration Back Review Group. *Spine, 25,* 2784–2796.

van Tulder, M. W., Scholten, R. J., Koes, B. W., & Deyo, R. A. (2000). Nonsteroidal anti-inflammatory drugs for low back pain: A systematic review within the framework of the Cochrane Collaboration Back Review Group. *Spine, 25,* 2501–2513.

Wandel., S., Juni, P., Tendal, B., Nuesch, E., Villiger, P. M., Welton, N. J., Trelle, S. (2010). Effects of glucosamine, chondroitin, or placebo in patients with osteoarthritis of hip or knee: Network meta-analysis. *British Medical Journal, 341,* c4675.

Weiner, D. K., Kim, Y. S., Bonino, P., & Wang, T. (2006). Low back pain in older adults: Are we utilizing healthcare resources wisely? *Pain Medicine, 7,* 143–150.

Weiner, D. K., Perera, S., Rudy, T. E., Glick, R. M., Shenoy, S., & Delitto, A. (2008). Efficacy of percutaneous electrical nerve stimulation and therapeutic exercise for older adults with chronic low back pain: A randomized controlled trial. *Pain, 140,* 344–357.

Weiner, D. K., Sakamoto, S., Perera, S., & Breuer, P. (2006). Chronic low back pain in older adults: Prevalence, reliability, and validity of physical examination findings. *Journal of the American Geriatric Society, 54,* 11–20.

Weinstein, J. N., Lurrie, J. D., Tosteson, T. D., Skinner, J. S., Hanscom, B., & Tosteson, A. N. (2007). Surgical vs. nonoperative treatment for lumbar disk herniation: The Spine Patient Outcomes Research Trial (SPORT) observational cohort. *Journal of the American Medical Association, 296,* 2451–2459.

Williams, K. A., Petronis, J., Smith, D., Goodrich, D., Wu, J., & Ravi, N. (2005). Effect of Iyengar yoga therapy for chronic low back pain. *Pain, 115,* 107–117.

World Health Organization (2004). *WHO scientific group on the assessment of osteoporosis at primary health care level.* Retrieved May, 14, 2011, from http://www .who.int/chp/topics/Osteoporosis.pdf

Zhang, X., Shu, X., Li, H., Yang, G., Li, Q., & Gao, Y. (2003). Prospective cohort study of soy food consumption and risk of bone fracture among postmenopausal women. *Archives of Internal Medicine, 165,* 1890–1895.

17

Neuropathic Pain Associated with Postherpetic Neuralgia and Diabetic Neuropathy

Acute nociceptive pain occurs in response to tissue damage through activation of the nociceptive system as discussed in Chapter 1. Neuropathic pain (NP) occurs through damage and changes in either the peripheral or the central nervous system, with the pain originating within the nervous system rather than outside it. In 1994, the International Association for the Study of Pain (IASP) defined NP as "pain initiated or caused by a primary lesion or dysfunction in the nervous system" (Merskey & Bogduk, 1994). More recently the Neuropathic Special Interest Group of the IASP (Haanpää et al., 2011) redefined NP as "pain arising as a direct consequence of a lesion or disease affecting the somatosensory system" that includes the following:

- Mechanoreception
- Thermoreception
- Nociception
- Proprioception
- Visceroreception

These provide sensory information arising from the skin, viscera, and musculoskeletal system (Treede et al., 2008). This revised definition stresses that NP

- encompasses both the central and the peripheral nervous systems
- is caused by a disease rather than changes resulting from nociceptive pain
- is different than pain caused by lesions in different parts of the nervous system (i.e., central motor pathways)

There is substantial variation in prevalence reports of NP. This variation is due, at least in part, to variation in definition, subject identification, and assessment techniques (Haanpää et al., 2011). What may be a conservative estimate is that 3.8 million Americans suffer with NP, with a greater estimated prevalence in the United Kingdom and France (Fine, 2009). Characteristics of NP are that it

- advances over time (days to months)
- is inconsistent with the amount of tissue damage
- can be spontaneous in onset
- continues even when there is no longer noxious stimulation
- continues beyond the anticipated time for healing
- is pain that can occur in areas different from the injury
- is neurological sensory sensation that occurs in varying measures
- is often manifested to varying degrees in one or more of the following:
  - paresthesia (an abnormal sensation)
  - paroxysms (sudden onsets or episodes of pain)
  - hyperalgesia (increased response to painful stimulus)
  - allodynia (pain elicited by gentle touching, brushing, or application of cool or warm stimuli that normally is not considered painful)
  - hyperpathia ("associated with an increased reaction to a stimulus, especially a repetitive stimulus, and a decreased threshold"; pain is often described as explosive) (Fine, 2009; Sips & Karapas, 2010)
- generally does *not* respond well to opioids (Backonja, 2003; Fine, 2009; Nicholson & Verma, 2004; Zhang & Baccei, 2009)

Although the underlying pathologies may differ among the various NP syndromes, the pain symptomatology is similar. In addition to the pain itself, marked interference with quality of life (QOL) is common, impacting energy, sleep, appetite, mobility, activity, socialization, concentration and affect, and outlook on life. Depression and anxiety are common comorbidities (Backonja, 2003; Nicholson & Verma, 2004; Sadosky, McDermott, Brandenburg, & Strauss, 2008). Postherpetic neuralgia (PHN) and painful diabetic neuropathy (DN) are included under the umbrella of NP syndromes. Because PHN and DN are commonly seen among older adults, they are discussed in this chapter.

IMPACT OF NP ON QOL

NP compromises QOL, including function, interpersonal relationships, and socialization. Areas negatively impacted include the following:

- Physical activities and function (including mobility, exercise)
- Emotional functioning
- Integrity/quality of sleep
- Usual roles in life (O'Connor, 2009)

Economic Impact of NP

The societal costs of NP are incurred as a result of
- Direct medical care costs, with annual estimated costs for
  - DN and PHN ranging from $1,600 to $7,000 per person
  - Excess costs with DN and PHN ranging from $1,000 to $8,000
  - PHN-specific costs ranging from $2,100 to more than $5,000
  - Diagnostic and care, including medications and interventional procedures
- Inability of caregivers to continue to work
- Possible more frequent institutionalization
- Increased costs related to assistance with living (Dworkin, Panarites, Armstrong, Malone, & Pham, 2011; Dworkin, White, O'Connor, Baser, & Hawkins, 2007; O'Connor, 2009)

Clinical Assessment of NP

In the absence of a gold standard for diagnosing NP, the Neuropathic Pain Special Interest Group (NeuPSIG) recently (2011) published guidelines for clinical assessment of NP that include patient interview, validated screening tools specific to NP in general, clinical evaluation/examination, quantitative sensory testing, pain assessment, psychological assessment, and functional assessment. The following information is based on those guidelines.

- *Patient interview* is the starting point. Ask the older adult to describe symptoms and pain. The OLD CARTS (Chapter 3) pneumonic can be helpful. In addition to the location, intensity, onset, and any potential originating factors (i.e., illness, trauma) can be important.

> *Pearl* Words frequently used to describe NP are "shooting," "tingling," and "burning."

- *Screening of NP* is important and can be done using one of several screening tools. It is important to remember that not all tools are validated in all languages. In addition, approximately 10% to 20% of patients clinically diagnosed with NP are not identified through screening tools. Table 17.1 includes screening tools discussed in the NeuPSIG guidelines (see also Chapter 4).

■ *Clinical evaluation/examination* is a basic and important part of assessment.

Attal et al. (2008) reported that, with the exception of PHN, clinical manifestations were "trans-etiological" (similar regardless of differing etiologies). They found that burning pain and allodynia particularly in response to brush strokes were present in 90% of the subjects with PHN, but they did not demonstrate deep pain or parasthesia or dysesthesia. These differences may account for differences in response of PHN to some medications used for NP. PHN responds well to capsaicin but does not respond well to some oral preparations.

■ Although no clinical examination can prove pain to be neuropathic in origin, it is important to identify support that there is an alteration in function of the nervous system. Clinical exam should include *assessment of somatosensory function* in the various dermatomes that includes the following:
  ■ Tactile (hypoesthesia is discriminant)
  ■ Pinprick (hypoalgesia is discriminant)
  ■ Thermal (hot and cold)
  ■ Vibration via tuning fork
  ■ Changes from normal can be demonstrated as
    ■ quantitative (hyposensitivity or hypersensitivity)
    ■ qualitative
      ■ allodynia: sensitivity to painless stimuli especially brush and cold
      ■ dysesthesia: unpleasant abnormal sensation
      ■ hyperalgesia: increased sensitivity to painful stimuli
    ■ temporal (after sensations or summations)
    ■ spatial (dyslocalization or radiation of sensations)

■ All atypical findings should be compared with the contralateral area, yet it is not uncommon for there to be bilateral sensory abnormalities (i.e., PHN). *Quantitative sensory testing* can be included in the clinical evaluation but cannot be used to estimate the location of a lesion or malfunction. (Arnstein, 2010; Bennett, 2001; Bennett, et al, 2007; Bouhassira, et al, 2004; Bouhassira, et al, 2005; Cox & Karapas, 2010; Gilron, et al, 2006; Haanpää, et al., 2011.)

Table 17.1 ■ *Neuropathic Pain Assessment Tools*

Tool	Description	Psychometric Information	Miscellanous
Leeds Assessment of Neuropathic Symptoms and Signs (LANSS)	5 symptom items; 2 clinical exam items	Specificity 82%–91% compared with clinical diagnosis; Sensitivity 80%–94% compared with clinical diagnosis	The S-LANSS is a self-report version of this tool
The Neuropathic Pain Questionnaire (NPQ)	10 sensation or sensory questions; 2 questions regarding affect	Research suggests that it may differentiate between neuropathic and nonneuropathic pain; Sensitivity is 66% Specificity is 74%	Tool is long; computations are complicated
Doleur neuropathique en 4 questions (DN4)	7 items related to symptoms; 3 items related to clinical examination	Validated in French, Spanish, Thai Sensitivity is 83% Specificity is 90%	Widely used in research and clinical settings; Easy to score; Translated into 15 languages including English
painDE-TECT	Self-report 9 items (7 weighted sensory descriptor and 2 spatial and temporal); no clinical component	Validated in German	Translated into 22 languages, including English
ID-Pain	5 sensory descriptor items; 1 question regarding joint in; no clinical component		

Sources: This information is based upon information found in the following: From Arnstein, 2010; "The LANSS Pain Scale: The Leeds assessment of neuropathic symptoms and signs," by M. I. Bennett, 2001, *Pain, 92*, pp. 147–157; "Using screening tools to identify neuropathic pain," by M. I. Bennett, N. Attal, M. M. Backonja, R. Baron, D. Bouhassira, R. Freynhagen, T. S. Jensen, 2007, *Pain, 127*, pp. 199–203; Bouhassira et al., 2005; and "NeuPSIG guidelines on neuropathic pain assessment," by M. Haanpää, N. Attal, M. Backonja, R. Baron, M. Bennett, D. Bouhassira, R. D. Treede, 2011, *Pain, 152*, pp. 14–27.

■ A thorough *pain assessment* as outlined in Chapter 3 must be part of the assessment of any NP. Consideration should also be given to the *psychosocial, functional,* and *QOL impacts* (see Chapter 2) (Cox & Karapas, 2010; Haanpää et al., 2011).

■ *Reassessment* of the older person following treatment should be done on a regularly scheduled basis
  ■ with time intervals depending on the pharmacokinetics of medications used
  ■ to determine response to interventions
  ■ to detect adverse effects so that early intervention can be accomplished

MULTIMODAL NP MANAGEMENT

NP is very difficult to manage. The challenges in managing it in older adults include the following:

■ Identification of particular NP mechanisms
■ Selection of appropriate analgesia with the particular pain mechanism
■ Evaluation and consideration of current medications and potential interactions
■ Evaluation and consideration of the side effect profiles of medications
■ Assess and treat associated comorbidities (Nicholson & Verma, 2004).

Medications need to be used cautiously with older adults. Safety has not been established for long-term use of some medications in older adults who have NP. Although methadone and tramadol must be used guardedly in older adults (see Chapter 7), small doses of these opioids have been effective in the treatment of NP (American Geriatrics Society [AGS], 2009; Fine, 2009; McGeeney, 2009).

In 2010, the NeuPSIG of the IASP supported development of evidenced-based guidelines for the pharmacological treatment of NP. That same year, the European Federation of Neurological Societies (EFNS) Task Force updated their pharmacological treatment guidelines for NP. In 2011, the American Academy of Neurology (AAN) published guidelines. The pharmacological management information for PHN and DN outlined in this chapter are based on those guidelines in conjunction with the 2009 AGS Guidelines for Management of Persistent Pain in Older Adults. Additional resources are cited as appropriate.

Pearl	In older adults, it is imperative to assess for comorbidities, concomitant medications, and potential side effects when administering medications for NP.

POSTHERPETIC NEURALGIA

PHN is pain that continues or recurs at the site of a healed herpes zoster (HZ) rash. The rash and subsequent neuralgia can occur along any dermatome but is most common in the mid to low thoracic region or along the ophthalmic branch of the trigeminal nerve. Diagnosis is made when pain continues after the HZ rash disappears. PHN is often described as pain that occurs 1 month or 3 months following the onset of the rash or at the time of healing of the rash. It has also been considered to be a continuation of HZ pain rather than as a separate pain entity. Once it develops, PHN can last for months or even years. PHN can be refractory to usual treatments and is recognized as one of the most challenging pain conditions to treat.

Prevalence reports vary, depending on the definition of PHN from time and severity perspectives. It is estimated that, in the United States, approximately 1 million people are diagnosed with HZ. As many as 30% will develop HZ at some point in time and 50% among those who are 65 years of age or older. The range of PHN prevalence among patients 3 months after HZ is from 7% to 27%. Prevalence increases with age, with as many as 50% of those who are 70 years of age and older having PHN lasting at least 1 year (Christo, Hobelmann, & Maine, 2007; Dworkin & Schmader, 2003; Dworkin et al., 2007; Oster, Harding, Dukes, Edelsberg, & Cleary, 2005; Sadosky et al., 2008; Schmader, 2002).

Frequently agreed upon risk factors for developing PHN include the following:
- Older age
- Limitation in usual activities before developing HZ
- More severe pain during the acute phase of HZ
- More severe rash

- In addition, the risk of developing PHN increases markedly with age:
  - Risk among those younger than 60 is 5%.
  - Risk among those 60 to 69 is 10%.
  - Risk among those 70 and older is 19%.

Less frequently identified risk factors are prodromal pain, being female, living alone, socializing less, and more somatic symptoms (Drolet et al., 2010; Jung, Johnson, Griffin, & Dworkin, 2004; Katz et al., 2005).

Pharmacological Management of PHN Pain

Frequently acetaminophen, nonsteroidal anti-inflammatory drugs, and opioids are not considered effective in controlling the pain involved with PHN (Oster et al., 2005).

Antiviral therapy is the treatment of choice for HZ. It is also found to be prophylactic to manage the severity and duration of PHN. Prompt antiviral therapy, within 72 hours of onset of the HZ lesions, with acyclovir, famciclovir, or valacyclovir has been associated with less severe illness and less severe pain over time and a shorter duration of PHN among older patients. Even when treatment is begun later than 72 hours, evidence indicates that there is benefit (Christo et al., 2007; Drolet et al., 2010; Katz et al., 2005; Li et al., 2009). The most common antiviral medications are outlined in Table 17.2.

In 2010, the EFNS Task Force updated the pharmacological recommendations for treatment of PHN. The medications recommended by the EFNS as first-, second- and third-line medications are listed in Table 17.3.

Although the EFNS listed the category of tricyclic antidepressants (TCAs) as the first medication for use with PHN, they did

Table 17.2 ■ *Antiviral Medications Used to Treat HZ*

Name of Antiviral	Dose (mg)	Daily Frequency	Duration (Days)
Valaciclovir	1,000	3×	7
Famiclovir	500	3×	7
Acyclovir	800	5×	7–10

Source: From "Post-herpetic neuralgia in older adults," by P. J. Christo, G. Hobelmann, & D. N. Maine, 2007, *Drugs Aging, 24*, pp. 1–19.

Table 17.3 ■ *Medications with EFNS Level of Efficacy Recommended by the EFNS for Treatment of PHN*

Recommended As First-, Second-, or Third-Line Use	Medication	Cautions	Miscellanous
First	Gabapentin		FDA approved for NP[a]; Few drug–drug interactions
First	Pregabalin	Can cause dizziness, somnolence, and dry mouth	FDA approved for NP[a]; Few drug–drug interactions
First	Lidocaine Topical 5% patch		FDA approved for NP[a]
First	TCA[b]	Nortriptyline and desipramine are the safest TCAs to use with older adults	
Second	Capsaicin cream or patches		
Second	Opioids		

Sources: From "The management of persistent pain in older adults," by American Geriatrics Society, 2002, *Journal of the American Geriatrics Society, 50*, pp. S205–S224; "Pharmacological management of persistent pain in older adults," by American Geriatrics Society, 2009, *Journal of the American Geriatrics Society, 57*, pp. 1331–1346; "EFNS guidelines on the pharmacological treatment of neuropathic pain: 2010 revision," by N. Attal, G. Cruccu, R. Baron, M. Haanpää, P. Hansson, T. S. Jensenand, & T. Nurmikko, 2010, *European Journal of Neurology, 17*, pp. 1113–1123; "Pregabalin for peripheral neuropathic pain: A multicenter, enriched enrollment randomized withdrawal placebo controlled trial," by I. Gilron, D. Wajsbrot, F. Therrien, & J. Lemay, 2011, *Clinical Journal of Pain, 27*, pp. 185–193; "Pharmacological management of neuropathic pain in older adults: An update on peripherally and centrally acting agents," B. E. McGeeney, 2009, *Journal of Pain and Symptom Management, 38*, pp. S15–S27; and "Topical medications in the treatment of pain," by M. L. Moody, 2010, *Pain Medicine News, 8*, pp. 15–21.

[a]FDA= Food and Drug Administration; NP = Neuropathic Pain

[b]TCA must be used with caution in older adults; amitryptiline is not recommended for older adults

not specify medications. The anticholinergic effects of TCAs require them to be used with caution in older adults. The reader is referred to Chapters 8 and 9 for a detailed discussion of the medications and side effects. Of note are the anticholinergic effects of orthostatic hypotension that can lead to falls, cardiac arrhythmias, and constipation. If TCAs are used, nortriptyline and desipramine have been recommended as preferred agents in older adults (AGS, 2009; Attal et al., 2010; McGeeney, 2009).

The reader is referred to Chapters 7, 8, and 9 for specific information regarding the medications discussed in this chapter.

General points to consider regarding pharmacological treatment of PHN are as follows:

- Gabapentin and pregabalin have demonstrated effectiveness with PHN.
- Lidoderm patches were considered as a first-line intervention for PHN in older adults, despite the need for further research.
- TCAs are also listed as first-line interventions for PHN;
  - however, they must be used with caution in older adults, and
  - if TCAs are used, nortriptyline and desipramine are preferred for older adults.
- Capsaicin cream and patches along with opioids are considered effective.
- When PHN pain is refractory the following may be considered:
  - corticosteroids, including administration via the epidural and intrathecal routes
  - sympathetic blockade (AGS, 2002, 2009; Attal et al., 2010; Christo et al., 2007; Duhmke, Cornblath, & Hollingshead, 2004; Fine, 2009; McGeeney, 2009; Skinner, Epstein, & Pappagallo, 2009)

Nonpharmacological Interventions for PHN

Interventional procedures utilized in the management of PHN include the following:

- Implantable medication delivery systems (see Chapter 10)
- Nerve and trigger point injections (see Chapter 10)
- Spinal cord stimulation (see Chapter 10)
- Transcutaneous electrical nerve stimulation (see Chapter 12)
- Acupuncture (see Chapter 10) (Dworkin et al., 2011)

Complementary Therapies for the Management of PHN

Many of the complementary modalities discussed in Chapter 11 can be used to help manage the pain of PHN. In addition, benzydamine, geranium, and peppermint oil used topically have been used to manage PHN. Although they are thought to be low-risk interventions, there is no evidence to support their use with PHN (Christo et al., 2007).

Pearls

An important caution is that all topical preparations should be used only as directed and should be tried cautiously in small amounts on small areas of skin in older adults.

Many aromatherapy oils should not be applied directly to skin.

DIABETIC NEUROPATHY

DN can be manifested in an acute presentation but is most commonly seen as a chronic pain condition. It occurs in older adults living with diabetes who are not dependent on insulin as well as those who are dependent on insulin. From the National Health and Nutrition Examination Survey, it is estimated that 16% to 47% of people with diabetes have DN and that in the United States, 28.5% of middle- and older-aged adults who live with diabetes have peripheral neuropathy (AAN, 2011; Gregg et al., 2004).

The most common of the chronic DNs is painful diabetic peripheral neuropathy for which there has been the most focus and data. Available data suggest that the incidence of DN increases with

- age
- duration of diabetes
- worsening of glucose tolerance (Davies, Brophy, Williams, & Taylor, 2006; Sadosky et al., 2008)

In 2010, the EFNS Task Force updated the pharmacological recommendations for treatment of DN. The medications recommended by the EFNS as first-, second-, and third-line medications are listed in Table 17.4. The reader is referred to Chapters 7, 8, and 9 for specific information regarding use of the medications with older adults AGS, 2002, 2009; Attal et al., 2010; Davies et al., 2006; Duhmke et al., 2004; McGeeney, 2009; Skinner et al., 2009).

Table 17.4 ■ *Medications with AAN and EFNS Levels of Efficacy Recommended by Both the AAN and the EFNS for Treatment of Diabetic NP[a]*

AAN Recommended As A or B	EFNS Recommended As First-, Second-, or Third-Line Use	Medication	AAN Recommended Dose[b]	Cautions	Miscellaneous
A	First	Pregabalin	300–600 mg/day	Can cause dizziness, somnolence, and dry mouth	FDA approved for NP[c]; Few drug–drug interactions
B	First	Duloxetine	60–20 mg/day	Use with caution in medications that are inhibited or metabolized by the CYP1A2 and CYPeD6 class of cytochrome P450 enzymes; Avoid in older adults with heavy alcohol consumption	FDA approved for NP[c]
B	First	Gabapentin	900–3600 mg/day		
B	First	TCA[c]		Nortriptyline and desipramine are the safest TCAs to use with older adults	FDA approved for NP[b]; Few drug–drug interactions

B	First	Venlafaxine ER	75–225 mg/day		
B	Second	Opioids			
B	Second	Tramadol	210 mg/day (EFNS recommended starting dose for older adults is 12.5–25 mg every 4–6 h)	Caution with older adults at risk for seizure activity or with history of seizure activity; To prevent development of serotonin syndrome, avoid in older adults being treated with selective serotonin reuptake inhibitors	Analgesic effect of tramadol can be reduced by administration of ondansetron, which is a selective serotonin-3 antagonist

Sources: From "Evidence-based guideline: Treatment of painful diabetic neuropathy," by American Academy of Neurology, 2011, *Neurology, 76,* pp. 1758–1765; From "The management of persistent pain in older adults," by American Geriatrics Society, 2002, *Journal of the American Geriatrics Society, 50,* pp. S205–S224; "Pharmacological management of persistent pain in older adults," by American Geriatrics Society, 2009, *Journal of the American Geriatrics Society, 57,* pp. 1331–1346; "EFNS guidelines on the pharmacological treatment of neuropathic pain: 2010 revision," by N. Attal, G. Cruccu, R. Baron, M. Haanpää, P. Hansson, T. S. Jensenand, & T. Nurmikko, 2010, *European Journal of Neurology, 17,* pp. 1113–1123; "Tramadol for neuropathic pain," by R. M. Duhmke, D. D. Cornblath, & J. R. Hollingshead, 2004, *Cochrane Database Systematic Review, 2,* CD003726; "Pregabalin for peripheral neuropathic pain: A multicenter, enriched enrollment randomized withdrawal placebo controlled trial," by I. Gilron, D. Wajsbrot, F. Therrien, & J. Lemay, 2011, *Clinical Journal of Pain, 27,* pp. 185–193; "Pharmacological management of neuropathic pain in older adults: An update on peripherally and centrally acting agents," by B. E. McGeeney, 2009, *Journal of Pain and Symptom Management, 38,* pp. S15–S27; and "Tramadol," by D. J. Skinner, J. Epstein, & M. Pappagallo, In *Current therapy in pain* (pp. 508–512), by H. S. Smith (Ed.), 2009, Philadelphia, PA: Saunders Elsevier. Adapted with permission.

[a] There are additional medications (sodium valporate, dexstromethrophan, capsaicin) that are recommended by the AAN but not recommended by the EFNS. and Dosages are those recommended by the AAN for DN pain and need to be adjusted for the individual older adult.

[b] FDA= Federal Drug Administration; NP = Neuropathic Pain.

[c] TCA must be used with caution with older adults; amitryptiline is not recommended.

The reader is referred to Chapters 7, 8, and 9 for specific information regarding the medications. Recommended first-line medications for the treatment of DN that are most appropriate for older adults include the following:

- Pregabalin
- Gabapentin alone or with morphine
- Duloxitine
- Venlafaxine ER

Recommended first-line medications that should be used with caution with older adults include

- TCAs (nortriptyline and desipramine are preferred with older adults)

Recommendations for second- or third-line medications include

- Opioids (cautions include dizziness, pruritus, sedation, respiratory depression)

  Tramadol alone or with acetaminophen (caution for dizziness, and contraindicated in individuals with a seizure history or at risk for seizures) (AAN, 2011; AGS, 2002, 2009; Attal et al., 2010).

Nonpharmacological Treatments for DN

Percutaneous electrical nerve stimulation (PENS) (Chapter 10) has been reported to have variable effects with DN. One study reported a marked (42%) reduction in pain, another study reported PENS plus amitryptiline had greater benefit than the medication alone but no effect was reported in a third study (AAN, 2011).

A low-fat, high-fiber diet combined with exercise is an important recommendation. In one small study, the majority of patients with DN who followed such a low fat, high fiber vegetarian diet no longer had NP at more than 1-year follow-up (Lee & Raja, 2011).

Alpha ipoic acid (ALA) is an antioxidant found in green vegetables (e.g., spinach, broccoli) as well as liver. It is believed to improve the pathophysiology of nerves. In one multicenter trial, ALA in dosage of 600 mg/day was found to be beneficial in alleviating pain of DN. It has been used in Germany for the treatment of DN for many years and is available over the counter in the United States. Side effects include gastrointestinal symptoms, pruritus, and rash (Lee & Raja, 2011).

INTERDISCIPLINARY TEAM MEMBERS AND CONSULTANTS

NP is complicated and challenging. Utilizing a variety of health care team members and consultants can be most helpful. Some specialists to involve in care are

- Pain management specialist
- Neurologist
- Rehabilitation experts
  - Physical therapists
  - Occupational therapists
- Psychiatry
- Complementary health care practitioners

GUIDELINES

American Academy of Neurology (AAN) (2011). Evidence-based guideline: Treatment of painful diabetic neuropathy. *Neurology, 76,* 1758–1765.

American Geriatrics Society (AGS) (2002). The management of persistent pain in older adults. *Journal of the American Geriatrics Society, 50,* S205–S224.

American Geriatrics Society (AGS) (2009). Pharmacological management of persistent pain in older adults. *Journal of the American Geriatrics Society, 57,* 1331–1346.

EFNS guidelines on the pharmacological treatment of neuropathic pain: 2010 revision. (2010). *European Journal of Neurology, 17,* 1113–1123.

NeuPSIG guidelines on neuropathic pain assessment. (2011). *Pain, 152,* 14–27.

Case Study

Mary Green is a 78-year-old woman. In addition to osteoarthritis in her knees and hypertension, 3 years ago she was diagnosed with a benign, slow-growing brain tumor. Today, Mary presents in the clinic complaining of "this terrible burning feeling in my left side and the middle of the left side of my back." She tells you that it hurts to have clothes touch that area. She tells you that the pain is awful and she does not understand why because the only thing she can see in the mirror are a few little pimples?

Questions

1. What do you think is going on with Mary?
2. What risk factors does Mary have for HPN?
3. What assessments are needed to determine a diagnosis?
4. What medications are appropriate for Mary to use for the pain in her rib area?
5. Should Mary be on other medications now?
6. What medications are appropriate for Mary if she develops PHN?
7. What concerns do you have for Mary using other medications? Why?

REFERENCES

American Academy of Neurology. (2011). Evidence-based guideline: Treatment of painful diabetic neuropathy. *Neurology, 76,* 1758–1765.

American Geriatrics Society. (2002). The management of persistent pain in older adults. *Journal of the American Geriatrics Society, 50,* S205–S224.

American Geriatrics Society. (2009). Pharmacological management of persistent pain in older adults. *Journal of the American Geriatrics Society, 57,* 1331–1346.

Arnstein, P. (2010). *Clinical coach for effective pain management.* Philadelphia, PA: F.A. Davis Company.

Attal, N., Cruccu, G., Baron, R., Haanpää, M., Hansson, P., Jensenand, T. S., & Nurmikko, T. (2010). EFNS guidelines on the pharmacological treatment of neuropathic pain: 2010 revision. *European Journal of Neurology, 17,* 1113–1123.

Attal, N., Fermanian, C., Fermanian, J., Lanteri-Minet, M., Alchaar, H., & Bouhassira, D. (2008). Neuropathic pain: Are there distinct subtypes depending on the aetiology or anatomical lesion? *Pain, 138,* 343–353.

Backonja, M. M. (2003). Defining neuropathic pain. *Anesthesia and Analgesia, 97,* 785–790.

Bennett, M. I. (2001). The LANSS Pain Scale: The Leeds assessment of neuropathic symptoms and signs. *Pain, 92,* 147–157.

Bennett, M. I., Attal, N., Backonja, M. M., Baron, R., Bouhassira, D., Freynhagen, R., Jensen, T. S. (2007). Using screening tools to identify neuropathic pain. *Pain, 127,* 199–203.

Bouhassira, D., Attal, N., Alchaar, H., Boureau, F., Brochet, B., Bruxelle, J., Vicaut, E. (2005). Comparison of pain syndromes associated with nervous somatic lesions and development of a new neuropathic pain diagnostic questionnaire (DN4). *Pain, 114,* 29–36.

Bouhassira, D., Attal, N., Fermanian, J., Alchaar, H., Gautron, M., Masquelier, E., Boureau, F. (2004). Development and validation of the Neuropathic Pain Symptom Inventory. *Pain, 108,* 248–257.

Christo, P. J., Hobelmann, G., & Maine, D. N. (2007). Post-herpetic neuralgia in older adults. *Drugs Aging, 24,* 1–19.

Cox, D. S., & Karapas, E. T. (2010). Taxonomy for pain management nursing. In B. St. Marie (Ed.), *Core curriculum for pain management nursing* (2nd ed., pp. 9–25). Dubuque, IA: Kendal Hunt.

Davies, M., Brophy, S., Williams, R., & Taylor, A. (2006). The prevalence, severity, and impact of painful diabetic peripheral neuropathy in type 2 diabetes. *Diabetes Care, 29,* 1518–1522.

Drolet, M., Brisson, M., Schmader, K., Levin, M., Johnson, R., Oxman, M., Mansi, J. A. (2010). Predictors of postherpetic neuralgia among patients with herpes zoster: A prospective study. *The Journal of Pain, 11,* 1211–1221.

Duhmke, R. M., Cornblath, D. D., & Hollingshead, J. R. (2004). Tramadol for neuropathic pain. *Cochrane Database Systematic Review, (2),* CD003726.

Dworkin, R. H., Panarites, C. J., Armstrong, E. P., Malone, D. C., & Pham, S. V. (2011). Healthcare utilization in people with postherpetic neuralgia and painful diabetic peripheral neuropathy. *Journal of the American Geriatrics Society, 59,* 827–836.

Dworkin, R. H., & Schmader, K. E. (2003). Treatment and prevalence of postherpetic neuralgia. *Clinics of Infectious Disease, 36,* 877–882.

Dworkin, R. H., White, R., O'Connor, A. B., Baser, O., & Hawkins, K. (2007). Healthcare costs of acute and chronic pain associated with a diagnosis of herpes zoster. *Journal of the American Geriatrics Society, 55,* 1168–1175.

Fine, P. (2009). Chronic pain management in older adults: Special considerations. *Journal of Pain and Symptom Management, 38,* S4–S14.

Gilron, I., Wajsbrot, D., Therrien, F., & Lemay, J. (2011). Pregabalin for peripheral neuropathic pain: A multicenter, enriched enrollment randomized withdrawal placebo controlled trial. *Clinical Journal of Pain, 27,* 185–193.

Gilron, I., Watson, P. N., Cahill, C. M., & Moulin, D. E. (2006). Neuropathic pain: A practical guide for the clinician. *Canadian Medical Association Journal, 175,* 265–275.

Gregg, E. W., Sorlie, P., Paulose-Ram, R., Gu, Q., Eberhardt, M. S., Wolz, M., Geiss, L. (2004). Prevalence of lower-extremity disease in the US adult population >=40 years of age with and without diabetes: 1999–2000 National Health and Nutrition Examination Survey. *Diabetes Care, 27,* 1591–1597.

Haanpää, M., Attal, N., Backonja, M., Baron, R., Bennett, M., Bouhassira, D., Treede, R. D. (2011). NeuPSIG guidelines on neuropathic pain assessment. *Pain, 152,* 14–27.

Jung, B. F., Johnson, R. W., Griffin, D. R., & Dworkin, R. H. (2004). Risk factors for postherpetic neuralgia in patients with herpes zoster. *Neurology, 62,* 1545–1551.

Katz, J., McDermott, M. P., Cooper, E. M., Walther, R. R., Sweeney, E. W., & Dworkin, R. H. (2005). Psychosocial risk factors for postherpetic neuralgia: A prospective study of patients with herpes zoster. *The Journal of Pain, 6,* 782–790.

Lee, F. H., & Raja, S. N. (2011). Complementary and alternative medicine in chronic pain. *Pain, 152,* 28–30.

Li, Q., Chen, N., Yang, J., Zhou, M., Zhou, D., Zhang, Q., & He, L. (2009). Antiviral treatment for preventing postherpetic neuralgia. *Cochrane Database Systematic Review, (2),* CD006866.

McGeeney, B. E. (2009). Pharmacological management of neuropathic pain in older adults: An update on peripherally and centrally acting agents. *Journal of Pain and Symptom Management, 38,* S15–S27.

Merskey, H., & Bogduk, N. (1994). *Classification of chronic pain: Descriptions of chronic pain syndromes and definitions of pain terms* (2nd ed.). Seattle, WA: IASP Press.

Moody, M. L. (2010). Topical medications in the treatment of pain. *Pain Medicine News, 8,* 15–21.

Nicholson, B., & Verma, S. (2004). Comorbidities in chronic neuropathic pain. *Pain Medicine, 5,* S9–S27.

O'Connor, A. B. (2009). Neuropathic pain: Quality-of-life impact, costs and cost effectiveness of therapy. *Pharmacoeconomics, 27,* 95–112.

Oster, G., Harding, G., Dukes, E., Edelsberg, J., & Cleary, P. D. (2005). Pain, medication use, and health-related quality of life in persons with postherpetic neuralgia: Results from a population-based survey. *The Journal of Pain, 6,* 356–363.

Sadosky, A., McDermott, A. M., Brandenburg, N. A., & Strauss, M. (2008). A review of the epidemiology of painful diabetic peripheral neuropathy, postherpetic neuralgia and less commonly studied neuropathic pain conditions. *Pain Practice, 8,* 45–56.

Schmader, K. E. (2002). Epidemiology and impact on quality of life of postherpetic neuralgia and painful diabetic neuropathy. *Clinical Journal of Pain, 18,* 350–354.

Skinner, D. J., Epstein, J., & Pappagallo, M. (2009). Tramadol. In H. S. Smith (Ed.), *Current therapy in pain* (pp. 508–512). Philadelphia, PA: Saunders Elsevier.

Treede, R. D., Jensen, T. S., Campbell, J. N., Cruccu, G., Dostrovsky, J. O., Griffin, J. W., Serra, J. (2008). Redefinition of neuropathic pain and a grading system for clinical use: Consensus statement on clinical and research diagnostic criteria. *Neurology, 70,* 1630–1635.

Zhang, J. M., & Baccei, M. L. (2009). Pathophysiology of pain. In H. S. Smith (Ed.), *Current therapy in pain* (pp. 4–8). Philadelphia, PA: Saunders Elsevier.

18

Central Poststroke Pain Syndrome

There is a common misconception that older adults who have experienced a cerebral vascular accident or stroke do not have pain, particularly if they have residual paralysis. Following a stroke, pain is common, with musculoskeletal and shoulder pain seen most frequently, followed by headache, spasticity, and central poststroke pain (CPSP) syndrome.

CPSP originates in the central nervous system (CNS) and is also known as Dejerine–Roussy syndrome, in recognition of those who first described it, and as thalamic pain-syndrome because the most common location for the pain inducing lesion is in the lateral thalamus. The current definition of CPSP is "pain arising as a direct consequence of a cerebrovascular lesion of the somatosensory system in the CNS" (Klit, Finnerup, Andersen, & Jensen, 2011, p. 818). CPSP is difficult to manage, interferes with rehabilitation efforts, socialization, function, and usual activities (Klit et al. 2011; Misra, Kalta, & Kumar, 2008).

EPIDEMIOLOGY

Epidemiology of CPSP is challenging to identify. It is estimated to occur in 1% to 12% of all patients who have had a stroke, but in as many as 18% of those who have sensory deficits (Klit, Finnerup, & Jensen, 2009). One Swedish study reported that among 140 older adults who had survived a stroke, 49% reported some pain, with 21% being related to the stroke and only 4 (3%) had CPSP (Lundström, Smits, Terént, & Borg, 2009). There are no relationships recorded with

- age,
- gender,

- time between stroke and CPSP,
- location of the lesion on the right or left, and
- if the lesion was hemorrhagic or ischemic.

Some studies indicate that when the lesion occurs in the thalamus or brain stem, pain is more severe, but other studies have negated those findings. As epidemiological information is scarce, it is not clear whether CPSP occurs rarely or if it is not well diagnosed (C 2009; Klit et al., 2009, 2011; Kumar, Kalita, Kumar, & Misra, 2009; Ramachandran, McGeoch, Williams, & Arcilla, 2007).

DIAGNOSIS

Diagnosis of CPSP is challenging and made by exclusion. Older adults who had a stroke often have comorbid diagnosis of chronic pain disorders, including neuropathic pain (NP), that complicate diagnosing CPSP. In one study, experts disagreed on diagnosis in 43% of the cases (Klit et al., & Jensen, 2011). The most severe presentation is considered by some as the classic one of harsh, never ending pain on the contralateral side. Even the location of pain is variable, with pain occurring in small isolated areas or an entire side of the body.

Although pain can be evoked during assessment, it frequently occurs spontaneously without warning. Approximately 85% of those afflicted by CPSP have spontaneous dysesthesia (abnormal and unpleasant sensation) or allodynia (pain in response to a stimulus that is not usually painful). When the spontaneous pain is prolonged, it has been described as burning, pricking, aching, freezing—compared with spontaneous pain that was intermittent, which was described as shooting or lacerating.

The following three conditions have been suggested as being essential to diagnose CPSP:

- History of a stroke with pain developing after the stroke onset
- Physiological pain that corresponds to a confirmed CNS lesion
- Nociceptive and peripheral NP unlikely causes

The following three additional factors are considered supportive to diagnose CPSP:

- Pain is not related primarily to movement, inflammation, or tissue damage.
- Description includes "burning," "painful cold," "electric shocks," "stinging," "pins and needles," "aching," and "pressing."

■ Touch or cold produce allodynia or dysesthesia (Greenspan, Ohara, Sarlani, & Lenz, 2004; Klit et al., 2009).

Multimodal analgesia management is important and similar to other NP syndromes. It is important to use multiple interventions because the few studies investigating the management of CPSP had small sample sizes but underscore that it is very difficult to treat. Currently, none of the medications or interventions listed is FDA-approved for CPSP. Further research is needed in this aspect. Many of the medications are not indicated for or should be used with caution in older adults. The reader is referred to Chapters 7, 8, and 9 for cautions using medications with older adults.

PHARMACOLOGICAL INTERVENTIONS

Currently, amitriptyline, lamotrigine, gabapentin, and pregabalin are considered first-line pharmacological treatments, with baclofen and selective serotonin reuptake inhibitors as secondary agents (Harvey, 2010).

■ *Tricyclic antidepressants (TCAs)* and amitriptyline in particular are considered a first-line medication with many NP situations and have been effective in treating CPSP (Dworkin et al., 2009); however, as previously noted (Chapters 8, 9, and 16), the anticholinergic effects of TCAs and amitriptyline in particular are a concern for older adults and amitriptyline is not recommended for use in older adults, (American Geriatrics Society, 2009).

■ *Anticonvulsants* have been effective in controlling peripheral NP, are promising with CPSP, and are suggested as being first-line medications along with TCAs for treatment of CPSP.

■ *Gabapentin* has not been officially studied with CPSP; however, one case study reported significant pain reduction after 2 weeks of therapy in a 45-year-old man whose CPSP had been refractory to other treatments (Stitik, Foye, Nadler, & Delisa, 2002).

■ *Pregabalin* was recently tested in a randomized placebo controlled study with 219 patients diagnosed with CPSP who averaged 59 years old. Although there was no statistically significant improvement in pain scores between the pregabalin and placebo groups, those who received pregabalin reported improved sleep, less anxiety, and sustained the pain relief they did report over at least 8 weeks compared with the placebo. That was comparable to earlier studies with amitriptyline (Kim et al., 2011). In an earlier study with 40 subjects with central NP pain, including some with CPSP, pregabalin was reported to relieve pain with statistical significance (Vranken et al., 2008).

■ *Lamotrigine* (200 mg/day) is an anti-glutaminergic preparation that is approved by the Federal Drug Administration as an anticonvulsant. It was reported to be effective in reducing pain intensity among 30 older adults diagnosed with CPSP. Reported side effects were generally mild (rash and headache), but severe pain was reported (Vestergaard, Andersen, Gottrup, Kristensen, & Jensen, 2001). In an earlier study it was given in higher doses (300 to 600 mg/day) with good results (Fese, Husstedt, Ringelstein, & Evers, 2006).

■ *Baclofen* administered in intrathecal (IT) boluses effectively relieved pain in four of five patients. Oral baclofen was not effective. Research is needed with IT baclofen infusions (Harvey, 2010).

■ *Intravenous lidocaine* has been effective in achieving reduction in pain for as long as 12 hours after infusion in small samples (Harvey, 2010). In another study, pain and allodynia were relieved for 45 minutes after infusion of lidocaine. A side effect of lightheadedness was common during and following infusion (Attal et al., 2000).

■ *Topical lidocaine* is **not** recommended to treat CPSP (Dworkin et al., 2009).

■ *Opioids* are generally not effective in managing CPSP, and they may even add to central sensitization (Willoch et al., 2004).

INTERVENTIONAL EFFORTS

■ *Vestibular caloric stimulation* (VCS) was effective in considerably reducing CPSP in two older patients for whom placebo interventions were not effective. The patients' ears were irrigated with water chilled to 4°C, and both had remarkable responses that lasted at least over several weeks. In a subsequent study with nine patients with CPSP, similar results in pain reduction were reported. It is believed that the benefit of VCS is an inhibition of pain generation in the anterior cingulate, through activation of the posterior insula. Replication and further research are needed in this aspect (McGeoch, Williams, Lee, & Ramachandran, 2008; Ramachandran et al., 2007).

■ *Deep brain stimulation (DBS)* was studied in 15 older adults who had refractory central NP averaging 5 years. Surgical stimulation was of the periventricular and periaqueductal gray areas and sensory thalamus. Average improvement in visual analog pain scores was 49%, with effectiveness seen in 70% of participants (Owen, Green, Stein, & Aziz, 2006). These results were more positive than a similar study of DBS in which benefit was noted in only 2 of 11 subjects and some had increased pain (Rasche, Rinaldi, Young, & Tronnier, 2006). Additional research is warranted.

- *Motor cortex stimulation (MCS)* has also had mixed results in patients with CPSP. Of seven older adults, three had reduction in pain that lasted from 1.5 to 4 years (Rasche, Ruppolt, Stippich, Unterberg, & Tronnier, 2006). These results were consistent with earlier studies. It is suggested that in CPSP, there may be an increased sensitivity of the motor cortex and perceptual system, thus complicating analgesia (Fukaya, Katayama, Kobayashi, Kasai, & Oshima, 2003). It is believed that MCS is more successful when motor function is intact, when the sensory threshold in the area of pain is not affected, and in patients with CPSP who have responded positively to infusions with ketamine but not IV morphine infusions (Harvey, 2010).

- *Spinal cord stimulation* (see Chapter 10) has had mixed results. A small study reported very favorable results with six patients of mixed ages (27 to 67) lasting 3 to more than 12 years. Additional research is needed (Lopez, Torres, Gala, & Iglesias, 2009).

- *Transcutaneous electrical nerve stimulation* (see Chapter 12) was tested in one study in which 4 of 15 participants reported reduction in pain averaging 42%, but five had increases in pain. Pain in the remaining six did not change (Harvey, 2010).

- *Acupuncture* has been used in rehabilitation efforts following a stroke, but it has rarely been used in older adults living with CPSP (Yen & Chan, 2003) (see Chapter 11).

NONPHARMACOLOGICAL AND COMPLEMENTARY INTERVENTIONS

- *Physical therapy (PT) and rehabilitation* are very important for the older adult suffering with CPSP (Klit et al., 2009). PT options are discussed in Chapter 12.

- *Stress management* through complementary techniques discussed in Chapter 11 can be beneficial to help manage the stress related to pain and disability. This is anticipated even though research may not have been conducted with the modality specifically with older adults living with PCSP. Music therapy, breathing, and relaxation techniques may be particularly helpful.

■ *Cognitive behavioral interventions*, including coping strategies, are recommended to augment other therapies (Klit et al., 2009).

Case Study

John Kane is a 72-year-old man who suffered a left-sided stroke 7 months ago. Since that time, he has sudden episodes of intense pain sporadically when anything touches his right arm. He describes the pain as being like very intense pins and needles, and it leaves a burning sensation that is the worst pain he has ever experienced. He has tried ibuprophen, hydrocodone with acetaminophen, morphine, and oxycodone, but none of them have helped the pain. His doctor has given him a prescription for pregabalin 75 mg to be taken three times a day.

Questions

1. What can you tell him about the pain he is experiencing?
2. How will you explain to him that the pregabalin may be helpful, even though the other medications were not helpful?
3. What cautions should you advise him about the pregabalin?

REFERENCES

American Geriatrics Society. (2009). Pharmacological management of persistent pain in older adults. *Journal of the American Geriatrics Society, 57,* 1331–1346.

Attal, N., Gaude, V., Brasseur, L., Dupuy, M., Guirim, F., Parker, F., & Bouhassira, D. (2000). Intravenous lidocaine in central pain: A double-blind, placebo-controlled, psychophysical study. *Neurology, 54,* 564–574.

Dworkin, R. H., O'Connor, A. B., Audette, J., Baron, R., Gourlay, G. K., Levy, R. M., & Wells, C. (2009). Recommendations for the pharmacological management of neuropathic pain: An overview and literature update. *Mayo Clinic Proceedings, 85,* S3–S14.

Fese, A., Husstedt, I. W., Ringelstein, E. B., & Evers, S. (2006). Pharmacologic treatment of central post-stroke pain. *Clinical Journal of Pain, 22,* 252–260.

Fukaya, C., Katayama, Y., Kobayashi, K., Kasai, M., & Oshima, H. (2003). Motor cortex stimulation in patients with post-stroke pain: Conscious somatosensory response and pain control. *Neurological Research, 25,* 153–156.

Greenspan, J. D., Ohara, S., Sarlani, E., & Lenz, F. A. (2004). Allodynia in patients with post-stroke central pain (CPSP) studied by statistical quantitative sensory testing within individuals. *Pain, 109,* 357–366.

Harvey, R. L. (2010). Central poststroke pain syndrome. *Topics in Stroke Rehabilitation, 17,* 163–172.

Kim, J. S., Bashford, G., Murphy, T. K., Martin, A., Dror, V., & Cheung, R. (2011). Safety and efficacy of pregabalin in patients with central post-stroke pain. *Pain, 152,* 1018–1023.

Klit, H., Finnerup, N. B., Andersen, G., & Jensen, T. S. (2011). Central poststroke pain: A population-based study. *Pain, 152,* 818–824.

Klit, H., Finnerup, N. B., & Jensen, T. S. (2009). Central post-stroke pain: Clinical characteristics, pathophysiology, and management. *Lancet Neurology, 8,* 857–868.

Kumar, B., Kalita, J., Kumar, G., & Misra, U. K. (2009). Central poststroke pain: A review of pathophysiology and treatment. *Anesthesia and Analgesia, 108,* 1645–1657.

Lopez, J. A., Torres, L. M., Gala, F., & Iglesias, I. (2009). Spinal cord stimulation and thalamic pain: Long-term results of eight cases. *Neuromodulation, 12,* 240–243.

Lundström, E., Smits, A., Terént, A., & Borg, J. (2009). Risk factors for stroke related pain 1 year after first-ever stroke. *European Journal of Neurology, 16,* 188–193.

Lušić, I. (2009). Central pain: Mechanisms, semiology and treatment. *Medical Sciences, 33,* 79–91.

McGeoch, P. D., Williams, L. E., Lee, R. R., & Ramachandran, V. S. (2008). Behavioral evidence for vestibular stimulation as a treatment for central post-stroke pain. *Journal of Neurology, Neurosurgery and Psychiatry, 79,* 1298–1301.

Misra, U. K., Kalta, J., & Kumar, B. (2008). A study of clinical magnetic resonance imaging, and somatosensory-evoked potential in central post-stroke pain. *Journal of Pain, 9*(12), 116–122.

Owen, S. L., Green, A. L., Stein, J. F., & Aziz, T. Z. (2006). Deep brain stimulation of post-stroke neuropathic pain. *Pain, 2006,* 202–206.

Ramachandran, V. S., McGeoch, P. D., Williams, L., & Arcilla, G. (2007). Rapid relief of thalamic pain syndrome induced by vestibular caloric stimulation. *Neurocase: The Neural Basis of Cognition, 13,* 185–188.

Rasche, D., Rinaldi, P. C., Young, R. F., & Tronnier, V. M. (2006). Deep brain stimulation for the treatment of various chronic pain syndromes. *Neurosurgical Focus, 21,* E8.

Rasche, D., Ruppolt, M., Stippich, C., Unterberg, A., & Tronnier, V. M. (2006). Motor cortex stimulation for long-term relief of chronic neuropathic pain: A 10 year experience. *Pain, 121,* 43–52.

Stitik, C. B., Foye, P. M., Nadler, S. F., & Delisa, J. A. (2002). Central post-stroke pain syndrome yet another use for gabapentin? *American Journal of Physical Medicine and Rehabilitation, 81,* 718–720.

Vestergaard, K., Andersen, G., Gottrup, H., Kristensen, B. T., & Jensen, T. S. (2001). Lamotrigine for central post-stroke pain: A randomized controlled trial. *Neurology, 56,* 184–190.

Vranken, J. H., Dijkgraaf, M. G., Kruis, M. R., van der Vegt, M. H., Hollmann, M. W., & Heesen, M. (2008). Pregabalin in patients with central neuropathic pain: A randomized double-blind, placebo-controlled trial of a flexible-dose regimen. *Pain, 136,* 150–157.

Willoch, F., Schindler, F., Wester, H. J., Empl, M., Straube, A., Schwaiger, M., Conrad, B., & Tölle (2004). Central poststroke pain and reduced opioid receptor binding within pain processing circuitries: A [^{11}C]diprenorphine PET study. *Pain, 108,* 213–220.

Yen, H. L., & Chan, W. (2003). An East-West approach to the management of central post-stroke pain. *Cerebrovascular Diseases, 16*(1), 27–30.

19

Facial Pain Associated with Temporal Arteritis or Trigeminal Neuralgia

Temporal arteritis (TA) is a panarteritis and the most frequent form of systemic vasculitis seen in older adults. Alternative names are giant cell arteritis (GCA) or cranial arteritis. It involves the adventitia, media, and intima of medium and large arteries. Etiology of this inflammatory disease is unknown, but *Chlamydia pneumoniae* was found in the majority of patients with TA in one small study, suggesting that it may play a role in the disease process (Wagoner et al., 2000).

Epidemiology is challenging to describe since there is little about TA in current literature, even when searched for the alternative names. In general, it is known that

- TA is rare; 18/100,000 or 0.00018% adults older than 50 years in the United States annually;
- US prevalence is 223/100,000 or 0.00223%;
- 72 years is the average age of onset;
- 95% of cases occur in those older than 50;
- older women are twice as likely to be diagnosed with TA; and
- incidence of TA in older patients who have polymyalgia rheumatica (PMR) but do not have clinical manifestations of TA is between 0% and 41% (American college of Rheumatology [ACR], 1990; Hellmann, 2002; Hoffman et al., 2002; Schmidt & Gromnica-Ihle, 2002).

Diagnosis of TA is based on symptoms, physical exam, and laboratory tests. Up to 40% have atypical presentations, including fever of unknown origin, respiratory symptoms (dry cough), and larger artery involvement. Prompt assessment and intervention are essential to prevent irreversible blindness.

- *Presenting symptoms* include new-onset localized (but at times diffused) headache, tender scalp, PMR, malaise, visual disturbances, claudication of the jaw and tongue, or deglutition. Visual impairment is a grave complication. Visual loss is not reversible.

- *Physical examination* reveals tender, indurated temporal artery with reduced pulse.
- *Laboratory tests* usually show
  - erythrocyte sedimentation rate greater than 50 mm/hour (in 89% of cases),
  - elevated platelet counts due to inflammation, and
  - normal values in other reports.
- *Surgically performed temporal artery biopsy* showing "necrotizing arteritis, characterized by a predominance of mononuclear cell infiltrates or granulomatous process with multinucleated giant cells" is diagnostic for TA (ACR, 1990, p. 1122).
- Ultrasonography has been reported as diagnostically effective for TA when concomitant with PMR (see Chapter 19) (Bruckenthal, 2009; British Society for Rheumatology and British Health Professionals in Rheumatology [BSR-BHPR], 2010; Hellmann, 2002; Schmidt & Gromnica-Ihle, 2002).
- *Treatment* for TA needs to be initiated promptly to prevent visual impairment and should be started empirically while diagnostics are pending.
- *Glucocorticosteroids* are the treatment for TA at least since Berger and Senders (1959) reported corticosteroid therapy was effective both to relieve symptoms and to stop progression of the process.
- *Recommended starting dose* is prednisone 40 to 60 mg daily as first-line treatment, to continue for at least 2 to 4 weeks before tapering.
- *Tapering* is recommended by Spiera and Spiera (2004) to be "approximately 3 mg every 3 days"; that can be slower if clinically indicated but not dependent on sedimentation rate that may be elevated for reasons other than TA.
- *Dose adjustment* may be needed for disease severity, side effects, and comorbidities.
- *Relapses* are reported in 27% to 62% of patients when dose is decreased, requiring glucocorticosteroids to continue for 1 to 5 years at same or increased dose; it is important to monitor older adults for indications of relapse.
- *Toxicity* concerns include fractures, infection, peripheral edema, myopathy, and cataracts; it can develop Cushing's syndrome and diabetes (Hoffman et al., 2002).
- *Precautions* include
  - screening for bone loss,
  - prophylactic calcium/vitamin D therapy,

■ possible bisphosphonate, and
■ monitor blood pressure, fluid retention, and glucose and cholesterol levels (American Geriatrics Society, 2009; BSR-BHPR, 2010; Spiera & Spiera, 2004).

Methotrexate (MTX) has been recommended as an adjuvant therapy (BSR-BHPR, 2010; Mahr et al., 2007; Spiera & Spiera, 2004). Although no evidence was found to support MTX effectiveness in two studies (Hoffman et al., 2002; Spiera et al., 2001), one placebo-controlled study reported some steroid-sparing benefit (Jover et al., 2001). A subsequent meta-analysis of the individual patients in those studies, however, concluded that low-dose MTX can be an effective corticosteroid-sparing addition for therapy with TA (Mahr et al., 2007) and is considered a second-line alternative when steroids are not an option (Kawasaki & Purvin, 2009).

Low-dose aspirin is recommended unless contraindicated (BSR-BHPR, 2010; Kawasaki & Purvin, 2009). It is important to note, however, aspirin is *not* advised for use in older adults (America Pain Society, 2003). Since aspirin and steroids are individually associated with gastrointestinal (GI) bleeding, the combination increases the risk (Carroll, Gaskin, & Danesh-Meyer, 2006).

Pain management was not specifically addressed in any of more than 100 references consulted using "TA," "GCA," or "cranial arteritis." It is presumed that this is because the documents focused on management and treatment of the disorder and that it is expected that as the corticosteroids improve the inflammation, the pain will subside. Pain relief is yet another reason that prompt steroid treatment is essential.

It is reasonable to treat the pain symptomatically, considering the type of pain described, comorbidities of the older patient, and potential side effects of medications.

Nonpharmacological and complementary interventions are also recommended. Possible benefit can be obtained through cold packs or heat, breathing exercises, progressive muscle relaxation, music therapy, distraction therapy, or other cognitive behavioral interventions. The reader is referred to Chapter 11 for more information on complementary options.

Trigeminal Neuralgia

Trigeminal neuralgia (TGN), which was previously known as tic douloureux, can either be "classical" or "symptomatic." In both cases TGN affects, and is experienced along, one or more divisions of the trigeminal nerve route. It is typically unilateral and character-ized by brief, "electric shock-like" pains that are unexpected in both starting and stopping. Onset can be spontaneous or triggered by normal activities of daily living involving the face. Trigger areas that may be particularly sensitive are in the nasolabial fold and chin. In older people, the most common cause (80%) of TGN is an artery or vein compressing the nerve root (IHS, 2005; Nurmikko & Eldridge, 2001).

EPIDEMIOLOGY

TGN is relatively rare and epidemiological data are scarce. The annual incidence of TGN is most frequently reported as 4 to 5 per 100,000 with a prevalence of 15 per 100,000 or 0.00015%. It occurs more frequently among women and older adults, with as many as 90% of the cases occurring in those who are 40 years of age or older; yet prevalence is higher (2%) among people diagnosed with multiple sclerosis. A study from the United Kingdom reported higher rates with 27 diagnoses of TGN per 100,000, again with the majority being older and female (Hall, Carroll, Parry, & McQuay, 2006). In a study with 82 subjects from six European countries, the average age was 63 but 46% were older than 65 years, and 67% were female (Devor, Amir, & Rappaport, 2001; Desimone et al., 2005; Rozen, 2001; Tolle, Dukes, & Sadosky, 2006).

Diagnosis

Diagnosis of TGN according to the International Headache Society [IHS] (2005) criteria includes the following:

- Paroxysmal pain lasts from 2 to 120 seconds and affects one or more divisions of the trigeminal nerve; there may or may not be aching between the paroxysms.
- Pain is "intense, sharp, superficial, or stabbing" and/or "precipitated from trigger areas by trigger factors."
- Episodes are always the same for each individual.
- No obvious neurological deficit exists clinically.

Classical TGN

■ Between paroxysms there are asymptomatic intervals.
■ No obvious neurological deficit exists.
■ There is no other etiology to account for the paroxysms and pain.
■ The pain frequently induces spasm of the facial muscle.

Symptomatic TGN

■ There are no symptomatic intervals between paroxysms.
■ "Causative lesion other than vascular compression," is identified.

Clinical evaluation, magnetic resonance imaging, and/or magnetic resonance angiography are needed to confirm diagnosis and rule out other etiologies, including TN, PHN, temporomandibular joint pain, dental pathology, cluster headaches, and "jabs and jolts syndrome." This is important because up to 30% of patients with TGN are misdiagnosed (Benoliel, Pertes, & Eliav, 2009; Bruckenthal, 2009; IHS, 2005; Nurmikko & Eldridge, 2001).

TREATMENT OPTIONS

Medications that have shown effectiveness, or that have been suggested to treat TGN, all have significant side effects that are of concern with older adults. Careful monitoring and intervention are needed when any of the medications are used.

■ *Carbamazepine* is considered as the first-line medication. Fifty-eight percent to 100% of study participants (see citations below) achieved marked to complete pain relief.

  ■ *Recommended daily dosing* is 200 mg/day initial dose and 400 to 1,200 mg/day maintenance; however, in older patients doses may need to be reduced.

  ■ It is *imperative* to consider the general condition, comorbidities, and sensitivities of the older adults and the side effects of sedation, cognitive impairment, ataxia, dizziness, leucopenia, diplopia, GI distress, Stevens–Johnson syndrome, and epidermal necrolysis.

■ *Oxcarbazepine* is reported as effective as carbamazepine in achieving relief.

  ■ *Recommended daily dosing* is 300 mg/day initial dose and 600 to 1800 mg/day maintenance; however, in older patients doses may need to be reduced.

  ■ Even though the side effects are less severe and not as significant as carbamazepine, consider the general condition, comorbidities, and sensitivities of the older adults and side effects of sedation, cognitive impairment, dizziness, and rash.

■ *Baclofen* was reported to be better than placebo in reducing the number of paroxysms daily. The side effects (sedation, ataxia, muscle weakness, and GI symptoms) are of concern.

■ *Lamotrigine* has shown benefit and promise. It is reported effective as an "add-on therapy"; however, side effects (somnolence, dizziness, and diplopia) are of concern in older adults.

■ *Levetiracetam* showed promise in one recent study but needs further investigation.

■ *Gabapentin, phenytoin, clonazepam, and valproate* have shown indications of being beneficial. They are recommended by some authors, but the American Academy of Neurology (AAN) and European Federation of Neurological Societies (EFNS) did not find adequate evidence to endorse their use (AAN & EFNS, 2010; Linn & Bajwa, 2009; Mitsikostas et al., 2010; Rozen, 2001).

SURGICAL INTERVENTIONS

■ *Microvascular decompression* is a surgical procedure in which the nerve is freed from the venous or arterial compression. In one retrospective study, pain relief and adverse event profile were identical for patients older than 70 years and those younger than 50 years. Pain relief ranges from 75% to 80% during the first 2 years and then 58% to 64% after 8 to 10 years. It is essential that older adults understand the risks and benefits of surgery prior to deciding on this option (Linn & Bajwa, 2009; Nurmikko & Eldridge, 2001).

■ *Percutaneous-controlled radiofrequency trigeminal rhizotomy* is a surgical procedure performed under sedation and analgesia since the cooperation of the patient is needed during the procedure. One of the three divisions of the trigeminal nerve is severed using thermistor electrodes. In one study of 1,600 patients (age 16 to 99 years), 76% required only one procedure, 98% of the participants had acute pain relief, and 58% of the half of the patients who were followed for 5 years continued to have pain relief. Pain control increased to 92% with multiple procedures. It is proposed to be safe and effective. Adverse events included impaired corneal reflex, keratitis, masseter dysfunction, chewing difficulties, painful dysesthesia, cranial nerve palsy, and cerebrospinal fluid leak (Kanpolat, Savas, Bekar, & Berk, 2001).

- *Balloon compression* is a percutaneous intervention in which the gasserian ganglion is compressed for 3 to 10 min with a catheter that is inflated. Immediate pain relief generally occurs, with approximately 91% continuing to have pain relief 6 months or longer and approximately 57% at 3 years. Complications involving cranial nerve and arterial injury, arteriovenous fistulae, and meningitis were more common than with other percutaneous procedures (Linn & Bajwa, 2009).
- *Cryotherapy* is a surgical procedure "in which a peripheral branch of the three major divisions of the trigeminal nerve is exposed and frozen by direct application of a cryoprobe." The results are not as effective as other surgical interventions. Infection and increased pain are complications. It is not a preferred intervention (Nurmikko & Eldridge, 2001, p. 126).

GUIDELINES AND RESOURCES

American Academy of Neurology and European Federation of Neurological Societies. (2010). Practice parameter: The diagnostic evaluation and treatment of TGN (an evidence-based review): Report of the Quality Standards Subcommittee of the American Academy of Neurology and the European Federation of Neurological Societies. *Neurology, 71,* 1183–1190.

British Society of Rheumatology and British Health Professionals in Rheumatology. (2010). BSR and BHP guidelines for the management of giant cell arteritis. *Rheumatology, 49,* 1594–1597.

International Headache Society. http://www.ihs-headache.org/

TNA the Facial Pain Association. http://www.fpa-support.org

Case Study

83-year-old Sue Vann presents today complaining of a sudden severe headache on the right side of her head for the last 2 days. She also reports some strange spasm-like pains on the right side of her face whenever she washes her face or brushes her teeth. She says that it hurts when she touches the right side of her face even lightly.

Questions

1. What examination and tests will you do to determine the cause of Sue's pain?
2. What medications, if any, will you start now?
3. Why will you start that/those medications?
4. What do you think is causing Sue's pain?
5. What long-term treatment is most appropriate for Sue?
6. What education will Sue and her family need?

REFERENCES

American Academy of Neurology and European Federation of Neurological Societies. (2010). Practice parameter: The diagnostic evaluation and treatment of trigeminal neuralgia (an evidence-based review): Report of the Quality Standards Subcommittee of the American Academy of Neurology and the European Federation of Neurological Societies. *Neurology, 71,* 1183–1190.

American College of Rheumatology. (1990). The American College of Rheumatology 1990 criteria for the classification of giant cell arteritis. *Arthritis & Rheumatism, 33,* 1122–1128.

American Geriatric Society. (2009). Pharmacological management of persistent pain in older adults. *Journal of the American Geriatric Society, 57,* 1331–1346.

American Pain Society. (2003). *Principles of analgesic use in the treatment of acute pain and cancer pain* (5th ed.). Glenview, IL: Author.

Benoliel, R., Pertes, R., & Eliav, E. (2009). Orofacial pain. In H. S. Smith (Ed.), *Current therapy in pain* (pp. 121–137). Philadelphia, PA: Saunders Elsevier.

Berger, E. H., & Senders, W. L. (1959). Temporal arteritis. *Journal of the American Medical Association, 171,* 1818–1822.

British Society of Rheumatology and British Health Professionals in Rheumatology. (2010). BSR and BHPR guidelines for the management of giant cell arteritis. *Rheumatology, 49,* 1594–1597.

Bruckenthal, P. (2009). Assessment of pain in the older adult. In H. S. Smith (Ed.), *Current therapy in pain* (pp. 14–24). Philadelphia, PA: Saunders Elsevier.

Carroll, S. C., Gaskin, B. J., & Danesh-Meyer, V. D. (2006). Giant cell arteritis. *Clinical and Experimental Ophthalmology, 34,* 159–173.

DeSimone, R., Marano, E., Brescia Morra, V., Raineri, A., Ripa, P., Esposito, M., & Bonavita, V. (2005). A clinical comparison of trigeminal neuralgic pain in patients with and without underlying multiple sclerosis. *Neurological Sciences, 26,* S150–S151.

Devor, M., Amir, R., & Rappaport, Z. H. (2001). Pathophysiology of trigeminal neuralgia: The ignition hypothesis. *The Clinical Journal of Pain, 18,* 4–13.

Hall, G. C., Carroll, D., Parry, D., & McQuay, H. J. (2006). Epidemiology and treatment of neuropathic pain: The UK primary care perspective. *Pain, 122,* 156–162.

Hellmann, D. B. (2002). Temporal arteritis: A cough, toothache, and tongue infarction. *Journal of the American Medical Association, 287,* 2996–3000.

Hoffman, G. S., Cid, M. C., Hellmann, D. B., Guillevin, L., Stone, J. H., Schousboe, J., Puechal, X. (2002). A multicenter, randomized, double-blind, placebo-controlled trial of adjuvant methotrexate treatment for giant cell arteritis. *Arthritis & Rheumatism, 46,* 1309–1318.

International Headache Society. (2005). *International classification of headache disorders* (2nd ed.). Retrieved June 13, 2011, from http://217.174.249.183/upload/CT_Clas/ICHD-IIR1final.pdf

Jover, J. A., Hernandez-Garcia, C., Morado, I. C., Vargas, E., Banares, A., & Fernandez-Guiterrez, B. (2001). Combined treatment of giant-cell arteritis with methotrexate and prednisone. A randomized double-blind, placebo-controlled trial. *Annals of Internal Medicine, 134,* 106–114.

Kanpolat, Y., Savas, A., Bekar, A., & Berk, C. (2001). Percutaneous controlled radiofrequency trigeminal rhizotomy for the treatment of idiopathic trigeminal neuralgia: A 25 year experience with 1600 patients. *Neurosurgery, 48,* 524–532.

Kawasaki, A., & Purvin, V. (2009). Giant cell arteritis: An updated review. *Acta Ophthalmologica, 87,* 13–32.

Linn, A., & Bajwa, Z. H. (2009). Trigeminal neuralgia. In H. S. Smith (Ed.), *Current therapy in pain* (pp. 256–261). Philadelphia, PA: Saunders Elsevier.

Mahr, A. D., Jover, J. A., Spiera, R. F., Hernandez-Garcia, C., Fernandez-Gutierrez, B., Lavalley, M. P., & Merkel, P. A. (2007). Adjunctive methotrexate for treatment of giant cell arteritis: An individual patient data meta-analysis. *Arthritis & Rheumatism, 56,* 1789–2797.

Mitsikostas, D. D., Pantes, G. V., Avramidis, T. G., Karageorgiou, K. E., Gatzonis, S. D., Stathis, P. G., & Vikelis, M. (2010). An observational trial to investigate the efficacy and tolerability of levetiracetam in trigeminal neuralgia. *Headache: The Journal of Head and Face Pain, 50,* 1371–1377.

Nurmikko, T. J., & Eldridge, P. R. (2001). Trigeminal neuralgia—pathophysiology, diagnosis and current treatment. *British Journal of Anaesthesia, 87,* 117–132.

Rozen, T. D. (2001). Antiepileptic drugs in the management of cluster headache and trigeminal neuralgia. *Headache: The Journal of Head and Face Pain, 41,* S25–S32.

Schmidt, W. A., & Gromnica-Ihle, E. (2002). Incidence of temporal arteritis in patients with polymyalgia rheumatica: A prospective study using colour Doppler ultrasonography of the temporal arteries. *Rheumatology, 41,* 46–52.

Spiera, R. F., Mitnick, H. J., Kupersmith, M., Richmond, M., Spiera, H., & Peterson, M. G. (2001). A prospective, double-blind, randomized, placebo controlled trial of methotrexate in the treatment of giant cell arteritis (GCA). *Clinical Experiments in Rheumatology, 19,* 218–223.

Spiera, R., & Spiera, H. (2004). Inflammatory disease in older adults: Cranial arteritis. *Geriatrics, 59,* 25–29.

Tolle, T., Dukes, E., & Sadosky, A. (2006). Patient burden of trigeminal neuralgia: Results from a cross-sectional survey of health state impairment and treatment patterns in six European countries. *Pain Practice, 6,* 153–160.

Wagoner, A. D., Gerard, H. C., Fresemann, T., Schmidt, W. A., Gromnica-Ihle, E., Hudson, A. P., & Zeidler, H. (2000). Detection of *Chlamydia pneumoniae* in giant cell vasculitis and correlation with the topographic arrangement of tissue-infiltrating dendritic cells. *Arthritis & Rheumatism, 43,* 1543–1551.

20

Rheumatological Conditions

Rheumatological or rheumatic conditions are considered "to be a large and growing public health problem" (National Arthritis Data Workgroup, 2008a, p. 15). Although older adults may suffer with the effects of many of these conditions, the two that are discussed in this chapter are rheumatoid arthritis (RA) and polymyalgia rheumatica, (PMR), because they are seen most frequently in older adults.

RHEUMATOID ARTHRITIS

RA is a chronic, systemic, inflammatory, destructive, autoimmune disorder that involves inflammatory cascades in multiple body systems. It is characterized by destructive synovitis, with swollen, tender joints, and damaged articular cartilage and bone. Consequences are pain, disability, and premature death. The disease course generally is one of painful acute episodes, alternating with periods of remission (Aletaha et al., 2010; American Pain Society [APS], 2002; Kennedy-Malone, Fletcher, & Plank, 2004; National Arthritis Data Workgroup, 2008a; Scott, Wolfe, & Huizinga, 2010; Watkins, Shifren, Park, & Morrell, 1999).

Epidemiology of RA

Approximately 0.5% to 1% of the population is afflicted with RA. Current estimates of the prevalence of RA in the United States is 1.3 million adults, which is significantly less than the 1995 estimate of 2.1 million. This reflects a continuation of a declining incidence that began in the early 1960s. In developed countries, the current incidence is estimated to be between 5 and 50 per 100,000 adults.

Although it is known to occur in all races, there is increased prevalence (3.5% to 5%) among Native Americans.

All indications are that it has evolved into a geriatric disorder. Although overall incidence and prevalence have declined in recent years, incidence increases with age, and prevalence is greatest in older women. The average age for prevalence of RA has increased from 66.3 years to 66.8 years (Aletaha et al., 2010; McAllister, Eyre, & Orozco, 2011; National Arthritis Data Workgroup, 2008a; Scott et al., 2010).

Etiology and Risk Factors of RA

The etiology of RA remains unknown; however, there seem to be complicated genetic factors involved. It is believed that these genetic factors combined with environmental risk factors lead to active disease.

Female gender is a significant risk factor. With age for both incidence and prevalence increasing, it has been suggested that perhaps hormonal features are involved in the pathology of RA.

The environmental risk factor for which there is the strongest evidence is smoking cigarettes. Other factors, that have been implicated, for which there is not much supporting confirmation, include coffee consumption, vitamin D status, oral contraceptive use, and low socioeconomic status (Lavelle, Lavelle, & Lavelle, 2009; McAllister et al., 2011; Scott et al., 2010; Symmons et al., 2002).

Diagnosis and Clinical Manifestations of RA

Early diagnosis is often challenging, and it is believed that if diagnosis could be made earlier, and treatment started earlier, much disability could be prevented. Diagnosis is generally based upon clinical presentation because there is no laboratory test that is diagnostic. However, there are generally a high number of white blood cells in aspirated synovial fluid. Generally, older patients who present with RA come with that diagnosis having been made previously.

With elderly onset RA, the older person may present with the following symptoms:

■ Gradually increasing morning stiffness
■ Pain and swelling in more than one joint
■ Larger joints (i.e., shoulders) more frequently involved
■ Low-grade fever

- Anorexia and weight loss
- Malaise

It is very important to ensure that an older person with new onset RA receives a timely referral to a rheumatologist. Initiation of disease-modifying antirheumatic drugs (DMARDs) is important with newly diagnosed RA. When begun within 3 months of diagnosis, DMARDs have been reported to modify the course of RA (Kennedy-Malone et al., 2004).

Clinical Manifestations

- Red, swollen, painful, stiff, warm joints, often with subcutaneous nodules
- Fatigue, malaise, and weakness
- Weight loss and wasting
- Anemia and thrombocytopenia
- Dry eyes and keratoconjunctivitis (Eliopoulos, 2001; Lavelle et al., 2009)

Pain Assessment in RA

As in all situations, a thorough pain assessment will guide the interventions that are most appropriate for the older person living with RA. Pain assessment needs to identify

- the location and intensity of the pain
- whether pain is chronic or part of an acute episode
- the words the older patient uses to describe the pain
- what has alleviated or aggravated the pain

The reader is referred to Chapters 3 and 5 for more specific information on pain assessment and tools that can be used.

The older patient with this disease must be carefully assessed not only for the characteristics and qualities of pain but also from a functional perspective. It is important to identify the effect of pain in such areas as

- what activities are limited
- how quality of life is impaired
- if anxiety and depression are comorbidities

Pharmacological Management

An important component of pain management is to ensure that the RA disease process is appropriately and adequately treated. Medications and pharmaceutical advances have dramatically improved the prognosis of RA during the last century. Generally, the approach to managing RA consists of DMARDs and biological agents, corticosteroids, and nonsteroidal anti-inflammatory drug (NSAID) medications (Kennedy-Malone et al., 2004).

■ *DMARDs* and *biological agents*, including TNF inhibitors (tumor necrosis factor inhibitors), are currently the cornerstone in treatment of RA. It is important to note that new medications are being introduced on a regular basis; consequently this may change in the future. Prescription, dosing, and management of those agents are beyond the scope of this chapter. When those medications are effective, pain is managed. For the older adult who is receiving those medications under the care of a rheumatologist, it is imperative for other HCPs to identify the medication and know the side effects and contraindications with any known comorbidities the older patient may have. The reader is referred to the American College of Rheumatology (2008) and the US Federal Drug Administration guidelines that are listed in the Resource and Guideline section in this chapter.

■ *Aspirin vs Acetaminophen:* Aspirin has been a basis for managing pain in people living with RA for years. Aspirin is not indicated for use with older adults because of side effects that include gastrointestinal (GI) bleeding. In agreement with the WHO ladder, the guidelines from the APS (2002) recommend acetaminophen for mild to moderate pain related to arthritis.

Cautions with acetaminophen are as follows:

■ It is imperative to remind all older adults and family members that there is a ceiling effect with acetaminophen and the total daily amount is restricted to no more than 4 g.

■ In the frail elderly, it is recommended that the total daily amount is 3 g.

■ Acetaminophen is contraindicated in older adults who
   ■ have comorbid liver disease
   ■ consume alcohol on a regular basis (American Geriatrics Society, 2009; APS, 2002)

■ *NSAIDs* are central to management of RA because a significant component of pain is due to inflammation. That can be challenging with older patients for whom NSAID use may be problematic. The reader is referred to Chapters 7 and 9 for more detailed information on analgesic medications and side effects.

NSAIDs are used for their anti-inflammatory action through the inhibition of prostaglandin synthesis. Although this is an important role in managing pain related to RA, the NSAIDs all have side effects that are problematic with older adults. Of particular concern are GI irritation, dizziness, blurred vision, and cardiac and kidney toxicity.

If NSAIDs are prescribed for older adults, it is imperative to

- know the comorbidities of the older adults
- know the potential side effects of the NSAIDs
- monitor the older person for side effects
- educate the patient and family about side effects and signs to report
- intervene for the NSAID to be changed or discontinued when needed

Topical formulations of the NSAIDs as discussed in Chapter 7 are viable options for many older adults with RA (American College of Rheumatology Task Force [ACRTF], 2010; Meiner, 2006).

- *COX-2 Inhibitor:* Although there is risk of serious GI side effects with COX-2 inhibitors, the risk is considered lower than that with other NSAIDs. Celecoxib was found as effective as standard NSAIDs and had fewer GI side effects (Garner et al., 2002). It is important to remember that COX-2 agents do pose significant dose-related side effects that are concerning in older people. These include the following:
  - Renal failure
  - Cardiac issues
    - hypertension
    - myocardial infarction
    - intensity cardiac failure
    - stroke
  - Potential for thrombus

As with NSAIDs, carefully monitoring for potential side effects and educating the older adult and family about potential side effects is imperative (ACRTF, 2010; Bansal, Joshi, & Bansal, 2007; Meiner, 2006; Savage, 2005).

Celecoxib is one of the COX-2 inhibitor medications that is currently available in the United States.

Etodolac is considered somewhat COX-2 selective (likened to celecoxib) (Warner et al., 1999). It has reportedly shown promise when used in 100-mg doses for relieving pain following dental extractions, and the side effects were similar to those of the placebo. It has also been reported to be effective with pain related to osteoarthritis and RA (Tirunagari, Moore, & McQuay, 2009).

■ *Corticosteroids* are used for RA when symptoms are severe. They can be used either orally or intra-articularly. Orally, they should be used with caution for a short term only.

Side effects that are of particular concern with older adults are as follows:

■ Osteoporosis
■ Gastric ulcers
■ Increased susceptibility for infection
■ Hypokalemia
■ Hypertension
■ Hyperglycemia
■ Emotional lability

When caring for or working with an older person receiving corticosteroids, it is important to always

■ Monitor for side effects
■ Teach patient and family to
    ■ monitor for side effects
    ■ never discontinue the medication abruptly
■ Ensure that medication is tapered appropriately
■ Consider the need for calcium (1,500 mg) and vitamin D (400 IU)

Intra-articularly, corticosteroids are indicated only if one or two joints are involved. Pain can be relieved up to several months following injection. The joints that respond best are in the hands, shoulders, hips, knees, and ankles (Lavelle et al., 2009; Meiner, 2006).

■ *Opioid* use in the management of RA has been addressed with caution and ambivalence. Despite the need for additional research, opioids remain an option for managing pain in older adults with RA when other options analgesic options are

■ not possible
■ contraindicated
■ have not been effective

Opioid selection needs to be based upon

■ the degree of pain being experienced
■ comorbid illnesses
■ potential side effects of the opioid
■ potential interactions of the opioid with concomitant medications
■ the previous history of the older adult with opioids

The reader is referred to Chapters 7 and 9 for more information on opioid pain management in older adults and side effect management (American College of Rheumatology Task Force [ACRTF], 2010; APS, 2002; Chapman et al., 2010; Victor, Alvarez, & Gould, 2009).

Patient and Family Education

At a minimum, older adults living with RA and their families need to be educated in the following:

- RA as a disease process with exacerbations and remissions
- Treatment options that are available and their demonstrated efficacy
- Medications use with emphasis on
  - dosage recommendations and maximum limits
  - administration needs
  - potential side effects and how to manage them
- Ways to manage pain nonpharmacologically
- Importance of balancing rest and activity
- Exercise needs
- Safe walking and transferring
- Methods of protecting tender and painful joints
- Relationship between stress and anxiety with muscle tension and pain
- Ability to critically analyze or seek help to evaluate proposed "cures" that may be bogus
- Community resources such as the Arthritis Foundation (Eliopoulos, 2001; Kennedy-Malone et al., 2004)

Nonpharmacological and Complementary Interventions for RA

With the exception of marital support/couples counseling, the reader is referred to Chapter 11 for more information on the complementary interventions listed.

- *Ice packs* can be helpful during periods of acute inflammation, but caution needs to be observed to prevent damage to sensitive skin.
- *Moist heat* to painful joints and muscles may be helpful in relaxing surrounding muscles.
- *Progressive muscle relaxation* can be useful in facilitating relaxation, reducing stress and anxiety.
- *Guided imagery* serves as a distraction and relaxation technique with similar benefit to progressive muscle relaxation.
- *Therapeutic touch* can be helpful in relieving tension, stress, and pain.
- *Spirituality and prayer* are important coping strategies for RA-related pain among older people (Watkins et al., 1999).
- *Cognitive behavioral therapy (CBT)* is an important option for pain management. Sharpe et al. (2002) reported that older adults with RA

more frequently completed CBT programs than did their younger counterparts. Some CBT techniques used by older adults living with RA include

- diverting attention through cognitive activities, games, and leisure activities
- reframing or reinterpreting pain sensations (i.e., imagining or pretending the pain is a different sensation or outside of the body)
- coping self-affirmations
- deliberately ignoring painful sensations (Ignataicious, 2001; Watkins et al., 1999)

- *Marital support, including couples therapy,* can be an important component of pain management for married older adults who have RA. A recent study reported that being in a "well-adjusted or non-distressed marriage" was associated with less pain and disability (Reese, Somers, Keefe, Mosley-Williams, & Lumley, 2010). These results were consistent with earlier studies that positive marital relationships in people living with RA are correlated with enhanced mental health (Sterba et al., 2008; Van Lankveld, Ruiterkamp, Naring, & De Rooj, 2004). Another implication is that when an older person with RA experiences the death of a beloved, supportive spouse, pain management may be particularly challenging.

- *Aromatherapy* has been used in combination with light massage. The oils most frequently used with RA are German chamomile, lavender, peppermint, and frankincense. The reader is referred to Chapter 11 for precautions with aromatherapy. It is important to not use essential them unless they are diluted in a carrier oil or lotion for topical use. Even when diluted, it is always recommended to test the product on a small skin area (Halcón & Buckle, 2006; Ignataicious, 2001; Meiner, 2006; Watkins et al., 1999).

Referrals and Consultations

Referrals and consultations should be made to the following professionals:

- Rheumatologist
  - to initiate and medically manage the RA
  - to assess for and manage medications and potential side effects
  - for interventional therapies, including intra-articular injections
- Pain management specialists for medication management as well as interventional techniques (see Chapter 10)
- Physical therapist for mobility training, body mechanics, stretching, strengthening, and endurance exercises

- Occupational therapist for
  - splints to relieve pressure and pain in joints, protect painful joints, and improve joint function
  - assistive devices
  - home safety needs
- Nutritionist consultation
  - to improve nutrition
  - to maintain ideal weight to avoid added stress on painful weight-bearing knees and hips
  - for advice about antioxidant vitamins (A, C, and E) and supplements
  - for education about the role of omega 3 fatty acids in reducing inflammation
- Surgeon when pain is significant and loss of motion and function is high for assessment of possible surgical intervention/correction (ACRTF, 2010; Ignataicious, 2001; Kennedy-Malone et al., 2004; Meiner, 2006)

POLYMYALGIA RHEUMATICA

Polymyalgia rheumatica (PMR) is also a chronic inflammatory disease with unknown etiology. It is described as the most common inflammatory disorder among older adults. The characteristics symptoms are tenderness, muscle pain, and stiffness, particularly in the morning. There is typically a sudden onset affecting the hips, shoulders, and neck.

Traditionally, it has been closely associated with giant cell arteritis (GCA) (see Chapter 19). GCA is diagnosed in 10% to 30% of PMR cases and PMR has been noted in as many as 40% to 60% of people with GCA (Kennedy-Malone & Enevold, 2001; Meiner, 2006; Salvarani, Cantini, Boiardi, & Hunder, 2002; Salvarani, Cantini, Boiardi, & Hunder, 2004).

Epidemiology of PMR

PMR occurs primarily in people older than 50 years with a prevalence of one PMR diagnosis per 133 people in that age distribution. Additional epidemiological information include the following:

- The peak incidence is among those in their 70s.
- It is twice as prevalent in women as in men.
- Environmental or ethnic factors may be involved.

■ It is most common among older women of European descent.
■ PMR occurs more frequently at higher latitudes.

Although older adults generally respond well to treatment, spontaneous exacerbations occur in approximately 33% of patients (British Society for Rheumatology and British Health Professionals in Rheumatology Standards, Guidelines and Audit Working Group [BSR-BHPR SGAWG], 2010; Dasgupta et al., 2008; Kennedy-Malone & Enevold, 2001; Kreiner, Langberg, & Galbo, 2010; Lawrence et al., 2008; Salvarani et al., 2002, 2004).

Etiology and Risk Factors of PMR

The etiology is unknown but is most likely polygenic involving a number of environmental and genetic features that influence both vulnerability to and severity of the disorder once it is acquired. As with GCA, *Chlamydia pneumoniae* has been implicated in the etiology of PMR as has *Mycoplasma pneumoniae,* and Parvovirus B19 (Salvarani et al., 2002, 2004).

Diagnosis and Clinical Manifestations of PMR

The 2010, BSR-BHPR SGAWG developed guidelines for the management of PMR that follow a four-tiered approach:
■ Core inclusion criteria
  ■ Age older than 50 years
  ■ Duration of symptoms 2 weeks or longer
  ■ Shoulder and/or pelvic girdle aching bilaterally
  ■ Morning stiffness lasting more than 45 minutes
  ■ Evidence of response during an acute phase
■ Exclusion criteria
  ■ Core exclusion criteria are as follows:
    ■ Active infection
    ■ Active cancer diagnosis
  ■ Additional exclusion criteria that make the diagnosis of PMR unlikely include the following:
    ■ Other inflammatory rheumatic disorders
    ■ Drug-induced myalgia
    ■ Chronic pain syndromes
    ■ Endocrine diseases
    ■ Neurological disorders (i.e., Parkinsonism)
■ Assessment for comorbid GCA, which *necessitates urgent intervention* to prevent blindness (see Chapter 19).

- Assessment of response to standardized steroid therapy
  - Prednisone 15 mg orally per day is considered standard.
  - If global improvement is 70% or more in 1 week of starting steroid, therapy is indicative of a diagnosis of PMR.
  - Inflammatory markers should normalize in 4 weeks.
  - Monitor blood count, ESR/CRP (erythrocyte sedimentation rate and C-reactive protein), urea, glucose, and electrolytes.
  - Follow-up evaluations are essential to assess progress and for other conditions (BSR-BHPR SGAWG, 2010).

Pharmacological Management

Steroid therapy with prednisone is the standard intervention. A common treatment plan is to

- start with 10 to 20 mg prednisone orally per day for approximately 1 month
- then reduce the prednisone by 2.5 to 5 mg/day/month until 10 mg/day
- then reduce the prednisone by 1 to 2.5 mg/day/month

Therapy may be required for 1 to 3 years, but some older adults may require small doses for longer periods of time (Salvarani et al., 2004).

Pain Management

Pain is generally relieved with steroid therapy.

If pain is not relieved with steroid therapy, pain should be treated symptomatically, beginning with acetaminophen for mild to moderate pain and as outlined in the RA section.

Patient and Family Education for PMR

Medication education regarding prednisone should include awareness of side effects including

- risk of osteoporosis
- increased likelihood of infections, fractures, diabetes, and stomach ulcers
- probable weight gain
- possible depression or labile emotions

Diet should include adequate calcium.

Signs of GCA are important to teach, because GCA frequently occurs in conjunction with PMR. Signs include visual changes, headache, tenderness in temporal area of head/face, and jaw pain.

Table 20.1 ■ *Comparison of RA with Polymyalgia Rheumatica*

	RA	*Polymyalgia Rheumatica*
Prevalence	5–50 per 100,000 total population	21 per 100,000 over 50 years
Age factors	Onset can be in 30 or 40 year age group	Onset almost always after 50 years with peak in the 70s
Gender	Predominantly female	Predominantly female
Etiology	Unknown; genetic and environmental factors implemented	Unknown; genetic and environmental factors implemented
Muscle stiffness	Upon awakening	Upon awakening lasting 45–60 min
Distal edema	Present	Present
Joints involved	Hands, feet, knees, shoulders, and hips	Shoulders, neck, and hips
Joint erosion	Characteristic	None
Extra articular nodules	Characteristic	None
Joints range of motion	Limited range of motion	No limitation in range of motion
Possible systematic symptoms	Fever, malaise, anorexia, and weight loss	Fever, malaise, anorexia, and weight loss
Response to medication	Slow	Quick response to steroids with improvement in symptoms in 1–2 days
Association with GCA	No to minimal correlation	Close correlation
Medication management	DMARDs and Biological agents; corticosteroids, NSAIDs	Corticosteroids, NSAIDs
Duration of disease	Life long	1–3 years

Sources: Information derived from various references cited in this chapter.

Nonpharmacological and Complementary Interventions for PMR

The reader is referred to the section on nonpharmacological, complementary interventions for RA and to Chapter 11 for more information on the complementary interventions.

Referrals and Consultations for PMR

Ophthalmologist referral for visual disturbances or indications of GCA is appropriate only if the older adult can be seen immediately. If that is not possible then referral to the *emergency department* is needed. Prompt and aggressive treatment is necessary to prevent blindness.

Rheumatologist referral is appropriate when older adults do not respond as expected to the standard treatment or if there is a comorbid diagnosis of GCA.

Physical therapy is appropriate to maintain optimal function and learn exercise that promotes function without damaging joints.

Nutritionist can be helpful in preventing additional weight gain beyond that associated with prednisone and to learn dietary sources of calcium (Kennedy-Malone & Enevold, 2001) (Table 20.1).

RESOURCES AND GUIDELINES

American College of Rheumatology. http://www.rheumatology.org

American College of Rheumatology (ACR) (2008). American College of Rheumatology 2008 recommendations for the use of nonbiologic and biologic disease-modifying antirheumatic drugs in RA. *Arthritis and Rheumatism, 59,* 762–784.

American College of Rheumatology Task Force (ACRTF) (2010). Report of the American College of Rheumatology Pain Management Task Force. *Arthritis Care & Research, 62,* 590–599.

American Pain Society (APS) (2002). *Guideline for the management of pain in osteoarthritis, RA, and juvenile chronic arthritis.* Glenview, IL: American Pain Society.

Arthritis Foundation. http://www.arthritis.org

Arthritis Foundation. 800–283–7800

Arthritis & Rheumatism. *59,* 762–784. Able to download these guidelines from: http://www.rheumatology.org/practice/clinical/guidelines/recommendations.pdf

British Society for Rheumatology and British Health Professionals in Rheumatology Standards, Guidelines and Audit Working Group. (2010). BSR and BHPR guidelines for the management of polymyalgia rheumatica. *Rheumatology, 49,* 186–190.

The American College of Classification Criteria for PMR. Dasgupta, B., Salvaran, I. C., Schrimer, M., Crowson, C. S., Maradit-Kremers, H., Matteson, E. L., Members of The American College of Classification Criteria for PMR. (2008). Development of classification criteria for polymyalgia rheumatica (PMR): Results from an expert work group meeting and wider survey. *Journal of Rheumatology, 35,* 270–277.

US Food and Drug Administration Information on Rheumatology Therapeutics. http://www.fda.gov/Drugs/ResourcesForYou/Health-Professionals/ucm103200.htm

US Food and Drug Administration. http://www.fda.gov/NewsEvents/Newsroom/PressAnnouncements/default.htm

Case Study

Delores Cardinal is a 79-year-old woman from Danish descent. She is being admitted to the hospital with a fever of unknown origin, no appetite, and "soreness" in her shoulders and neck for the last 4 days. She says that it is particularly hard to get up in the morning and for the first hour or so, her hips really hurt. Although she is talking, you notice that she holds her hands tightly in a downward position so that you cannot really see them. When you ask her to sign the admission papers, you notice that there are three nodules on her right hand.

Questions

1. What do you think is the underlying disease that is causing the symptoms Ms. Cardinal is reporting?
2. What additional information do you need to collect?
3. Is there a potential need for urgent care of Ms. Cardinal's condition?
4. If so, what is the basis of the emergency need?

5. What medical treatment is indicated for Ms. Cardinal?
6. What patient and family education will you need to prepare for her and her family?
7. What referrals are indicated for Ms. Cardinal?
8. Are there complementary interventions that you could share with or teach Ms. Cardinal?

REFERENCES

Aletaha, D., Neogi, T., Silman, A. J., Funovits, J., Felson, D. T., Bingham, C. O., Hawker, G. (2010). 2010 RA classification criteria: An American College of Rheumatology/European League Against Rheumatism collaborative initiative. *Arthritis & Rheumatism, 62,* 2569–2581.

American College of Rheumatology (ACR). (2008). American College of Rheumatology 2008 recommendations for the use of nonbiologic and biologic disease-modifying antirheumatic drugs in RA. *Arthritis and Rheumatism, 59,* 762–784.

American College of Rheumatology Task Force (ACRTF). (2010). Report of the American College of Rheumatology Pain Management Task Force. *Arthritis Care & Research, 62,* 590–599.

American Geriatrics Society (AGS). (2009). Pharmacological management of persistent pain in older persons: American Geriatrics Society Panel of the Pharmacological Management of Persistent Pain in Older Adults. *Journal of the American Geriatrics Society, 57,* 1331–1346.

American Pain Society (APS). (2002). *Guideline for the management of pain in osteoarthritis, RA, and juvenile chronic arthritis.* Glenview, IL: Author.

Bansal, S. S., Joshi, A., & Bansal, A. K. (2007). New dosage formulations for targeted delivery of cyclo-oxygenase-2 inhibitors. *Drugs Aging, 24,* 441–451.

British Society for Rheumatology and British Health Professionals in Rheumatology Standards, Guidelines and Audit Working Group (BSR-BHPR SGAWG). (2010). BSR and BHPR guidelines for the management of polymyalgia rheumatica. *Rheumatology, 49,* 186–190.

Chapman, C. R., Lipshitz, D. L., Angst, M. S., Chou, R., Denisco, R. C., Donaldson, G. W., Weisner, C. M. (2010). Opioid pharmacotherapy for chronic non-cancer pain in the United States: A research guideline for developing an evidence-base. *The Journal of Pain, 11,* 807–829.

Dasgupta, B., Salvaran, I. C., Schrimer, M., Crowson, C. S., Maradit-Kremers, H., Matteson, E. L., & Members of the American College of Classification Criteria for PMR (2008). Development of classification criteria for polymyalgia rheumatica (PMR): Results from an expert work group meeting and wider survey. *Journal of Rheumatology, 35,* 270–277.

Eliopoulos, C. (2001). *Gerontological nursing.* Philadelphia, PA: Lippincott.

Garner, S. E., Fidan, D. D., Frankish, R. R., Judd, M., Shea, B., Towheed, T., Wells, G. A. (2002). Celecoxib for RA. *Cochrane database of systematic reviews,* (4), CD003831.

Halcón, L. L., & Buckle, J. (2006). Aromatherapy. In M. Snyder & R. Lindquist (Eds.), *Complementary/Alternative therapies in nursing* (5th ed., pp. 335–350). New York, NY: Springer.

Ignataicious, D. D. (2001). Rheumatoid arthritis and the older adult. *Geriatric Nursing, 22,* 139–142.

Kennedy-Malone, L., & Enevold, G. L. (2001). Assessment and management of polymyalgia rheumatica in older adults. *Geriatric Nursing, 22,* 152–154.

Kennedy-Malone, L., Fletcher, K. R., & Plank, L. M. (2004). *Management guidelines for nurse parishioners: Working with older adults* (2nd ed.). Philadelphia, PA: F. A. Davis Company.

Kreiner, F., Langberg, H., & Galbo, H. (2010). Increased muscle interstitial levels of inflammatory cytokines in polymyalgia rheumatica. *Arthritis & Rheumatism, 62,* 3768–3775.

Lavelle, L. A., Lavelle, W. F., & Lavelle, E. D. (2009). Rheumatoid Arthritis. In H. S. Smith (Ed.), *Current therapy in pain* (pp. 245–250). Philadelphia, PA: Saunders Elsevier.

Lawrence, R. C., Felson, D. T., Helmick, C. G., Arnold, L. M., Choi, H., Deyo, R. A., & Wolfe, F. (2008). Estimates of the prevalence of arthritis and other rheumatic conditions in the United States. *Arthritis & Rheumatism, 58,* 26–35.

McAllister, K., Eyre, S., & Orozco, G. (2011). Genetics of Rheumatoid Arthritis: GWAS and beyond. *Rheumatology: Research and Reviews, 3,* 31–46.

Meiner, S. E. (2006). Musculoskeletal function. In S. E. Meiner & A. G. Luekenotte (Eds.), *Gerontologic nursing* (3rd ed., pp. 596–629). St. Louis, MO: Mosby Elsevier.

National Arthritis Data Workgroup (2008a). Estimates of the prevalence of arthritis and other rheumatic conditions in the United States—Part 1. *Arthritis and Rheumatism, 58,* 15–25.

Reese, J. B., Somers, T. J., Keefe, F. J., Mosley-Williams, A., & Lumley, M. A. (2010). Pain and functioning of RA patients based on marital status: Is a distressed marriage? *The Journal of Pain, 11,* 958–964.

Salvarani, C., Cantini, F., Boiardi, L., & Hunder, G. G. (2002). Polymyalgia and giant-cell arteritis. *New England Journal of Medicine, 347,* 261–271.

Salvarani, C., Cantini, F., Boiardi, L., & Hunder, G. G. (2004). Polymyalgia rheumatica. *Best Practice & Research Clinical Rheumatology, 18,* 705–722.

Savage, R. (2005). Cyclo-oxygenase-2 inhibitors when should they be used in the elderly? *Drugs Aging, 22,* 185–200.

Scott, D. L., Wolfe, F., & Huizinga, T. W. (2010). Rheumatoid Arthritis. *Lancet, 376,* 1094–1108.

Sharpe, L., Senski, T., Timberlake, N., Ryan, B., Brewin, C. R., & Allard, S. (2002). A blind, randomized, controlled trial of cognitive-behavioral intervention for patients with recent onset rheumatoid arthritis: Preventing psychological and physical morbidity. *Pain, 89,* 275–283.

Sterba, K. R., Devellis, R. F., Lewis, M. A., Devellis, B. M., Jordan, J. M., & Baucom, D. H. (2008). Effect of couple illness perception congruence on psychological adjustment in women with RA. *Health Psychology, 27,* 221–229.

Symmons, D., Turner, G., Webb, R., Asten, P., Barrett, E., Lunt, M., & Silman, A. (2002). The prevalence of Rheumatoid Arthritis in the United Kingdom—new estimates for a new century. *Rheumatology, 41,* 793–800.

Tirunagari, S. K., Moore, R. A., & McQuay, H. J. (2009). Single dose of oral etodolac for acute postoperative pain in adults. *Cochrane Database of Systematic Reviews,* (3), CD007357.

van Lankveld, W., Ruiterkamp, G., Naring, G., & de Rooj, D. J. (2004). Marital and sexual satisfaction in patients with Rheumatoid Arthritis and their spouses. *Scandinavian Journal of Rheumatology, 33,* 405–408.

Victor, T. W., Alvarez, N. A., & Gould, E. (2009). Opioid prescribing practices in chronic pain management: Guidelines do not sufficiently influence clinical practice. *The Journal of Pain, 10,* 1051–1057.

Warner, T. D., Giuliano, F., Vojnoivc, I., Bukasa, A., Mitchell, J. A., & Vane, J. R. (1999). Nonsteroid drug selectivities for cyclo-oxygenase-1 rather than cyclo-oxygenase-2 are associated with human gastrointestinal toxicity: A full in vitro analysis. *Proceedings of the National Academy of Sciences of the United States of America, 96,* 7563–7568.

Watkins, K. W., Shifren, K., Park, D. C., & Morrell, R. W. (1999). Age, pain, and coping with rheumatoid arthritis. *Pain, 82,* 217–228.

21

Fibromyalgia

Fibromyalgia syndrome (FMS) is a chronic, idiopathic, nonarticular, pain-amplification syndrome that is characterized by severe, spontaneous, widespread muscular pain, reduced pain threshold, generalized tender points, and fatigue. As it is known currently, FMS has a recent history. Classification criteria were first introduced in 1990 and have evolved since then (Staud, 2008; Staud, 2009; Wolfe et al., 1990; Wolfe et al., 2010).

EPIDEMIOLOGY OF FMS

Even though the incidence and prevalence estimates for FMS are more abundant than for many chronic pain situations, there is the possibility that available figures are an underestimation of the true prevalence of FMS. This is because FMS is common among those who have other chronic illnesses, and epidemiological figures may not reflect people with FMS as a diagnosis secondary to another chronic illness.

Currently, it is estimated that

- between 2% and 4% of the general population suffer with FMS,
- prevalence in 2005 was estimated as 5 million adults in the United States,
- 3.4% of adult women and 0.5% of adult men have FMS,
- approximately 80% of those with FMS are women,
- the mean age is reported as 49 years,
- prevalence increases with age, and it is estimated that 8% of the female population between 55 and 64 years has FMS,
- it is believed that 15% of hospitalized patients have FMS,

- there are approximately 5.5 million ambulatory care encounters related to FMS,
- annual medical costs per person are estimated as $5,945, and
- people living with FMS are 3.4 times more likely to have major depression (American college of Rheumatology [ACR], 2009; CDC, 2011; Lawrence et al., 2008; Staud, 2009).

ETIOLOGY AND FACTORS ASSOCIATED WITH FMS

The etiology of FMS is unknown; however, several associations and possible risk factors have been suggested.

Genetic Factors Associated with FMS

- It is believed that genetics may be involved and result from polymorphisms that occur in receptors and signaling pathways that are involved in pain perception (American College of Rheumatology, 2010; Dadabhoy, Crofford, Spaeth, Russell, & Clauw, 2008).
- In the "Family Study of Fibromyalgia" it was found that first-degree relatives of someone with FMS had an eight times greater chance of also developing FMS (Arnold et al., 2004).
- FMS also occurs more frequently among relatives of people with FMS (Chakrabarty & Zoorob, 2007; Neumann & Buskila, 2003).
- FMS and major depressive disorder have been reported as having "shared familial risk factors" (Staud, 2009).

Demographic and Social Factors Associated with FMS

- Female gender
- Divorced marital status
- Less than high-school education
- Lower income (Chakrabarty & Zoorob, 2007).

Psychological Factors Associated with FMS

- Somatization disorder
- Anxiety
- Personal or family history of depression (Chakrabarty & Zoorob, 2007; Staud, 2009).

Conditions Frequently Seen as Comorbid with FMS that Increase Likelihood of FMS

It is thought that individuals who suffer with other rheumatic disorders (i.e., rheumatoid arthritis [RA], ankylosing spondylitis, systemic lupus erythematosus, and osteoarthritis [OA]) are more likely to develop FMS (ACR, 2009).

Conditions frequently comorbid with FMS are as follows:

- Anxiety occurs at some point in time in 35% to 62% of people with FMS.
- Depression
  - Depression with major depressive disorder occurs at some point in 58% to 86% of people with FMS.
  - Bipolar disorder occurs in up to 11% of people with FMS.
- Sleep disturbances are common among people with FMS.
- Headaches occur in more than 50% of people with FMS.
- Irritable bowel syndrome is a common codiagnosis.
- Other common coexisting conditions include irritable bladder, restless leg syndrome, temporomandibular joint pain, Raynaud's syndrome, Sjögren's syndrome, and noncardiac chest pain (Arnold, Clauw, & McCarberg, 2011; Chakrabarty & Zoorob, 2007).

PATHOPHYSIOLOGY ASPECTS OF FMS

The specific factors involved in pain amplification with FMS are not fully understood; however, it is believed that peripheral and central pain amplification with a corresponding absence of descending central nervous system (CNS) pain inhibition may be responsible for the particular pain exhibited in FMS. Thus, the experience of FMS pain involves peripheral sensitization, central sensitization, and impaired descending inhibition of pain.

Peripheral sensitization occurs following tissue damage and/or "upregulation of nociceptor expression in peripheral nerve endings," when the peripheral nociceptors become progressively more sensitive. When this happens, and the nociceptors are again activated, there is enhanced firing and pain. In addition, when there is repeated stimulation by the long C-fiber of the second-order neurons in the CNS, a swell of electrical discharges from these neurons with stimulation and amplification of pain in the dorsal horn and spinal cord can result. These result in "second pain" or "wind up" that is often described as dull, burning, aching pain.

It is believed that NMDA (N-Methyl-D-aspartic acid) receptors are also involved in this process.

Central sensitization subsequently develops. It involves neuroplasticity changes involving multiple neurochemical interactions, with neurotransmitters and neuromodulators occurring within the CNS. This can occur as an initial response at the time of injury or it can occur at some later time. There is increased excitability of the neurons of the dorsal horn that transmit pain information to the brain. This results in slight stimulation being perceived as intense pain. These functional changes in the CNS result in

- heightened excitability of spinal cord neurons following trauma
- extension of the receptive fields of those neurons
- decrease in pain threshold
- "recruitment of novel afferent inputs" (Staud, 2008)

Sharp, lancinating pain and allodynia (pain experienced in response to a usually nonpainful stimuli) are manifestations of central sensitization. In addition, with central sensitization, the heightened sensitivity to pain occurs in body areas that were not associated with the original pain situation.

These processes result in an amplification of pain with increased pain sensitivity in response to stimulation that often is not perceived as painful, such as pressure, heat, or cold. Not only are these sensations perceived as painful, but the pain related to them is often widespread (Dadabhoy et al., 2008; Desmeules et al., 2003; Staud, 2008; Staud, 2009).

Impaired descending inhibition of pain is due to deficiency in diffuse noxious inhibitory control (DNIC). It is an impairment of the descending pain inhibitory system that is believed to be the third aspect of the FMS pain process. The DNIC-like mechanisms normally function as a barricade preventing pain from becoming widespread and unbearable. DNIC-like mechanisms maintain pain to a localized area where it can be managed. It is believed that in FMS, there is a deficiency in the descending pathway inhibitory control that is responsible for suppression of some of the pain messages (mediated by the C-fibers). It is characterized by the release of less serotonin and norepinephrine. In this way, the diminished DNIC is pathogenic.

There is support for this in that people living with FMS often have low serum concentration of serotonin and noradrenalin while having increased levels of substance P. Even though it is not clear how unique this process is to FMS, it is possible that DNIC deficiency or impairment is a potential biomarker for this disorder.

Furthermore, there is evidence that the descending pathway has bidirectional influence in pain enhancement and inhibition, as well as psychological stress and fear. This influence occurs through ON-cell (descending pain facilitation) and OFF-cell (descending pain inhibition) neurons. It is believed that descending facilitation contributes to *central sensitization* and subsequently extensive hyperalgesia (Dadabhoy et al., 2008; Heinricher, Tavares, Leith, & Lumb, 2009; Julien, Goffaux, Arsenault, & Marchand, 2005; Kinder, Bennett, & Jones, 2011; Pielsticker, Haag, Zaudig, & Lautenbacher, 2005).

DIAGNOSIS AND CLINICAL
MANIFESTATIONS OF FMS

Diagnosis of FMS is generally made based upon clinical criteria. There is no definitive test to confirm the clinical diagnosis of FMS. There is generally no evidence of damage or inflammation in the affected tissues that would support the degree of pain.

The 1990 ACR criteria for FMS diagnosis required

- tenderness in response to pressure in a minimum of 11 of 18 specified sites or "tender points" and
- presence of widespread pain (US Federal Drug Administration [US FDA], 2008; US FDA, 2009; Wolfe et al., 1990).

In 2010, the ACR provisionally approved revised criteria for FMS diagnosis to require clinical evaluation that satisfies the following three criteria:

1. "The widespread pain index (WPI) is ≥7 and the symptom severity (SS) scale score is ≥5 or the WPI is 3 to 6 and the SS scale score is ≥9."
2. "Symptoms have been present at a similar level for at least 3 months."
3. "The patient does not have a disorder that would otherwise explain the pain."

- To determine the WPI, the clinician establishes whether the pain has been present in any of the 19 specific physical locations during the past week. Presence of pain in each area contributes one point to the WPI score that can thus range from 0 (no areas of pain) to 19 (pain in all areas).

■ To determine the SS scale, the clinician rates the severity on a 0 to 3 scale of fatigue, waking unrefreshed, and cognitive symptoms and adds those scores. To that score is added a 0 to 3 score that describes the severity of somatic symptoms in general. The somatic symptoms that can be reflected in the general score are wide ranging (i.e., muscle pain, fatigue, muscle weakness, headache, dizziness, hives, hair loss, constipation, depression, dry eyes, etc.) (Wolfe et al., 2010. p. 607).

■ Cognitive difficulties are common and frequently referred to as "fibro-fog" or "decognition." This may include forgetfulness, slow processing of information, difficulty in concentrating, disorganization in thinking, and impaired executive function (Arnold et al., 2011; Williams & Schilling, 2009).

FMS assessment tools

■ *FMS assessment tools* have been developed, and there are a variety of tools available. Two that have reported validity and reliability are briefly described. In addition a more generic tool that assesses change is frequently used in the assessment of FMS and is also described.

■ *The Fibromyalgia Impact Questionnaire* (FIQ) (Figure 21.1) is reported as the most frequently used tool to quantify the severity of FMS disease. Validity, reliability for FMS, and internal consistency have been reported as acceptable. It was originally developed in 1997 and was modified in 2002. The FIQ is a self-administered test that generally takes between 3 and 5 minutes for the older adult to complete. The FIQ consists of a total of 20 questions that are distributed in three sections:

  ■ Eleven question address challenges with activities of daily living.

  ■ Two questions ask about the impact of FMS on life during days in the previous week.

  ■ Seven questions assess symptoms on a visual analog scale (VAS) (Bennett, 2005; Burkhardt, Clark, & Bennett, 1991; Meyer & Lemley, 2000).

■ *The Revised Fibromyalgia Impact Questionnaire* (FIQR) (Figure 21.2) is a 2009 revision of the FIQ. There are fewer questions and the symptom impact section carries greater weight than in the original FIQ. Rather than using the VAS as the original FIQ did, the revised tool uses a numeric scale with boxes numbered 0–10. Reportedly, the FIQR can be completed by patients in less than 2 minutes. Scoring by the health care provider (HCP) is reportedly easier and takes approximately 1 minute. Scoring is comparable to the original FIQ,

Fibromyalgia Impact Questionnaire (FIQ)

Last name:	First name:	Age :	Todays date :
Duration of FM symptoms (years):		Years since diagnosis of FM:	

Directions: For questions 1 through 11, please check the number that best describes how you did over all for the *past week*. If you don't normally do something that is asked, place an 'X' in the 'Not Applicable' box.

Were you able to:	Always	Most	Occasionally	Never	Not Applicable
1. Do shopping?	$\square_0$	$\square_1$	$\square_2$	$\square_3$	$\square_4$
2. Do laundry with a washer and dryer?	$\square_0$	$\square_1$	$\square_2$	$\square_3$	$\square_4$
3. Prepare meals?	$\square_0$	$\square_1$	$\square_2$	$\square_3$	$\square_4$
4. Wash dishes/ cooking utensils by hand?	$\square_0$	$\square_1$	$\square_2$	$\square_3$	$\square_4$
5. Vacuum a rug?	$\square_0$	$\square_1$	$\square_2$	$\square_3$	$\square_4$
6. Make beds?	$\square_0$	$\square_1$	$\square_2$	$\square_3$	$\square_4$
7. Walk several blocks?	$\square_0$	$\square_1$	$\square_2$	$\square_3$	$\square_4$
8. Visit friends or relatives?	$\square_0$	$\square_1$	$\square_2$	$\square_3$	$\square_4$
9. Do yard work?	$\square_0$	$\square_1$	$\square_2$	$\square_3$	$\square_4$
10. Drive a car?	$\square_0$	$\square_1$	$\square_2$	$\square_3$	$\square_4$
11. Climb stairs?	$\square_0$	$\square_1$	$\square_2$	$\square_3$	$\square_4$
Sub-total scores (*for internal use only*)	$\square$	$\square$	$\square$	$\square$	$\square$
Total score (*for internal use only*)	$\square$				

12. Of the 7 days in the past week, how many days did you feel good?   Score

$\square_0$ $\square_1$ $\square_2$ $\square_3$ $\square_4$ $\square_5$ $\square_6$ $\square_7$ $\square$

13. How many days last week did you miss work, including house work, because of fibromyalgia?   Score

$\square_0$ $\square_1$ $\square_2$ $\square_3$ $\square_4$ $\square_5$ $\square_6$ $\square_7$ $\square$

Directions: For the remaining items, mark the point on the line that best indicates how you felt overall for the past week.

14. When you worked how much did pain or other symptoms of your fibromyalgia interfere with your ability to do your work, including housework?   (for internal use only)

No problem with work ├─────────────┤ Great difficulty with work Score $\square$ Score

15. How bad has your pain been?

No pain ├─────────────┤ Very severe pain $\square$ Score

16. How tired have you been?

No tiredness ├─────────────┤ Very tired $\square$ Score

17. How have you felt when you get up in the morning?

Awoke well rested ├─────────────┤ Awoke very tired $\square$ Score

18. How bad has your stiffness been?

No stiffness ├─────────────┤ Very stiff $\square$ Score

19. How nervous or anxious have you felt?

Not anxious ├─────────────┤ Very anxious $\square$ Score

20. How depressed or blue have you felt?

Not depressed ├─────────────┤ Very depressed $\square$ Score

$\square$ **Sub-total**

$\square$ **FIQ total**

Figure 21.1 ■ Fibromyalgia Impact Questionnaire. Used with permission of R. Bennett, MD

Revised Fibromyalgia Impact Questionnaire (FIQR)

Last name:	First name:	Age :

Duration of FM symptoms (years):

Time since FM was first diagnosed (years):

Directions: For each of the following 9 questions, check the box that best indicates how much your fibromyalgia made it difficult to perform each of the following activities during the past 7 days. If you did not perform a particular activity in the last 7 days, rate the difficulty for the <u>last time</u> you performed the activity. If you can't perform an activity, check the last box.

Brush or comb your hair	No difficulty	□□□□□□□□□□□	Very difficult
Walk continuously for 20 minutes	No difficulty	□□□□□□□□□□□	Very difficult
Prepare a homemade meal	No difficulty	□□□□□□□□□□□	Very difficult
Vacuum, scrub or sweep floors	No difficulty	□□□□□□□□□□□	Very difficult
Lift and carry a bag full of groceries	No difficulty	□□□□□□□□□□□	Very difficult
Climb one flight of stairs	No difficulty	□□□□□□□□□□□	Very difficult
Change bed sheets	No difficulty	□□□□□□□□□□□	Very difficult
Sit in a chair for 45 minutes	No difficulty	□□□□□□□□□□□	Very difficult
Go shopping for groceries	No difficulty	□□□□□□□□□□□	Very difficult

Subtotal *(for internal use only)* ☐

Directions: For each of the following 2 questions, check the box that best describes the overall impact of your fibromyalgia over the last 7 days.

Fibromyalgia prevented me from accomplishing goals for the week.	Never	□□□□□□□□□□□	Always
I was completely overwhelmed by my fibromyalgia symptoms.	Never	□□□□□□□□□□□	Always

Sub-total *(for internal use only)* ☐

Directions: For each of the following 10 questions, select the box that best indicates your intensity of these common fibromyalgia symptoms over the past 7 days.

Please rate your level of pain	No pain	□□□□□□□□□□□	Unbearable pain
Please rate your level of energy	Lots of energy	□□□□□□□□□□□	No energy
Please rate your level of stiffness	No stiffness	□□□□□□□□□□□	Severe stiffness
Please rate the quality of your sleep	Awoke rested	□□□□□□□□□□□	Awoke very tired
Please rate your level of depression	No depression	□□□□□□□□□□□	Very depressed
Please rate your level of memory problems	Good memory	□□□□□□□□□□□	Very poor memory
Please rate your level of anxiety	Not anxious	□□□□□□□□□□□	Very anxious
Please rate your level of tenderness to touch	No tenderness	□□□□□□□□□□□	Very tender
Please rate your level of balance problems	No imbalance	□□□□□□□□□□□	Severe imbalance
Please rate your level of sensitivity to loud noises, bright lights, odors, and cold	No sensitivity	□□□□□□□□□□□	Extreme sensitivity

Sub-total *(for internal use only)* ☐

FIQR total *(for internal use only)* ☐

Figure 21.2 ■ Fibromyalgia Impact Questionnaire Revised. Used with permission of R. Bennett, MD so research results using the FIQR can be compared with earlier results using the FIQ. Initial validity and reliability testing were adequate, but further testing needs to be done in larger and more diverse populations (Bennett et al., 2009).

A very recent revision of the FIQR called the Symptom Impact Questionnaire has been pilot tested. This variant of the FIQR is intended to distinguish between FMS and rheumatoid arthritis and systemic lupus erythematosus. Early psychometric testing is very promising (Friend & Bennett, 2011).

■ *Patient's global impression of change* (PGIC) (Figure 21.3) is valid and considered the gold standard for assessing change that has occurred over time. It is a simple, categorical scale on which the older adult selects the option that best describes the degree of improvement over time, from the last clinic visit, commencement of medication, beginning a complementary therapy, and so forth (Farrar, Young, Lamoreaux, Werth, & Poole, 2001; Field, Newell, & McCarthy, 2010; Hurst & Bolton, 2004).

The PGIC is not specific to FMS but has been widely used to assess change in FMS symptoms, including change after initiation of medications (Crofford et al., 2005; Crofford et al., 2008; Mease et al., 2009).

MULTIMODAL TREATMENT APPROACH

This approach is imperative when working with older adults with FMS.

PHARMACOLOGICAL MANAGEMENT

General Guidelines for Medication Management of FMS

1. Factors to consider when identifying/selecting a medication to treat FMS include the
   ■ symptom that is most problematic for the older adult (pain, fatigue, etc.)
   ■ adverse effect profile of the medications
   ■ comorbidities of the older adult
   ■ concomitant medications required for the older adult
   ■ preferences of the older adult
2. *Start low and go slow* in dosing.
3. Monitor carefully for adverse reactions
4. Reassess effectiveness of the medication at regular intervals (Hauser, Petzke, & Sommer, 2010).

Patient's Global Impression of Change (PGIC) Scale

Since _____(i.e. date, starting medicine, starting therapy, etc.),
how would you describe the change (if any) in _____(i.e. activity,
change, symptoms, quality of life, etc) related to your _____
(i.e. pain, FMS, etc)?

	(tick ONE box)
No change (or condition worse)	☐₁
Almost the same, hardly any change at all	☐₂
A little better, but no noticeable change	☐₃
Somewhat better, but the change has not made any real difference	☐₄
Moderately better, and a slight but noticeable change	☐₅
Better and a definite improvement that has made a real and worthwhile difference	☐₆
A great deal better, and a considerable improvement that has made all the difference	☐₇

Figure 21.3 ■ Patient's Global Impression of Change (PGIC) Scale

US FDA Approved Medications to Treat FMS

Currently, there are three medications (pregabalin, duloxetine hydrochloride, and milnacipran hydrochloride) that have received FDA approval for the treatment of FMS. Other medications are commonly used but their use is not FDA approved.

Pregabalin (Lyrica) was approved in 2007 as the first medication specifically to treat FMS. Reports are inconsistent regarding the effectiveness of pregabalin in managing pain related to FMS (Siler, Gardner, Yanit, Cushman, & McDonagh, 2010).

Dosing is recommended at 150–300 mg per day in two divided doses.

Action is through reduction of calcium influx nerve terminals with inhibition of neurotransmitters (glutamate and substance P).

Side effects, which appear to be dose related, and are of concern for older adults include

■ mild to moderate dizziness
■ sleepiness
■ blurred vision
■ weight gain and increased appetite
■ swelling of the extremities

- constipation
- fatigue (US FDA, 2008)

Duloxetine Hydrochloride (Cymbalta): It has been approved as a medication to treat FMS since 2008.

Dosing is suggested at 60 mg per day

Action is primarily through dual inhibition of the reuptake of serotonin and norepinephrine (SNRI).

Side effects that pose concern for older adults include

- drowsiness
- constipation
- dizziness
- insomnia
- nausea
- fatigue
- liver damage
- pneumonia
- agitation and restlessness
- depressed mood and suicide ideation/behavior (US FDA, 2010)

Milnacipran Hydrochloride (Savella): It is a selective SNRI. It is the most recent medication approved by the FDA for treatment of FMS. It is available in 12.5, 25, 50, and 100 mg tablets.

Dosing is recommended at 100 mg per day in two divided doses. The FDA recommends starting at 50 mg twice per day and may be increased to 100 mg twice per day.

Cautions when using with older adults:

With the exception of clinically significant hyponatremia, preliminary studies indicated that milnacipran hydrochloride has similar safety profile in older adults as in younger adults.

- Since it is excreted predominantly unchanged from the kidneys, renal function must be assessed in older adults prior to initiating this medication.
- Dosing should be initiated low and increased slowly.
- Renal function needs to be monitored.

Contraindications include

- older adults taking monoamine oxidase inhibitor medications
- uncontrolled narrow-angle glaucoma

FDA warning

- *FDA warning* is for potentially life-threatening serotonin syndrome or neuroleptic malignant syndrome–like reactions, requiring careful monitoring.

- Symptoms of serotonin syndrome include mental status changes, autonomic instability, neuromuscular aberrations, and gastrointestinal (GI) symptoms.
- Symptoms of neuroleptic malignant syndrome include hyperthermia, muscle rigidity, autonomic instability, and mental status changes.

Other warnings include
- severe hypertension
- tachycardia
- increased bleeding risk (use with caution with nonsteroidal anti-inflammatory drugs (NSAIDs), aspirin, and anticoagulants)
- genitourinary difficulties
- chronic liver disease or substantial alcohol intake

Side effects include
- nausea and vomiting
- headache
- constipation
- dizziness
- insomnia
- hyperhidrosis
- palpitations
- tachycardia
- hypertension
- dry mouth (Forest Laboratories & Inc, 2009; US FDA, 2010)

Pearls	Caution with older adults is to start low and go slow. Carefully monitor older adults for side effects.

Other Medications Used in the Treatment of FMS

Several medications were used prior to pregabalin, duloxetine hydrochloride, and milnacipran hydrochloride receiving FDA approval. Alternate medications are used less frequently now. The following medications have been used to manage the symptoms of FMS but currently do not have FDA approval as such:

- Amitriptyline; although there is strong efficacy for using this in FMS, it is not recommended for use in older adults (see Chapter 8)
- Cyclobenzaprine (Flexeril) 10–30 mg at bedtime

- Gabapentin at 1200–2400 mg per day
- Effexor at 150 mg per day
- Mirtazapine at 15 mg per day
- Fluoxetine hydrochloride (Prozac) at 20–60 mg per day
- Tramadol 50 mg twice per day (may need to be reduced in older people)
- NSAIDs have limited evidence of effectiveness

As with all medications, each of these has side effects and potential interactions with other medications and contraindications with certain comorbidities. These factors for each medication need to be considered with the situation of individual older adult prior to use (American Geriatrics Society, 2009; Arnold et al., 2007; Goldenberg, 2007; Goldenberg, Burckhardt, & Crofford, 2004; Rao & Bennett, 2003; Staud, 2009).

No Evidence to Support Effectiveness with FMS of
- opioids other than tramadol
- steroids
- benzodiazepines (Goldenberg, Burckhardt, & Crofford, 2004; Rao & Bennett, 2003)

On the Horizon
Sodium oxybate is a sodium salt of GHB (gamma hydroxybutyrate) that is a metabolite of γ-aminobutyric acid. In doses of 4.5–6 mg each night, sodium oxybate reportedly showed promising results in significantly reducing pain and other symptoms when compared with placebo. Currently it is not approved for treatment of FMS. Further research is needed in this aspect (Russell, Perkins, & Michalek, 2009).

PATIENT AND FAMILY EDUCATION

Education is a critical component of managing pain in older adults living with FMS.

Formal education generally occurs in group settings ranging from 6 to 17 classes, but occasionally may be intense education occurring over 1–2 days. Data show that there is generally immediate benefit and that benefit is sustained over time (Goldenberg, Burckhardt, & Crofford, 2004).

NON-PHARMACOLOGICAL AND COMPLEMENTARY INTERVENTIONS FOR RA

The reader is referred to Chapter 11 for more information on the complementary interventions listed.

Exercise

The goal of exercise is to improve the general condition, flexibility, and balance. The American Pain Society Guideline Panel (2005) strongly recommended "moderately intense aerobic exercise at least two or three times a week." The panel stressed that it is important to start low and increase slowly.

In one 30-week study, combining supervised exercise with motivational interviewing in a study with middle-aged and older women resulted in significant reductions in pain severity, pain interference, and physical impairment (Ang, Kesavalu, Lydon, Lane, & Bigatti, 2007).

Aerobic exercise has been the focus of numerous research studies among patients with FMS, and there is strong evidence to support using it to manage the symptoms of FMS (Goldenberg, Burckhardt, & Crofford, 2004; Hauser et al., 2010). Some of the aerobic forms of exercise that have been effectively used in older adults with FMS are pool aerobics, cycling, aerobic dance, and walking indoors (Goldenberg, Burckhardt, & Crofford, 2004).

A meta-analysis of various aerobic exercise studies involving a total of 2,494 people living with FMS concluded that land or water aerobic exercise is beneficial in reducing pain and improving mood. The concluding recommendations were that aerobic exercise for people living with FMS should

- be either land- or water-based exercise
- be mild to moderate intensity
- occur 2–3 times per week
- last at least 4 weeks
- encourage participants to continue participation at the end of the 4 weeks (Hauser et al. 2010)

Aerobic endurance exercise was effective in significantly reducing pain in one German study (Meiworm, Jakob, Walker, Peter, & Keul, 2000).

- *Cognitive behavioral therapy (CBT)* is an important option for FMS symptom management and has strong evidence to support the use of this intervention (Goldenberg, Burckhardt, & Crofford, 2004; Hauser et al., 2010; Williams, 2003). CBT has been used with FMS in a variety of ways ranging from individual therapy to group therapy. As a small example, it has been used effectively to

- improve coping skills
- change from an internal to external locus of control (see Chapter 2)
- reframe negative thought patterns
- improve sleep

Cognitively, CBT can also be used to divert attention through cognitive activities, games, and leisure activities.

One multidisciplinary 12-week intervention with sociotherapy, physiotherapy, psychotherapy, and creative arts therapy in the Netherlands resulted in significant improvement in the FIQ and quality of life (QOL) scores (Kroese et al., 2009).

- *Hypnosis* can be helpful in managing the FMS disease process.
- *Relaxation techniques have been effective in progressive muscle relaxation (PMR)* that can be useful in facilitating relaxation and reducing stress and anxiety.
- *Guided imagery* serves as a distraction and relaxation technique with similar benefit to PMR.
- *Combining education and relaxation techniques* was effective in one study. Pain and depression were reduced following a 10-week program of 90-minute group sessions (Nicassio et al., 1997).
- *Therapeutic touch* can be helpful in relieving tension, stress, and pain. In one small study it was found effective in relieving pain and improving QOL (Denison, 2004; Monroe, 2009).
- *Massage* twice a week was effective in relieving anxiety, reducing the number of tender points and improving sleep (Field et al., 2002). Massage has moderate evidence for efficacy as an intervention for FMS (Hauser et al., 2010).
- *Spirituality, prayer, and meditation* are important coping strategies for older adults living with FMS.

REFERRALS AND CONSULTATIONS

Referrals and consultations should be made to the following professionals:

- Physical therapist for mobility training, body mechanics, stretching, strengthening, and endurance exercises

■ Nutritionist to maintain ideal weight and identify the best food options; design an elimination diet if food allergies are a concern (Smith, Terpening, Schmidt, & Gums, 2001)

■ Psychologist or psychiatrist for assessment and intervention for anxiety and depression (America Pain Society, 2005)

RESOURCES AND GUIDELINES

American Pain Society Guideline for the Management of Fibromyalgia Syndrome in Adults and Children. (2005). Glenview, IL.

Guidelines on the management of fibromyalgia syndrome—A systematic review of the guidelines of the American Pain Society, European League Against Rheumatism, and the Association of the Scientific Medical Societies in Germany. (2010). *European Journal of Pain, 14,* 5–10.

The American College of Rheumatology preliminary diagnostic criteria for fibromyalgia and measurement of severity index. (2010). Wolfe, F., Clauw, D. J., Fitzcharles, M. A., Goldenberg, D. L., Katz, R. S., Mease, P., Yunus, M. B. (2010). *Arthritis Care and Research, 62,* 600–610.

> *Case Study*
>
> Caroline Byrd is a 68-year-old woman who has recently moved to your area. She was referred to clinic today by her new neighbor. Caroline tells you that she is always tired and has no energy. When you ask her about pain, she replies "oh, yes, everywhere" "I hurt everywhere, but some places are always more sensitive than others." She tells you that she treats the pain with ibuprophen but it does not seem to help. She says that she does not think anything will, because when she was in the hospital a couple of years ago when she had her gall bladder removed, they gave her morphine and that helped the pain from her gall bladder but did not do anything for the pain that she always has all over. She tells you that she does not do much of anything because of the pain and fatigue. She also does not sleep well most nights. She tells you that she does not think that anyone can help her with this pain. You ask her if she feels sad and depressed. She replies, "yes, wouldn't you if you had to live with this?" Besides, she tells you that with the pain and tiredness she has gained weight and hates to wear such a large dress size.

Questions

1. What indications are there that Caroline has FMS?
2. What other assessment is needed to make a diagnosis?
3. What assessment tool/s seem most appropriate to use with Caroline?
4. If she has FMS, what medication will most likely be effective for her?
5. What things do you need to consider regarding medication choice, administration, and follow up?
6. What nonpharmacological interventions would be helpful for Caroline?
7. What will you include in an educational plan for her?

REFERENCES

American College of Rheumatology (ACR). (2009, June). *American College of Rheumatology- Fibromyalgia*. Retrieved May 22, 2011, from http://www.rheumatology.org

American College of Rheumatology Pain Management Task Force (ACRPMTF). (2010). Report of the American College of Rheumatology Pain Management Task Force. *Arthritis Care and Research, 62,* 590–599.

American Geriatrics Society (AGS). (2009). Pharmacological management of persistent pain in older persons: American Geriatrics Society Panel of the Pharmacological Management of Persistent Pain in Older Adults. *Journal of the American Geriatrics Society, 57,* 1331–1346.

American Pain Society. (2005). *American Pain Society releases new clinical practice guideline for fibromyalgia pain*. Glenview, IL: Author.

Ang, D., Kesavalu, R., Lydon, J. R., Lane, K. A., & Bigatti, S. (2007). Exercise-based motivational interviewing for female patients with fibromyalgia: A case series. *Clinical Rheumatology, 26,* 1843–1849.

Arnold, L. M., Clauw, D. J., & McCarberg, B. H. (2011). Improving the recognition and diagnosis of fibromyalgia. *Mayo Clinic Proceedings, 86,* 457–464.

Arnold, L. M., Goldenberg, D. L., Stanford, S. B., Lalonde, J. K., Sandhu, H. S., Keck, P. E., Hudson, J. I. (2007). Gabapentin in the treatment of fibromyalgia. *Arthritis & Rheumatism, 56,* 1336–1344.

Arnold, L. M., Hudson, J. I., Hess, E. V., Ware, A. E., Fritz, D. A., Auchenbach, M. B., Keck, P. E Jr. (2004). Family study of fibromyalgia. *Arthritis and Rheumatism, 50,* 944–952.

Bennett, R. (2005). The Fibromyalgia Impact Questionnaire (FIQ): A review of its development, current version, operating characteristics and uses. *Clinical and Experimental Rheumatology, 23*(Suppl. 39), S154–S162.

Bennett, R. M., Friend, R., Jones, K. D., Ward, R., Han, B. K., & Ross, R. L. (2009). The revised Fibromyalgia Impact Questionnaire (FIQR) validation and psychometric properties. *Arthritis Research & Therapy, 11,* R120. Retrieved from http://arthritis-research.com/content/11/4/R120

Burkhardt, C. S., Clark, B. D., & Bennett, R. M. (1991). The fibromyalgia impact questionnaire: Development and validation. *Journal of Rheumatology, 18,* 728–733.

Centers for Disease Control, (CDC). (2011). *Fibromyalgia.* Retrieved October 3, 2011, from http://www.cdc.gov/arthritis/basics/fibromyalgia.htm

Chakrabarty, S., & Zoorob, R. (2007). Fibromyalgia. *American Family Physician, 76,* 247–254.

Crofford, L. J., Mease, P. J., Simpson, S. L., Young, J. P., Martin, S. A., Haig, G. M., & Sharma, U. (2008). Fibromyalgia relapse evaluation and efficacy for durability of meaningful relief (FREEDOM): a 6 month, double-blind, placebo-controlled trial with pregabalin. *Pain, 136,* 419–431.

Crofford, L. J., Rowbotham, M. C., Mease, P. J., Russell, I. J., Dworkin, R. H.. Corbin, A. E., & the Pregabalin 1008-105 Study Group. *Arthritis & Rheumatism, 52,* 1264–1273.

Dadabhoy, D., Crofford, L. J., Spaeth, M., Russell, I. J., & Clauw, D. J. (2008). Biology and therapy of fibromyalgia—evidence-based biomarkers for fibromyalgia syndrome. *Arthritis Research & Therapy, 10,* 211. doi:http://arthritis-research.com/content/10/4/211

Denison, B. M. (2004). Touch the pain away: A new research on Therapeutic Touch and persons with fibromyalgia syndrome. *Holistic Nursing Practice, 18,* 142–150.

Desmeules, J. A., Cedraschi, C., Rapiti, E., Baumgartner, A., Finckh, A., Cohen, P., & Vischer, T. L. (2003). Neurophysiologic evidence for a central sensitization in patients with fibromyalgia. *Arthritis & Rheumatism, 48,* 1420–1429.

Farrar, J. T., Young, J. P., Lamoreaux, L., Werth, J. L., & Poole, R. M. (2001). Clinical importance of changes in chronic pain intensity measured on an 11-point numerical pain rating scale. *Pain, 94,* 149–151.

Field, T., Diego, M., Cullen, C., Hernandez-Reif, M., Sunshine, W., & Douglas, W. (2002). Fibromyalgia pain and substance P decrease and sleep improves after massage therapy. *Journal of Clinical Rheumatology, 8,* 72–76.

Forest Laboratories, Inc. (2009). *Savella (milnacipran HCl) Tablets Prescribing Information* [Brochure]. St. Louis, MO: Author.

Friend, R., & Bennett, R. M. (2011). Distinguishing fibromyalgia from rheumatoid arthritis and systemic lupus in clinical questionnaires: An analysis of the revised Fibromyalgia Impact Questionnaire (FIQR) and its variant, the Symptom Impact Questionnaire (SIQR), along with pain locations.

Arthritis Research & Therapy, 13, Retrieved from http://arthritis-research .com/content/13/2/R58

Goldenberg, D. L. (2007). Pharmacological treatment of fibromyalgia and other chronic musculoskeletal pain. *Best Practice & Research Clinical Rheumatology, 21,* 499–511.

Goldenberg, D. L., Burckhardt, C., & Crofford, L. (2004). Management of fibromyalgia syndrome. *Journal of the American Medical Association, 292,* 2388–2395.

Hauser, W., Klose, P., Langhorst, J., Steinbach, M., Schiltenwolf, M., & Busch, A. (2010). Efficacy of different types of aerobic exercise in fibromyalgia syndrome: A systematic review and meta-analysis of randomised controlled trials. *Arthritis Research & Therapy, 12,*(R79), 1–14.

Hauser, W., Petzke, F., & Sommer, C. (2010). Comparative efficacy and harms of duloxetine, milnacipran, and pregabalin in fibromyalgia syndrome. *The Journal of Pain, 11,* 505–521.

Heinricher, M. M., Tavares, I., Leith, J. L., & Lumb, B. M. (2009). Descending control of nociception: Specificity, recruitment and plasticity. *Brain Research Reviews, 60,* 214–225.

Hurst, H., & Bolton, J. (2004). Assessing the clinical significance of change scores recorded on subjective outcome measures. *Journal of Manipulative and Physiological Therapeutics, 27,* 26–35.

Julien, N., Goffaux, P., Arsenault, P., & Marchand, S. (2005). Widespread pain in fibromyalgia is related to deficit of endogenous pain inhibition. *Pain, 114,* 295–302.

Kinder, L. L., Bennett, R. M., & Jones, K. D. (2011). Mounting pathophysiologic evidence to link fibromyalgia with other common chronic pain disorders. *Pain Management Nursing, 12,* 15–24.

Kroese, M., Schulpen, G., Bessems, M., Nijhuis, F., Severens, J., & Landewe, R. (2009). The feasibility and efficacy of a multidisciplinary intervention with aftercare meetings for fibromyalgia. *Clinical Rheumatology, 28,* 923–929.

Lawrence, R. C., Felson, D. T., Helmick, C. G., Arnold, L. M., Choi, H., Deyo, R. A., Wlofe, F. (2008). Estimates of the prevalence of arthritis and other rheumatic conditions in the United States. *Arthritis & Rheumatism, 58,* 26–35.

Mease, P. J., Clauw, D. J., Gendreau, R. M., Rao, S. G., Kranzler, J., Chen, W., & Palmer, R. H. (2009). The efficacy and safety of milnacipran for treatment of fibromyalgia. A randomized, double-blind, placebo-controlled trial. *The Journal of Rheumatology, 36,* 398–409.

Meiworm, L., Jakob, E., Walker, U. A., Peter, H. H., & Keul, J. (2000). Patients with fibromyalgia benefit from aerobic endurance exercise. *Clinical Rheumatology, 19,* 253–257.

Meyer, B. B., & Lemley, K. J. (2000). Utilizing exercise to affect the symptomatology of fibromyalgia: A pilot study. *Medicine & Science in Sports & Exercise, 15,* 1691–1697.

Monroe, C. M. (2009). The effects of Therapeutic Touch on pain. *Journal of Holistic Nursing, 27,* 85–92.

Neumann, L., & Buskila, D. (2003). Epidemiology of fibromyalgia. *Current Pain and Headache Reports, 7,* 362–368.

Nicassio, P. M., Radojevic, V., Weisman, M. H., Schuman, C., Schoenfeld-Smith, K, & Krall, T (1997). A comparison of behavioral and educational interventions for fibromyalgia. *Journal of Rheumatology, 24,* 2000–2007.

Pielsticker, A., Haag, G., Zaudig, M., & Lautenbacher, S. (2005). Impairment of pain inhibition in chronic tension-type headache. *Pain, 118,* 215–223.

Rao, S. G., & Bennett, R. M. (2003). Pharmacological therapies in fibromyalgia. *Best Practice & Research Clinical Rheumatology, 17,* 611–627.

Russell, R. J., Perkins, A. T., Michalek, J. E., & The Oxybate SXB-26 Fibromyalgia Syndrome Study Group. (2009). Sodium oxybate relieves pain and improves function in fibromyalgia syndrome. *Arthritis & Rheumatism, 60,* 299–309.

Siler, A. C., Gardner, H., Yanit, K., Cushman, T., & McDonagh, M. (2010). Systematic review of the comparative effectiveness of antiepileptic drugs for fibromyalgia. *The Journal of Pain ,* 1–9. doi: www.sciencedirect.com

Smith, J. D., Terpening, C. M., Schmidt, S. O., & Gums, J. G. (2001). Relief of fibromyalgia symptoms following discontinuation of dietary excitotoxins. *Annals of Pharmacotherapy, 35,* 702–706.

Staud, R. (2008). Biology and therapy of fibromyalgia: Pain in fibromyalgia syndrome. *Arthritis Research & Therapy, 8,* 208. doi:http://arthritis-research.com/content/8/3/208

Staud, R. (2009). Fibromyalgia syndrome. In H. S. Smith (Ed.), *Current therapy in pain* (pp. 233–241). Philadelphia, PA: Saunders Elsevier.

US Food and Drug Administration. (2008). *Living with fibromyalgia, drugs approved to manage pain.* Retrieved October 3, 2011 from http://www.fda.gov/ForConsumers/ConsumerUpdates/ucm107802.htm

US Food and Drug Administration. (2010, February). *Savella (milnacipran HCl) tablets—Safety labeling changes approved.* Retrieved June 17, 2011, from http://google2.fda.gov/search?q=milnacipran+hcl&x=5&y=12&client=FDAgov&proxystylesheet=FDAgov&output=xml_no_dtd&sort=date%253AD%253AL%253Ad1&site=FDAgov-MedWatch-Safety

US Food and Drug Administration. (2010, July). *Sodium oxybate oral solution NDA 22–531.* Retrieved from http://www.fda.gov/downloads/AdvisoryCommittees/CommitteesMeetingMaterials/Drugs/ArthritisDrugsAdvisoryCommittee/UCM222888.pdfhttp://

US Food and Drug Administration. (2010). *FDA approves first drug for treating fibromyalgia.* Retrieved June 17, 2010, from http://www.fda.gov/NewsEvents/Newsroom/PressAnnouncements/2007/ucm108936.htm

US Food and Drug Administration. (2011). *FDA news release: FDA clears Cymbalta to treat chronic musculoskeletal pain*. Retrieved June 17, 2011, from http://www.fda.gov/NewsEvents/Newsroom/PressAnnouncements/2010/ucm 232708.htm

Williams, D. A. (2003). Psychological and behavioral therapies in fibromyalgia and related syndromes. *Best Practice & Research in Clinical Rheumatology, 17,* 649–665.

Williams, D. A. & Schilling, S. (2009). Advances in the assessment of fibromyalgia. *Rheumatic Disease Clinics of North America, 35,* 339–357

Wolfe, F., Clauw, D. J., Fitzcharles, M. A., Goldenberg, D. L., Katz, R. S., Mease, P., Yunus, M. B. (2010). The American College of Rheumatology preliminary diagnostic criteria for fibromyalgia and measurement of severity index. *Arthritis Care and Research, 62,* 600–610.

Wolfe, F., Smythe, H. A., Yunus, M. B., Bennett, R. M., Bombardier, C., Goldenberg, D. L., Clark, P. (1990). The American College of Rheumatology 1990 criteria for the classification of fibromyalgia: Report of the Multicenter Criteria Committee. *Arthritis and Rheumatism, 33,* 160–172.

22

Anxiety and Depression with Pain in Older Adults

We know that pain is a multiphasic experience that involves the mind, emotions, and spirit of the older adult, as well as genetics and the many experiences the older person has had with pain (Gatchel, Peng, Peters, Fuchs, & Turk, 2007; Keefe, Lumley, Anderson, Lynch, & Carson, 2001; Keefe, Rumble, Scipio, Giordano, & Perri, 2004; Merskey, 2009; Pasero & Portenoy, 2011).

The *Gate Control Theory of Pain* was initiated by Melzack and Wall almost 50 years ago. In that theory, they offered a multidimensional model that explained that centers in the brain had the ability to "open the gates," allowing full pain perception or to "close the gates," reducing pain perception. They proposed that this modulation system involves the

- traditional rapid versus slow conduction of pain via the spinal pathways
- central brain processing of pain signals
- descending signals from the brain, which interrupt ascending signals at the spinal cord (Figure 22.1)

The *Neuromatrix Theory of Pain* was proposed by Melzack in 2001 as a refinement of the gate control theory. The neuromatrix theory describes the complexity of the interactions of the body with emotions, cognition, motivation, and experience in the perception, processing, and management of pain.

A full discussion of the interconnected involvement of emotional and psychological factors involved in pain that is experienced by older people is beyond the scope of this chapter. Since depression and anxiety are common comorbid diagnosis with chronic pain in older adults (McWilliams, Goodwin, & Cox, 2004; Smith & Zautra, 2008), they will be the focus of this chapter.

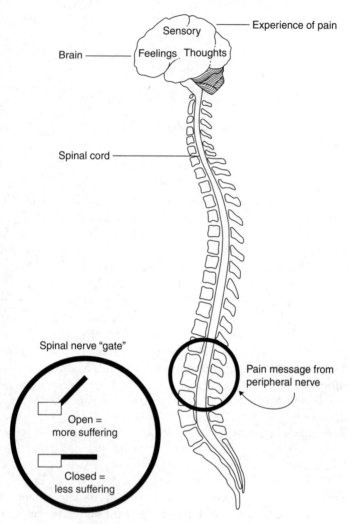

Figure 22.1 ■ Gate control theory of pain.

I. DEPRESSION

Depression is described by the World Health Organization (WHO) (2011) as "a common mental disorder that presents with depressed mood, loss of interest or pleasure, feelings of guilt or low self-worth, disturbed sleep or appetite, low energy, and poor concentration."

Epidemiological Information

Depression is a significant health care need of older adults in all areas of society. Approximation of depression in older adults varies widely. It is estimated that between 17% and 37% of community-dwelling older adults live with depression and 30% of them have a major depressive disorder. Estimates for hospitalized elders are 11% to 12% for major depression and 25% for less severe depression.

Among those living in nursing homes, it is believed that 12% suffer with major depression and 30% have less severe forms of depression; however, in some reports, estimates are as high as 78% among elders in nursing homes. Two studies noted that Caucasian, non-Hispanic, women, with good cognitive function, comorbid physical illness, married currently or previously, and of younger old age in the nursing home were at highest risk for depression (Gaboda, Lucas, Siegel, Kalay, & Crystal, 2011; Reed, 2006).

Information regarding the prevalence of comorbid chronic pain and depression is scarce. It is estimated that in general 6% of all people without chronic pain have depression, and approximately 16% have chronic pain. It is also estimated that between 30% and 54% of people living with chronic pain also have depression (Campbell, Clauw, & Keefe, 2003; Gatchel et al., 2007). Since the estimates of depression among older adults are significantly higher than those for the general population, it is reasonable to deduce that depression among older adults who are living with chronic pain is also higher.

In one epidemiological study involving almost 119,000 Canadians, who were predominantly middle aged and older, 9% reported chronic back pain. Of the participants without pain, 6% were estimated to have major depression, but those with both major depression and chronic back pain were estimated to be markedly higher at 20%. The authors also noted that men were more likely to have major depression associated with pain and those with comorbid back pain and major depression had the greatest disability (Currie & Wang, 2004) (Table 22.1).

The Depression and Chronic Pain Relationship

The relationship of depression with chronic pain is similar to the conundrum of which came first the chicken or the egg. Additional factors that contribute to the conundrum include stress, negative thought

Table 22.1 ■ *Comparison of General Population Estimates with Canadian Study*

	Estimates of Chronic Pain and Depression Compared with Currie and Wang Study	
Condition	*Estimated General (%)*	*Currie and Wang Canadian Study (%)*
Depression	6	6
Chronic Pain[a]	16	9
Comorbidity of Depression with Chronic Pain	30–54	20

Sources: Developed from information in Campbell et al. (2003) and Currie and Wang (2004).

[a]Chronic pain in the estimated general population is all chronic pain compared with the Currie and Wang study that only reported on chronic back pain.

processing, and catastrophizing (Gatchel et al., 2007; Keefe et al., 2001, 2004; Lee, Chan, & Breven, 2007).

Some research studies indicate that depression causes chronic pain. The findings of one prospective study showed that depression was predictive of developing low back pain (LBP). In fact people diagnosed with depression were 2.3 times more likely to have LBP (Jarvik et al., 2005). Others studies indicate that chronic pain causes depression and still others that chronic pain and depression mutually occur in a symbiosis-like relationship. The nature of the involvement more probably is dependent upon the particular chronic pain syndrome. Pain related to osteoarthritis (OA) tends to be of a peripheral nature with little central pain involvement and psychosocial affect. Pain related to fibromyalgia and irritable bowel tend to have central pain contribution with significant psychosocial affect and neuroplasticity changes (see Chapter 21) (Clauw & Crawfford, 2003; Campbell et al., 2003; Gatchel et al., 2007).

Using structural equation modeling analysis Lee et al. (2007) found that perceived severity of pain, interference of pain with activity, stress, and catastrophizing contributed to depression in people with chronic pain. That was in contrast to less depression seen among people with chronic pain who used active pain coping skills and had support from family and friends. Researchers in another study with older adults found that pain and major depressive disorder were strongly associated. These participants rarely sought treatment for symptoms of depression but were likely to seek treatment for pain (Bonnewyn et al., 2009).

Physiology of Depression and Pain

A recent study found that the brain responded with a cascade of activities in various cerebral areas when a depressed mood was provoked. In contrast, these responses were not activated when a neutral mood was elicited. There was also a proportional effect noted with greater frontal gyrus and amygdale activity corresponding with greater pain affect (Berna et al., 2010).

Four neurotransmitters (serotonin, norepinephrine [NE], substance P, and corticotrophin-releasing factor or CRF) (Table 22.2) seem to be engaged in the processes of depression and pain:

- Serotonin
  - In depression, serotonin is generally found in reduced levels in the cerebrospinal fluid (CSF). This is also true in people who are suicidal.
  - In pain processing, it is believed that serotonin has
    - a *pronociceptive* role with the perception of pain in the periphery with the 5-HT3 receptor.
    - an *antinociceptive* role with pain modulation through the central descending 5-HT1A and 5-HT2 receptors.
  - Antidepressant and electroconvulsive therapy (ECT) increase serotonin levels.
- Norepinephrine
  - NE levels are also known to be lower in individuals who are depressed.
  - In pain processing, the primary role of NE is
    - *antinociceptive,* selectively acting on the alpha-2 adrenoceptors of the descending modulation pathway.
    - NE may also have a secondary *pronociceptive* role in peripheral pain perception.
    - When NE is at low levels, it is suggested that substance P is able to function without opposition.
    - It is noteworthy that depression often responds to medications that are designed for NE reuptake.
- Substance P release is crucial in responses to stress and noxious stimuli:
  - It is believed that in the absence of noxious stimuli, release of substance P can lead to anxiety, psychological distress, and depression.
  - It is involved in central sensitization of pain.
  - Substance P antagonist agents can be involved in reversing pathological conditions; however, in at least one experimental study a substance P antagonist was not effective for treating depression.

Table 22.2 ■ *Neurotransmitter Roles in Depression and Pain*

Neurotransmitter	Role in Depression	Role in Pain
Serotonin	Low serum levels with depression; Antidepressants increase levels	Pronociceptive in peripheral pain perception; Antinociceptive role in central descending modulation of pain
NE	Low serum levels with depression; Depression often responds to medications that reuptake NE	Antinociceptive role in central descending modulation of pain; May be pronociceptive in peripheral pain perception; May inhibit release of Substance P
Substance P	Release can lead to anxiety and psychological distress	Release can lead to pain and inflammation; Involved in central sensitization of pain; Substance P antagonists are involved in reversing pathology
CRF	Increased levels are involved in melancholic depression	Antinociceptive in the CNS; Antinociceptive in peripheral inflammation

Source: Based on information in Campbell et al. (2003).

- Corticotrophin-releasing factor
  - CRF elevations are associated with melancholic depression.
  - In the pain process, CRF is involved with antinociception in the central nervous system (CNS) and with inflammatory situations in the periphery (Campbell et al., 2003; Keller et al., 2006) (Table 22.2).

Psychosocial Mechanisms of Pain and Depression

A number of psychological-based characteristics and behaviors have been identified among people living with chronic pain who have high pain severity and are comorbidly depressed. These include

- pain catastrophizing (always assuming the worst, extremely negative concept of painful situation, interpretation of minor situations as catastrophes)
- perceived helplessness about pain situation (believing there is nothing that can be done to change or improve the pain experienced)
- poor self-efficacy or ability to self-manage pain (believing there is nothing that the older adult can do to manage, improve, or change the pain experienced)

- processing information with negative connotations and information recall negatively biased
- dichotomous or polarized thought processes (i.e., "all or nothing," "perfect or failure," "in extreme pain or in no pain")
- over-generalizing with a single perhaps minor painful event being perceived as an overwhelming, never ending problem with pain (Campbell et al., 2003; Okifuji & Skinner, 2009)

Differentiating Depression from Dementia and Delirium

Distinguishing between the "3Ds" (depression, dementia, and delirium) of psychological aging can be challenging:

- Onset
    - depression onset can be sudden (situation related) or slower more insidious
    - delirium has a rapid onset that is situation related
    - dementia has a very slow onset over months or years
- Mood
    - depression is consistently sad, anxious, irritable
    - delirium is labile with mood swings and suspicion common
    - dementia fluctuates with apathy and disinterest common
- Communication
    - depression may be slow but speech and language are normal for the older person
    - delirium may be rambling or forced or slurred or incoherent
    - dementia may be disordered; identifying words can be difficult
- Cognition
    - depression is characterized by hopelessness, helplessness, self-depreciation; pseudodementia with cognitive deficits may occur
    - delirium is disorganized, unable to maintain concentration or attention
    - dementia is characterized by progressively impaired abstract thinking, thought processes, and judgment
- Level of consciousness
    - not altered in depression
    - altered in delirium
    - not altered in dementia

Interventions, both pharmacological and complementary, can be effective with all. Depression and delirium can be reversed but the dementia process can only be slowed (Eliopoulos, 2001; Reed, 2006).

Assessment of Depression in Older Adults

Assessment of depression in older patients needs to include clinical evaluation, as well as patient and family report for signs and symptoms of depression, evaluation to rule out physiological causes, and testing with the geriatric depression scale (GDS).

Possible Signs and Symptoms of Depression in Older Adults

Older adults who experience depression may experience the following:

- Dysphoria, depressed (sad) mood either self-endorsed or observed by others
- Apathy
- Anhedonia, significant loss of interest in pleasurable and other activities
- Withdrawal from family and friends
- Alterations in weight (gain or loss) and appetite (increased or decreased)
- Changes in sleep pattern (insomnia or hypersomnia)
- Changes in psychomotor activity (increased/agitated or reduced/retarded)
- Fatigue or low energy
- Subjective feelings of low self-worth, uselessness, helplessness, and/or guilt
- Feeling hopeless
- Increased dependency on others
- Reduced ability to focus, think, or concentrate
- Vague physical complaints
- Ruminating thoughts about death and/or suicide (American Psychiatric Association, 2000; Reed, 2006)

Differential Diagnosis of Depression in Older Adults

Differential diagnosis of depression in older adults should include

- organic mood disorders caused by illness or medications
- other mental illness (i.e., schizophrenia)
- grief related to loss of a family member, beloved friend, pet animal, home, or loss of independence through loss of ability to drive an automobile
- substance abuse (see Chapter 23)
- dementia or pseudodementia (Kennedy-Malone, Fletcher, & Plank, 2004).

Assessing Depression in Older Adults

There are no diagnostic laboratory tests to confirm depression. The GDS (see Figure 22.2) has been used effectively to assess depression in older adults (Brown & Schinka, 2005; Kurlowicz, 2001). The reader is referred to the discussion of this tool in Chapter 5.

Multimodal Management of Depression in Older Adults

Management of depression in older adults with or without chronic pain is best done from a multimodal approach under the supervision of a mental health care provider with specialty expertise in geriatric mental health, psychiatry, or psychology. The multimodal approach and options are important because older adults are often reluctant

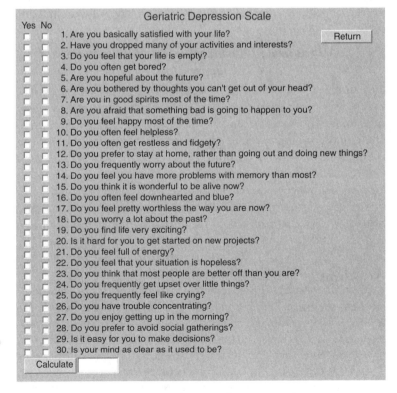

Figure 22.2 ■ Geriatric depression scale.

to take antidepressant medications, and many prefer psychotherapy (Laidlaw, Thompson, & Gallagher-Thompson, 2004). The following points are intended to guide the care of older patients with depression.

Appropriate Management of Coexisting Chronic Pain

Appropriate management of coexisting chronic pain is an essential first step. This will depend upon the etiology of the pain as discussed in preceding chapters. For some pain situations the, first- or second-line medication of choice is an antidepressant. This could either be a tricyclic antidepressant (TCA), such as nortriptyline, or a selective serotonin reuptake inhibitor (SSRI), such as duloxetine. The latter category is more commonly used in the treatment of older adults with comorbid chronic pain and depression and do not have the anticholinergic side effects seen with the TCAs (see Chapters 8 and 9) (American Geriatrics Society, 2009; Campbell et al., 2003; Carter & Sullivan, 2002).

Appropriate Pharmacological Management of Depression

Not all older people need pharmacological intervention for depression; however, generally those who present with moderate to severe symptoms will benefit from antidepressant medication. Selection of the most appropriate medication for an individual older person is best done by a mental health provider who specializes in geriatric care. Consideration must include the psychiatric diagnosis, comorbid medical diagnoses, required medications for comorbid conditions, side effect profiles of other medications and antidepressants, and history of previous reactions to medications. In general, SSRI and atypical antidepressants are more frequently prescribed, particularly for older adults. Again, TCAs are generally avoided because of the anticholinergic side effects (Kennedy-Malone et al., 2004).

Some *important points* to remember when caring for an older adult receiving pharmacological antidepressant therapy are the following:

- Start with low doses (generally 50% of the usual recommended dose).
- Assess for interactions with required medications for comorbid illnesses.
    - Antidepressants can increase the effects of some medications while decreasing the effects of other medications.
    - Antidepressant effects can be increased by thiazide diuretics and alcohol.

- Educate older patients and families about dosage of medication and any special precautions.
- Educate the older patients and families that generally one full month of consistently taking the medication is needed to notice a beneficial effect.
- Educate about and monitor for side effects, especially sedation, constipation, hypotension, blurred vision, urinary retention, diaphoresis, appetite, and weight changes (Eliopoulos, 2001).

Pearl	The general rules for pharmacology with older adults are: Start low and go slow! Monitor response and side effects

Therapeutic Interventions

There are a variety of different types of psychotherapy that are effective for older adults. A meta-analysis assessing the various types of therapy concluded that all psychological therapies that are considered legitimate (bona fide) are effective at a similar or same level (Warmpold, Minami, Baskin, & Tierney, 2002). The type of therapy depends upon the availability of therapists, the specialty focus of therapists, and the preference of the older adult.

Cognitive behavioral therapy (CBT) is a vital component, with proven effectiveness for helping older people who suffer from depression as well as from chronic pain. The general concepts of CBT are that it is a structured, problem-solving intervention occurring over a specified time period involving education designed to change behavior. Frequently, CBT is offered in group settings; however, the principles can be used individually with older adults (Keefe, Beaupre, & Gil, 2002; Laidlaw et al., 2004). An innovative approach to CBT in the Netherlands was Internet based. When the Internet CBT was compared with standard group CBT, it was found to be as effective among almost 300 older adults. This is an option for older adults with depression for whom transportation issues are challenging (Spek et al., 2007).

Interpersonal psychotherapy is based upon depression in a social framework. A number of techniques can be utilized, including communication analysis and role playing. It has been effective with older adults. It was also found that older adults are often more compliant with interpersonal therapy than with medications because therapy does not have the untoward physical side effects. Yet, this therapy has particularly positive results with geriatric patients when combined with antidepressant medications (Bruce et al., 2004; Lynch & Smoski, 2009).

Problem-solving therapy (PST) is one type of cognitive therapy that has been used successfully with older adults. The older person learns to develop a positive approach toward problem solving and is actively engaged with "homework assignments." It has been effective with older people. PST has been used effectively in a home care format that is useful for elders who have challenges with transportation (Gellis & Bruce, 2010; Gellis, McGinty, Horowitz, Bruce, & Misener, 2007; McClintock, Staub, & Husain, 2011). In one small study, PST was found to be more effective than supportive therapy in older adults with major depression. The elders who received PST had effective remissions and fewer depressive symptoms following treatment (Alexopoulos, Raue, & Arean, 2003).

Other psychotherapy interventions have been used with older adults with mixed results. They include psychodynamic psychotherapy, life review and reminiscence psychotherapy, group psychotherapy, and bibliotherapy (Lynch & Smoski, 2009).

ECT is considered the most effective treatment for older adults who have severe depression. It is safe, with a speedy response rate and low relapse rate in older adults. One meta-analysis of 22 studies reported that ECT and maintenance ECT (continuation of ECT treatments) most likely have the same effectiveness as antidepressant medications. Further research is needed in this area (Van Schalik et al., 2011). Determination of this therapy would be made by a psychiatrist managing depression in the older person.

Pearls	Psychotherapy is a good and effective intervention for older adults.
	Traditional psychotherapy may need to be modified for older adults.
	It is best to refer the older adult to a geriatric mental health professional.

Suicidality in Chronic Pain and Depression Among Older Adults

Suicide is a significant risk among depressed individuals and it is twice as common among people who live with chronic pain than among their pain-free counterparts. Approximately 20% of people who live with chronic pain have suicide ideation (SI) and between 5% and 14% attempt suicide. The incidence of suicide increases with age, with approximately 23% of all suicides being accomplished by older adults. Among Caucasians, African Americans, and Hispanics, older males suicide more than their female counterparts, and older Caucasian males have the highest suicide rate of all groups. Most elders who attempt suicide have seen a primary care provider in the recent past. Older suiciders tend to use more violent methods. There was a higher prevalence of hospitalizations in general, and of prior hospitalizations specifically for depression among the older group, but there were also many who had no history or indication of depression.

It is imperative to listen carefully to older adults and take any indication of SI very seriously. Indications of older people at risk for suicide may be subtle. Some indications include

- misusing medications either through excessive use or by omitting required medications
- not adhering to therapeutic treatment plans (diet, exercise, therapy)
- not eating or drinking
- high-risk behaviors such as drunk driving

When there is a concern for or indication of SI, it is imperative to assess for any changes in the life of the older person. With caring concern, ask the older person if he or she currently or have ever considered suicide. If the answer is affirmative or indicates that there is a risk of suicide, the person needs to be monitored and further evaluated immediately by a mental health professional (Bruce et al., 2004; Corna, Cairney, & Streiner, 2010; Eliopoulos, 2001; Heok & Ho, 2008; Koponen et al., 2007; Tadros & Salib, 2007).

Pearl | Take all references to suicide or "ending it all" very seriously. When there is a risk of suicide, monitor the person and seek immediate mental health evaluation.

II. ANXIETY

Anxiety is a condition that is characterized by increased worry about what will or might occur. The types of anxiety include panic disorder (PD), social phobia, agoraphobia, obsessive–compulsive disorder, generalized anxiety disorder (GAD), acute stress disorder, and posttraumatic stress disorder. Fear, arousal (either autonomic or situational), and avoidance are common in most types. In addition, there is subthreshold anxiety in which older adults do not satisfy full, formal diagnostic criteria of the American Psychiatric Association Diagnostic and Statistical Manual-IV (APA DSM-IV), but demonstrate some signs of anxiety (American Psychiatric Association, 2000; Greiner et al., 2011; Lenze & Wetherell, 2009).

Epidemiology of Anxiety Among Older Adults

Despite anxiety disorders among the geriatric population not being followed, studied, or researched as well as depression, it is considered a public health concern. There is very little information available regarding incidence and prevalence of anxiety in any age group. Complicating this is that different criteria are used for determining prevalence, resulting in wide variations in reports. Estimates have ranged from 0.1% to 28% among older people but are generally considered to be close to the 10% that is seen in other age groups. In a recent study, prevalence rates of anxiety among older adults varied from 5.6%, when strict APA DSM-IV criteria were used, to 26.2%, when subthreshold anxiety was considered (Greiner et al., 2011). One review of the literature reported that the prevalence of anxiety symptoms is as high as 52% in community settings and 56% in clinical settings (Bryant, Jackson, & Ames, 2008). It is possible that the formal diagnostic inclusion criteria for anxiety disorders may not include criteria that are more relevant to older adults. In one study involving170 middle-aged and older women (42 to 76 years) with OA and rheumatoid arthritis (RA), the direct effect of anxiety was almost double the effect of depression, and when anxiety was controlled for, the effect of depression became nonsignificant (Greiner et al., 2011; Kessler, Keller, & Wittchen, 2001; Lenze & Wetherell, 2009; Smith & Zautra, 2008; Stanley & Novy, 2000; Troller, Anderson, Sachdev, Brodaty, & Andrews, 2007).

There is also a lack of agreement as to when anxiety disorders most frequently begin in older adults. Some researchers believe that anxiety disorders generally develop during youth and young adulthood and continue with aging. Others believe anxiety disorders frequently develop during later years. Still others believe that approximately 66% develop early and continue with age, and the other approximately 33% have an onset later in life. Differences may be related to the aging process, chronic illnesses, and medications (Kessler et al., 2007; Le Roux, Gatz, & Wetherell, 2005; Lenze et al., 2005; Sheikh, Swales, Carlson, & Lindley, 2004).

Anxiety in older people has been associated with

- having an external locus of control (see Chapter 2)
- dysfunctional coping strategies
- history of experiencing traumatic events
- never having a child
- lower income (Vink, Aartsen, & Schoevers, 2008)

Anxiety and Pain

Like pain and depression, the relationship between pain and anxiety can be considered a conundrum of which came first. There is very little data that specifically address pain and anxiety in older patients. The research that has been done has been primarily with younger adults. One study did investigate anxiety, depression, and anger among 100 older patients in a postsurgical rehabilitation unit. In that sample, only state anxiety was a significant predictor of acute pain (Feeney, 2004).

Anxiety is believed to intensify both the perception of pain and the estimation of pain intensity. A circular effect can develop between pain and anxiety, when older adults who experience chronic or persistent pain develop anxiety or fear about pain or fear of reinjury. Fear of pain at baseline has been reported to be predictive of more severe pain when pain occurs. With pain anxiety or fear of pain, there is a tendency to

- be extra vigilant to pain sensation
- expect that they will experience higher levels of pain
- self-report disability high
- perform physical activities and participate in the physical exam slowly
- avoid participation in social, work, or leisure activities (Feeney, 2004; Keefe et al., 2004).

Physiology and the Anxiety–Pain Relationship

There is very little known about the physiological issues affecting anxiety among older adults. It is suggested that there may be a relationship between GAD among older people and the age-related changes that occur in the hypothalamic–pituitary–adrenocortical axis. Diurnal cortisol levels are reported to be 40% to 50% greater among elders with GAD than in their nonaffected counterparts. Interestingly these stress-related cortisol levels reduce in response to diazepam in older adults, but not in their younger counterparts with GAD (Lenze & Wetherell, 2009; Meiner, 2006; Pomara, Willoughby, Sidtis, Cooper, & Greenblatt, 2005).

Physiological factors associated with an increased risk of older adults having anxiety symptoms and disorders include

- cognitive impairment
- hypertension
- sensory loss (either visual or hearing)

Anxiety and Depression as Comorbidities with Pain

The relationship with pain is more involved when considering the frequent comorbidity of anxiety and depression, which have been closely associated in the literature. In fact, it has been suggested that anxiety may be a risk factor for developing geriatric depression.

One Spanish study with more than 7,100 middle-aged and older adults (mean age 51) found that participants diagnosed with GAD (59%) were twice as likely as the controls (28%) to have painful physical symptoms (PPS). Interestingly, although 59% of those diagnosed with GAD had PPS, 78% of participants who had both GAD and major depressive disorder had PPS. These differences were statistically significant (Romera et al., 2010). Those findings were consistent with an earlier international study of adults (~20% over 60 years) in which chronic pain compared with other chronic conditions had the strongest correlation with anxiety and depression individually. The correlation between chronic pain with both anxiety and depression was significantly stronger (Scott et al., 2007).

Researchers from the Longitudinal Aging Study Amsterdam reported that 48% of older adults who were diagnosed with major depressive disorder also had anxiety disorders. That is consistent with clinical studies in which approximately half of older patients had both depression and anxiety (Lenze & Wetherell, 2009).

Studies in a variety of settings demonstrate that anxiety, rather than depression, was predictive of pain. Researchers in one study assessed the relationship between three psychopathologies (anxiety, depression, and panic attacks) with three chronic pain conditions (arthritis, migraines, and back pain). Among more than 3,000 adult participants between 25 and 74 years, the associations were greatest among anxiety with the three pain variables (McWilliams et al., 2004). In a study with 170 older women with OA and RA, anxiety and depression were both predictive of current and future pain, but the effects for anxiety were nearly twice that of depression (Smith & Aautra, 2008). These findings are consistent with earlier findings in a study of older adults who were institutionalized in a multilevel facility. Interestingly, anxiety, not depression, was significantly related to pain (Casten, Parmelee, Kleban, Lawton, & Katz, 1995).

Assessment of Anxiety in Older Adults

This is based upon what has occurred in the recent history, patient's chief complaint, observation, and interview.

Possible Signs and Symptoms of Anxiety in Older Adults

Key elements to assess include
- Objective indicators of anxiety
    - patient self-report of anxiety (often described as "feeling nervous," "inability to relax," "trembling," "jumpiness," "feeling edgy")
    - behavioral indicators such as pacing, wringing hands, fidgeting
    - reports of worry, or anticipating something negative will happen
- Short-term and delayed memory
- Changes in sleep patterns
- Changes in eating patterns
- Physical complaints (i.e., sweating, gastrointestinal disturbances, palpitations, dizziness, headache, tremor, dry mouth, polyuria, pain, hot/cold spells)
- Cognitive complaints (i.e., difficulty concentrating or easily distracted) (Kennedy-Malone et al., 2004; Mantella et al., 2007; Reed, 2006)

Tools for Assessing Anxiety in Older Adults

The Geriatric Anxiety Scale was specifically designed to assess anxiety in older adults. It has good reliability and validity (Segal, June, Payne, Coolidge, & Yochim, 2010). It is a 30-item self-report instrument that could conceivably be used as an admission (hospital, long-term care, rehabilitation center) screening tool or annual evaluation (primary care office or clinic) screening tool (Figure 22.3).

Hospital Anxiety and Depression Scale is also a self-rating scale. It is shorter than the geriatric anxiety scale, consisting of only 14 items. It has good validity and reliability for assessing both anxiety and depression in patients hospitalized for both somatic and psychiatric illnesses in different age groups, including older adults. It has extensive use and documentation in a number of languages (Bjelland, Dahl, Haug, & Neckelmann, 2002; Crawford, Henry, Crombie, & Taylor, 2001; Olsson, Mykletun, & Dahl, 2005).

Multimodal Management of Anxiety in Older Adults

Anxiety in older adults is best managed from a multimodal perspective. As with pain and depression, using therapy interventions in addition to medication helps to keep dosages lower and minimize side effects.

Appropriate management of coexisting chronic pain is an essential component of managing anxiety. As discussed, pain can be a trigger for anxiety or for worsening anxiety.

Appropriate Pharmacological Management of Anxiety

There is very little research or evidence to guide pharmacological management of anxiety in older adults. As with major depression, GAD is best managed by a mental health professional.

Buspirone is an atypical anxiolytic medication that can take 4 to 6 weeks to become effective. During that period, it may be necessary to cautiously use a short-acting benzodiazepine (as described below).

The usual adult starting does of buspirone is 7.5 mg twice daily, but it can be started as low as 2.5 mg twice daily in older adults. In addition to assessing potential interactions of buspirone with each medication concomitantly taken by individual older adults, some general cautions and contraindications include the following:

■ Avoid with renal or hepatic impairment
■ Avoid with

- alcohol
- Monoamine oxidase inhibitors
- other CNS depressants
- Use with caution with psychotropic medications
- Major side effects that could pose problems to older adults are
  - dizziness
  - nervousness and/or restlessness
  - lightheadedness
  - fatigue
  - restless leg syndrome

Antidepressants, especially the SSRIs (i.e., sertraline) and the serotonin–norepinephrine-reuptake inhibitors (i.e., duloxetine), have been used as first-line treatment with young adults, but there are limited small studies in the geriatric community. The reader is referred to Chapters 8 and 9 for more information on these medications and side effects.

Benzodiazepines (alprazolam, lorazepam, or oxazepam) have been reported as effective in some studies; however, the concern is that this class of medications needs to be used very cautiously with older adults. If one of these medications is needed for symptom management, it is imperative to consider

- the comorbidities of the older adult
- concomitant medications (including over-the-counter and herbal products)
- potential for misuse of the medication (see Chapter 23)
- side-effect profile of the benzodiazepine medication options

Primary concerns are for the older adult falling and developing cognitive deterioration

Risperidone was studied in one small Spanish study but there was insufficient evidence to evaluate clinical use in older adults. The investigators reported very good efficacy and recommended further investigation. (Lenze et al., 2005; Lenze & Wetherell, 2009; Morinigo, Blanco, Labrador, Martin, & Noval, 2005; Schurmans et al., 2006).

Therapeutic Interventions

CBT has very effective outcomes when used with older adults with GAD. Outcomes were best for elders who were consistently involved in doing the homework between sessions (Stanley & Novy, 2000; Wetherell et al., 2005).

Below is a list of common symptoms of anxiety or stress. Please read each item in the list carefully. Indicate how often you have experienced each symptom during the PAST WEEK, INCLUDING TODAY by checking under the corresponding answer.

	Not at all	Sometimes	Most of the time	All of the time
1. My heart raced or beat strongly.				
2. My breath was short.				
3. I had an upset stomach.				
4. I felt like things were not real or like I was outside of myself.				
5. I felt like I was losing control.				
6. I was afraid of being judged by others.				
7. I was afraid of being humiliated or embarrassed.				
8. I had difficulty falling asleep.				
9. I had difficulty staying asleep.				
10. I was irritable.				
11. I had outbursts of anger.				
12. I had difficulty concentrating.				
13. I was easily startled or upset.				
14. I was less interested in doing something I typically enjoy.				
15. I felt detached or isolated from others.				

	Not at all	Sometimes	Most of the time	All of the time
16. I felt like I was in a daze.				
17. I had a hard time sitting still.				
18. I worried too much.				
19. I could not control my worry.				
20. I felt restless, keyed up, or on edge.				
21. I felt tired.				
22. My muscles were tense.				
23. I had back pain, neck pain, or muscle cramps.				
24. I felt like I had no control over my life.				
25. I felt like something terrible was going to happen to me.				
26. I was concerned about my finances.				
27. I was concerned about my health.				
28. I was concerned about my children.				
29. I was afraid of dying.				
30. I was afraid of becoming a burden to my family or children.				

Figure 22.3 ■ Geriatric Anxiety Scale. (Segal et al., 2010)

Stanley, Diefenbach, and Hopko (2004) identified the following as important elements when using CBT for treatment of GAD in older adults:

- Motivational exercises addressing goals and realistic expectations
- Education
  - about anxiety (physical, emotional, and behavioral manifestations)
  - about CBT
  - relaxation (breathing exercises)
  - problem solving
  - coping skills (i.e., thought stopping)
- Develop awareness of anxiety and how it feels
- Practice
  - relaxation
  - problem solving
- Exposure exercises (the person being exposed to what creates anxiety for them)
- Sleep management

Muscle relaxation therapy or *progressive muscle relaxation* has been successfully used to manage GAD and PD even though the mechanisms of action are not known. The older adult is guided first to tense muscles and then to progressively relax muscles (Conrad & Roth, 2007). Once it is learned, older adults can practice it at their convenience and use the technique whenever needed or desired.

Pearl	Anxiety among older adults must be taken seriously. Management of anxiety is an important aspect of pain management in older adults who have comorbid pain and anxiety.

RESOURCES AND GUIDELINES

American Psychiatric Association. http://www.psych.org/

APA practice guideline for the treatment of patients with major depressive disorder (3rd ed.). http://www.psychiatryonline.com/content.aspx?aID=654034

Case Study

Sally Green is a pleasant 81-year-old woman who is being seen for her presurgical screening visit prior to having a total hip replacement next month. You notice that she looks down at the floor most of the time and continually smooths the wrinkled skirt of her dress and turns her wedding band. She slowly tells you that she is a widow and never had any children, and she still very much misses her husband who died 5 years ago. After she tells you what medicines she is taking for her arthritis (etodolac and oxycodone), diabetes, and migraine headaches, she tells you that she is "a bit nervous" about the surgery. She also tells you that she is very afraid that things will not go well during surgery. She has tears in her eyes when she tells you that nothing seems to go right for her since her husband died, and she cannot stand for one more thing to go wrong. She says, "it just is not worth all the trouble anymore." As she tells you this, she moves her ring more and shakes her head side to side.

Questions

1. What is your assessment of Sally Green?
2. What are the most important things to address right now?
3. What other things may be going on with her?
4. What referrals should be made for her?
5. What medication options are best for her?
6. What education does she need?
7. What nonpharmacological interventions might be good for her?

REFERENCES

Alexopoulos, G., Raue, P., & Arean, P. (2003). Problem-solving therapy versus supportive therapy in geriatric major depression with executive dysfunction. *American Journal of General Psychiatry, 11,* 46–52.

American Geriatric Society. (2009). Pharmacological management of persistent pain in older adults. *Journal of the American Geriatric Society, 57,* 1331–1346.

American Psychiatric Association. (2000). *Diagnostic and statistical manual of mental disorders Fourth Edition Text Revision*. Washington, DC: American Psychiatric Association.

Berna, C., Leknes, S., Holmes, E. A., Edwards, R. R., Goodwin, G. M., & Tracey, I. (2010). Induction of depressed mood disrupts emotion regulation neurocircuitry and enhances pain unpleasantness. *Biological Psychiatry, 67,* 1083–1090.

Bjelland, I., Dahl, A. A., Haug, T. T., & Neckelmann, D. (2002). The validity of the Hospital Anxiety and Depression Scale. An updated literature review. *Journal of Psychosomatic Research, 52,* 69–77.

Bonnewyn, A., Katona, C., Bruffaerts, R., Haro, J. M., De Graaf, R., Alonso, J., & Demyttenaere, K. (2009). Pain and depression in older people: Comorbidity and patterns of help seeking. *Journal of Affective Disorders, 117,* 193–196.

Brown, L. M., & Schinka, J. A. (2005). Development and initial validation of a 15-item informant version of the Geriatric Depression Scale. *International Journal of Geriatric Psychiatry, 20,* 911–918.

Bruce, M. L., Ten Have, T. R., Reynolds, C. F., Katz, I. L., Schulberg, H. C., Mulsant, B. H., Alexopoulos, G. S. (2004). Reducing suicide ideation and depressive symptoms in depressed older primary care patients: A randomized controlled trial. *Journal of the American Medical Association, 291,* 1081–1091.

Bryant, C., Jackson, H., & Ames, D. (2008). The prevalence of anxiety in older adults: Methodological issues and a review of the literature. *Affective Disorders, 109,* 233–250.

Campbell, L. C., Clauw, D. J., & Keefe, F. J. (2003). Persistent pain and depression: A biopsychosocial perspective. *Biological Psychiatry, 54,* 399–409.

Carter, G. T., & Sullivan, M. D. (2002). Antidepressants in pain management. *Current Opinion in Investigational Drugs, 2,* 454–458.

Casten, R. J., Parmelee, P. A., Kleban, M. H., Lawton, M. P., & Katz, I. R. (1995). The relationships among anxiety, depression, and pain in a geriatric institutionalized sample. *Pain, 61,* 271–276.

Clauw, D. J., & Crawfford, L. J. (2003). Chronic widespread pain and fibromyalgia: What we know and what we need to know. *Best Practice in Research Clinical Rheumatology, 17,* 685–701.

Conrad, A., & Roth, W. T. (2007). Muscle relaxation therapy for anxiety disorders: It works but how. *Journal of Anxiety Disorders, 21,* 243–264.

Corna, L. M., Cairney, J., & Streiner, D. L. (2010). Suicide ideation in older adults: Relationship to mental health problems and service use. *The Gerontologist, 50,* 785–797.

Crawford, J. R., Henry, J. D., Crombie, C., & Taylor, E. P. (2001). Brief report: Normative data for the HADS from a large non-clinical sample. *British Journal of Clinical Psychology, 40,* 429–434.

Currie, S. R., & Wang, J. L. (2004). Chronic back pain and major depression in the general Canadian population. *Pain, 107,* 54–60.

Eliopoulos, C. (2001). *Gerontological nursing* (5th ed.). Philadelphia, PA: Lippincott.

Feeney, S. L. (2004). The relationship between pain and negative affect in older adults: Anxiety as a predictor of pain. *Anxiety Disorders, 18,* 733–744.

Gaboda, D., Lucas, J., Siegel, M., Kalay, E., & Crystal, S. (2011). No longer undertreated? Depression diagnosis and antidepressant therapy in elderly long-stay nursing home residents, 1999-2007. *Journal of the American Geriatrics Society, 59,* 673–680.

Gatchel, R. J., Peng, Y. B., Peters, M. L., Fuchs, P. N., & Turk, D. C. (2007). The biophysical approach to chronic pain: Scientific advances and future directions. *Psychological Bulletin, 133,* 581–624.

Gellis, Z. D., & Bruce, M. L. (2010). Problem-solving therapy for subthreshold depression in home healthcare patients with cardiovascular disease. *American Journal of Geriatric Psychiatry, 18,* 464–474.

Gellis, Z. D., McGinty, J., Horowitz, A., Bruce, M. L., & Misener, E. (2007). Problem-solving therapy for late-life depression in home care: A randomized field trial. *American Journal of Geriatric Psychiatry, 15,* 968–978.

Greiner, S., Preville, M., Boyer, R., O'Connor, K., Beland, S. G., Potvin, O., Scientific Committee of The ESA Study (2011). The impact of DSM-IV symptom and clinical significance criteria on the prevalence estimates of subthreshold and threshold anxiety in the older adult population. *American Journal of Geriatric Psychiatry, 19,* 316–326.

Heok, K. E., & Ho, R. (2008). The many faces of geriatric depression. *Current Opinions in Psychiatry, 21,* 540–545.

Jarvik, J. G., Hollingsworth, W., Heagerty, P. J., Haynor, D. R., Boyco, E. J., & Deyo, R. A. (2005). Three-year incidence of low back pain in an initially asymptomatic cohort. Clinical and imaging risk factors. *Spine, 30,* 1541–1548.

Keefe, F. J., Beaupre, P. M., & Gil, K. M. (2002). Group therapy for patients with chronic pain. In D. Turk & R. J. Gatchel (Eds.), *Psychological approaches to pain management: A practitioner's handbook* (pp. 259–282). New York, NY: Guilford Press.

Keefe, F. J., Lumley, M., Anderson, T., Lynch, T., & Carson, K. (2001). Pain and emotion: New research directions. *Journal of Clinical Psychology, 57,* 587–607.

Keefe, F. J., Rumble, M. E., Scipio, C. D., Giordano, L. A., & Perri, L M. (2004). Psychological aspects of persistent pain: Current state of the science. *The Journal of Pain, 5,* 195–211.

Keller, M., Montgomery, S., Ball, W., Morrison, M., Snavely, D., Liu, G., & Reines, S. (2006). *Biological Psychiatry, 59,* 216–223.

Kennedy-Malone, L., Fletcher, K. R., & Plank, L. M. (2004). *Management guidelines for nurse practitioners* (2nd ed.). Philadelphia, PA: F. A. Davis Company.

Kessler, R. C., Amminger, G. P., Aguilar-Gaxiola, S., Alonso, J., Lee, S., & Ustun, B. (2007). Age of onset of mental disorders: A review of recent literature. *Current Opinion in Psychiatry, 20,* 359–364.

Kessler, R. C., Keller, M. B., & Wittchen, H. U. (2001). The epidemiology of generalized anxiety disorder. *The Psychiatric Clinics of North America, 24,* 19–39.

Koponen, H. J., Villo, K., Hakko, H., Timonen, M., Meyer-Rochow, V. B., Sarkioja, T., Rasanen, P. (2007). Rates and previous disease history in old age suicide. *Geriatric Psychiatry, 22,* 38–46.

Kurlowicz, L. H. (2001). Benefits of psychiatric consultation-liaison nurse interventions for older hospitalized patients and their nurses. *Archives of Psychiatric Nursing, 15,* 53–61.

Laidlaw, K., Thompson, L. W., & Gallagher-Thompson, D. (2004). Comprehensive conceptualization of cognitive behaviour therapy for late life depression. *Behavioural and Cognitive Psychotherapy, 32,* 389–399.

Le Roux, H., Gatz, M., & Wetherell, J. L. (2005). Age at onset of generalized anxiety disorder in older adults. *American Journal of Geriatric Psychiatry, 13,* 23–30.

Lee, G., Chan, F., & Breven, N. L. (2007). Factors affecting depression among people with chronic musculoskeletal pain: A structural equation model. *Rehabilitation Psychology, 52,* 33–43.

Lenze, E. J., Mulsant, B. H., Mohlman, J., Shear, M. K., Dew, M. A., Schultz, R., & Reynolds, C. F. (2005). Generalized anxiety disorder in late life: Lifetime course and comorbidity with major depressive disorder. *American Journal of Geriatric Psychiatry, 13,* 77–80.

Lenze, E. J., Mulsant, B. H., Shear, M. K., Dew, M. A., Miller, M. D., & Pollock B. G. (2005). Efficacy and tolerability of citalopram in the treatment of late-life anxiety disorders: Results from an 8 week randomized, placebo-controlled trial. *American Journal of Psychiatry, 162,* 146–150.

Lenze, E. J., & Wetherell, J. L. (2009). Anxiety disorders. In D. G. Blazer & D. C. Steffens (Eds.), *The American Psychiatric Publishing textbook of geriatric psychiatry* (4th ed., pp. 333–345). Washington, DC: The American Psychiatric Publishing Company.

Lynch, T. R., & Smoski, M. J. (2009). Individual and group psychotherapy. In D. G. Blazer & D. C. Steffens (Eds.), *The American Psychiatric Publishing textbook of geriatric psychiatry* (4th ed., pp. 521–538). Washington, DC: American Psychiatric Publishing Company.

Mantella, R. C., Butters, M. A., Dew, M. A., Mulsant, B. H., Begley, A. E., Tracey, B. H., Lenze, E. J. (2007). Cognitive impairment in late-life generalized anxiety disorder. *American Journal of Geriatric Psychiatry, 15,* 673–679.

McClintock, S. M., Staub, B., & Husain, M. M. (2011). The effects of electroconvulsive therapy on neurocognitive function in elderly adults. *Annals of Long Term Care, 19,* 32–38.

McWilliams, L. A., Goodwin, R. D., & Cox, B. J. (2004). Depression and anxiety associated with three pain conditions: Results from a nationally representative sample. *Pain, 111,* 77–83.

Meiner, S. E. (2006). Theories of aging. In S. E. Meiner & A.G. Lueckenotte (Eds.), *Gerontologic Nursing* (pp. 19–32). St. Louis, MO: Mosby Elsevier.

Melzack, R. (2001). Pain and the neuromatrix of the brain. *Journal of Dental Education, 65,* 1378–1382.

Merskey, H. (2009). The taxonomy of pain. In H. S. Smith (Ed.), *Current therapy in pain* (pp. 1–4). Philadelphia, PA: Saunders Elsevier.

Morinigo, A., Blanco, M., Labrador, J., Martin, J., & Noval, D. (2005). Risperidone for resistant anxiety in elderly patients. *American Journal of Geriatric Psychiatry, 13*, 81–82.

Okifuji, A., & Skinner, M. (2009). Behavioral medicine approaches to pain management. In H. S. Smith (Ed.), *Current therapy in pain management* (pp. 513–518). Philadelphia, PA: Saunders Elsevier.

Olsson, I., Mykletun, A., & Dahl, A. A. (2005). The hospital anxiety and depression rating scale: A cross-sectional study of psychometrics and case finding abilities in general practice. *BMC Psychiatry, 5*(46), doi available on line at: http://www.biomedcentral.com/content/pdf/1471-244X-5-46.pdf

Pasero, C., & Portenoy, R. K. (2011). Neurophysiology of pain and analgesic and the pathophysiology of neuropathic pain. In C. Pasero and M. McCaggery (Ed.), *Pain assessment and pharmacologic management* (pp. 1–12). St. Louis, MO: Mosby Elsevier.

Pomara, N., Willoughby, L. M., Sidtis, J. J., Cooper, T. B., & Greenblatt, J. J. (2005). Cortisol response to diazepam: Its relationship to age, dose, duration of treatment, and presence of generalized anxiety disorder. *Psychopharmacology, 178*, 1–8.

Reed, M. J. (2006). Mental health. In S. E. Meiner & A. G. Lueckenotte (Eds.), *Gerontologic Nursing* (3rd ed., pp. 281–303). St. Louis, MO: Mosby Elsevier.

Romera, I., Fernandez-Perez, S., Montejo, A. L., Caballero, F., Caballero, L., Arbesu, J. A., Gilaberte, I. (2010). Generalized anxiety disorder, with or without co-morbid major depressive disorder, in primary care: Prevalence of painful somatic symptoms, functioning and health status. *Journal of Affective Disorders, 127*, 160–168.

Sheikh, J. L., Swales, P. J., Carlson, E. B., & Lindley, S. E. (2004). Aging and panic disorder: phenomenology, comorbidity, and risk factors. *American Journal of Psychiatry, 12*, 102–109.

Schurmans, J., Comijs, H., Emmelkamp, P. M., Gundy, C. M., Weijnen, I., van den Hout, M., & van Dyck, R. (2006). A randomized, controlled trial of the effectiveness of cognitive-behavioral therapy and sertraline versus a waitlist control group for anxiety disorders in older adults. *American Journal of Geriatric Psychiatry, 14*, 255–263.

Scott, K. M., Bruffaerts, R., Tsang, A., Ormel, J., Alonso, J., Angermeyer, M. C., von Korff, M. (2007). Depression - anxiety relationships with chronic physical conditions: Results from the World Mental Health surveys. *Journal of Affective Disorders, 103*, 113–120.

Segal, D. L., June, A., Payne, M., Coolidge, F. L., & Yochim, B. (2010). Development and initial validation of a self-report assessment tool for anxiety among older adults: The Geriatric Anxiety Scale. *Journal of Anxiety Disorders, 24*, 709–714.

Smith, B. W., & Zautra, A. J. (2008). The effects of anxiety and depression on weekly pain in women with anxiety. *Pain, 138*, 354–361.

Spek, V., Nyklicek, I., Smits, N., Cuijpers, P., Riper, H., Keyzer, J., & Pop, V. (2007). Internet-based cognitive behavioral therapy for subthreshold depression in people over 50 years old: A randomized controlled clinical trial. *Psychological Medicine, 2007,* 1797–1806.

Stanley, M. A., Diefenbach, G. J., & Hopko, D. R. (2004). Cognitive behavioral treatment for older adults with generalized anxiety disorder. *Behavior Modification, 28,* 73–117.

Stanley, M. A., & Novy, D. M. (2000). Cognitive-behavior therapy for generalized anxiety in late life: An evaluative overview. *Journal of Anxiety Disorders, 14,* 191–207.

Tadros, G., & Salib, E. (2007). Elderly suicide in primary care. *International Journal of Geriatric Psychiatry, 22,* 750–756.

Troller, J. N., Anderson, T. M., Sachdev, P. S., Brodaty, H., & Andrews, G. (2007). Prevalence of mental disorders in the elderly: The Australian National Mental Health Survey. *American Journal of Geriatric Psychiatry, 15,* 455–466.

van Schaik, A. M., Comijs, H. C., Sonnenberg, C. M., Beekman, A. T., Sienaert, P., & Stek, M. L. (2011). Efficacy and safety of continuation and maintenance electroconvulsive therapy in depressed elderly patients: A systematic review. *American Journal of Geriatric Psychiatry,* DOI: 10.1097/JGP.0b013e31820dcbf9.

Vink, D., Aartsen, M. J., & Schoevers, R. A. (2008). Risk factors for anxiety and depression in the elderly: A review. *Journal of Affective Disorder, 2008,* 29–44.

Warmpold, B. E., Minami, T., Baskin, T., & Tierney, S. C. (2002). A meta-analysis of the effects of cognitive therapy versus 'other therapies' for depression. *Journal of Affective Disorders, 68,* 159–165.

Wetherell, J. L., Hopko, D. R., Diefenbach, G. J., Averill, P. M., Beck, J. G., Craske, M. G., Stanley, M. A. (2005). Cognitive-behavioral therapy for late life generalized anxiety disorder: Who gets better? *Behavior Therapy, 36,* 147–156.

World Health Organization (WHO). (2011). *Mental health—depression—what is depression?* Retrieved June 21, 2011, from http://www.who.int/mental_health/management/depression/definition/en

23

Alcohol and Substance Use, Misuse, and Abuse

The "hidden plague" and "invisible epidemic" are terms used to describe alcohol and substance abuse among older adults (Brody, 2002; Widlitz & Martin, 2002). There are many reasons for this and many reasons that it is invisible or hidden. Many older adults who misuse or abuse substances do so in an effort to alleviate physical, psychological, emotional, or spiritual pain. Attempting to self-treat or manage pain is a common reason people become involved with the misuse or abuse of substances (Goebel et al., 2011).

EPIDEMIOLOGY OF ABUSE AND MISUSE OF SUBSTANCES BY OLDER ADULTS

As the number of people in the United States who are older than 55 years has increased, so has the prevalence of substance abuse with alcohol, nicotine, and prescription medications most frequently abused by older adults. In 2005, considering the increases during the previous two decades, it was estimated that by 2020, there would be 5 million older adults with substance abuse issues. Of that 5 million, it is estimated that 2.7 million older adults will involve nonmedical use of prescription medications. It is also estimated that in 2020, older adults will comprise 25% of the population. That would be twice the number of those older than 55 years with substance abuse issues in 1995 (Fleming, Manwell, Barry, Adams, & Stauffacher, 1999; Simoni-Wastila & Yang, 2006; US DHHS, 2005).

Now, it seems that may have been a significant underestimate for 2020. In 2008 it was estimated that 11% of older women misuse prescription medications. In 2009 it was estimated that 4.3 million (4.7%) adults older than 50 years used an illicit substance during the past year. This is a particular concern because earlier figures regarding substance abuse included alcohol, but these data did not include alcohol. Marijuana was the most common substance, representing 45% of usage, followed by nonmedical use of prescription type medications, representing 33% of usage. Marijuana was more common among those in their 50s, whereas nonmedical use of prescription type medications was more common in those 65 or older. In all categories, abuse reported by older men was higher than abuse by older women (Simoni-Wastila & Yang, 2006; US DHHS, 2009).

Admissions of older adults for substance abuse treatment steadily increased between 1995 and 2002. The 2002 rate for people 55 years or older who were admitted for substance abuse treatment was 107 per 100,000. Admissions increased 106% for older men and 119% for older women (US DHHS, 2005). Admissions increased 106% for older men and 119% for older women (US DHHS, 2005). Although that was marked lower than the 801 per 1000,000 rate for those less than 55 years, it is still significant. Alcohol was consistently the most frequent substance abused by older people who were admitted for treatment; however, the alcohol percentage of all substances abused by elders steadily declined from 86% in 1995 to 78% in 2002. During those same years, the percentage of other substances remained comparably small but steadily increased. Opiates, cocaine, marijuana, and stimulants all doubled in percentage. Opiates, which increased from 6.8% in 1995 to 12% in 2002, was second to alcohol in abuse.

There is a strong correlation between substance abuse, including alcoholism, with suicidality. Only depression is more closely correlated with suicide. Substance and alcohol abuse are also related to other factors (i.e., depression, illnesses, poor social support) that are involved in suicide. The reader is referred to Chapter 22 for a discussion of suicide in older adults (Blow, Brockmann, & Barry, 2004).

BARRIERS TO RECOGNIZING ALCOHOL AND SUBSTANCE MISUSE AND ABUSE IN OLDER ADULTS

There are numerous reasons that alcohol and substance misuse and abuse among older adults are not more openly recognized and addressed. The reasons, which are important for health care providers (HCPs) to appreciate, include the following:

- Substance abuse issues, addiction, and pain management often are not adequately covered in professional education (physicians, nurses, advanced practice nurses, and physician assistants).
- HCPs may be reluctant to discuss substance misuse or abuse, especially with older people.
- Ageism results in HCPs rarely asking elders about alcohol intake or substance use and misuse.
- Symptoms are attributed to comorbidities or common disorders of aging (i.e., dementia, depression).
- Older adults and family members do not recognize the abuse or misuse as a problem.
- When recognized, older adults may be less likely to seek help.
- Behaviors that call attention to alcohol and substance abuse and misuse (i.e., missed work) are not relevant for older people (Brody, 2002; Gourlay, Heot, & Almahrezi, 2005; Han, Gfroerer, Colliver, & Penne, 2009).

ALCOHOL USE, ABUSE, AND MISUSE AMONG OLDER ADULTS

Alcohol consumption is intrinsically part of socialization in many communities (Klein & Jess, 2002). In addition, during the past decade, there have been increasing reports that low or moderate alcohol consumption has positive health benefits. Although additional research is needed, red wine has been increasingly touted as beneficial and even protective against cardiovascular (CV) disease (Wollin & Jones, 2001). One report noted that people who drink wine tend to have healthier diets than those who drink beer or other alcoholic beverages (Barefoot et al., 2002). Another study report was that in addition to improvement in cholesterol and insulin sensitivity, ethanol itself provides CV benefit. It is stressed that any benefits are obtained through moderate alcohol consumption. Misuse or abuse of alcohol poses a threat to CV as well as general health (O'Keefe, Bybee, & Lavie, 2007).

In general, alcoholism is the number one cause of morbidity and mortality that could be prevented in the United States. Although alcoholism among the geriatric population is considered a "hidden issue," it is also a recognized public health problem, which is increasing more rapidly among older adults than other age groups. Alcohol misuse and abuse among older adults is costly. More than 20 years ago, when the prevalence was much less, Medicare paid more than $233 million dollars for hospital costs related to alcohol as a primary diagnosis. Approximately one-third of older adults who are alcoholic develop it in older age and two-thirds have grown older with alcoholism (Bradley et al., 2007; Fleming et al., 2002; Widlitz & Martin, 2002).

Emergency departments are often the first place that problems with alcohol are identified among older adults. Among 32,000 older adults with trauma, 50% had recently consumed alcohol and 72% were considered intoxicated based upon serum alcohol levels in excess of 80 mg/dL. In that study, the most frequent causes of trauma were falls and motor vehicle accidents (Zautcke, Cocker, Morris, & Stein-Spencer, 2002).

In one large study of nearly 4,800 older participants who were predominantly Caucasian (more than 90%) and very to moderately active (more than 87%) completed and returned survey questionnaires about their alcohol consumption, activities, and comorbid illnesses, the distributions of at-risk drinkers, abstainers, and not-at-risk drinkers were similar for education, income, activity level, marital status, and BMI. There were gender and smoking differences:

- Of those considered to be at-risk drinkers, 25% were older women and 75% were older men.
- Of those who abstained from alcohol, 66% were older women and 34% were older men.
- Of those deemed to be not-at-risk drinkers, 47% were older women and 53% were older men.
- Thirty-five percent of those at risk, 16% of the abstainers, and 27% of the not-at-risk drinkers were smokers (Moore et al., 2006).

Alcohol use in long-term care settings, including nursing homes, varies by the policy of the facility. At least since 1964, some nursing homes and long-term care settings have incorporated alcohol as part of the socialization efforts. It is important that screening efforts for risky alcohol use, appropriate interventions, and safety precautions be incorporated into plans of care (Klein & Jess, 2002).

ALCOHOL USE AMONG OLDER ADULTS WITH CHRONIC PAIN

The literature addressing the use of alcohol among older adults living with chronic pain is very scarce. In one U.S. study with 407 older adults, it was found that consumption of at least one drink of alcohol per week was associated with less pain and fewer reports of chronic pain (Ray, Lipton, Zimmerman, Katz, and Derby, 2011). The upper limits of alcohol consumption were not reported by the authors, so it is not known if there was any abuse of alcohol involved. It may be that these individuals consumed alcohol socially, and it was the socialization that was more closely related to lower pain reports.

The investigators in another study reported that older adults do use alcohol to manage chronic pain. While they found correlations between the amount of pain and amount of alcohol consumed, the correlation seemed to be mediated by the amount of alcohol the person consumed prior to developing chronic pain. They found that older people who had a history of risky behavior with alcohol were more likely to

- use alcohol to manage pain
- report greater pain
- consume more alcohol when using it to manage pain (Brennan, Schutte, & Moos, 2005).

A significant concern is for older adults living with chronic pain who consume alcohol while taking analgesic medication. All older adults, family members, and caregivers need to be educated about the risks of consuming alcohol while using analgesic medications (Moore, Whiteman, & Ward, 2007).

In one case, the staff in an assistive living facility was concerned that an older woman, who was prescribed opioids for chronic pain, needed to have the opioids reduced because of confusion and un-steadiness. Coincidentally, this woman was assessed during the evening meal and was observed swallowing her opioid while drinking her wine. Education about the risk of alcohol use with opioids was accepted and prevented future difficulties (personal experience of the author).

SCREENING AND DIAGNOSIS

The Substance Abuse and Mental Health Services Administration (SAMHSA) (2001) recommends that during annual physical examination, all people older than 60 years should be screened for alcohol and substance abuse/misuse. It is imperative that all screening efforts be sensitive and consider cultural beliefs and practices. Alcohol has many social implications and is frequently part of rituals and cultural practices (Barry & Blow, 1999).

In a study of nearly 4,700 older adults, correlations and hazard ratios were computed for at-risk alcohol consumption with comorbidities. Gout and ulcer disease were correlated with risky alcohol drinking in older men and ulcer disease and anxiety were correlated with it in older women. In both genders, analgesic products were the most common medication correlated with at-risk alcohol consumption (13% of older men and 22% of older women) (Moore et al., 2006).

Indications for concern of alcohol abuse among older adults include the following:

- Malnutrition and/or muscle wasting
- Abnormal liver function test results
- Social isolation or withdrawal
- Unmotivated or lack of energy
- Continual irritability, mood swings, anxiety, agitation, restlessness
- Confusion or memory blackouts
- Social isolation or withdrawal
- Unmotivated or lack of energy
- Poor personal hygiene
- Frequent injuries, falls, and clumsiness
- Using alcohol to relax or enhance mood (Eliopoulos, 2001; US DHHS, 2001).

Screening Tools for Risky Alcohol Behavior

The two most common tools to screen for risky alcohol consumption in older adults are the CAGE and the MAST-G (Reed, 2006). As screening tools they are used to identify older adults who are at risk for misuse or abuse of alcohol. If there are positive results from the screening, further assessment is needed.

CAGE is an acronym for four questions used to screen for history of or current problematic alcohol consumption. It was originally developed and validated in 1974. Based on validity and ease of use, it is considered by many to be the preferred screening tool to use with older adults. Generally, two or more positive responses indicate a concern for alcohol abuse. The four questions are

- Have you ever felt you should **C**ut down on your drinking?
- Have people **A**nnoyed you by criticizing your drinking?
- Have you ever felt **G**uilty about your drinking?

■ Have you **E**ver had a drink first thing in the morning to steady your nerves or to get rid of a hangover? (Berks & McCormick, 2008; Mayfield, McLeod, & Hall, 1974; Widlitz & Martin, 2002)

MAST-G, an acronym for The Michigan Alcohol Screening Test-Geriatric, is another excellent tool to screen for alcohol misuse or abuse among older adults. It has excellent sensitivity and good specificity. There are 24 questions that require a "yes" or "no" response. Each response has a different value that must be tallied and scored. The length of time to complete and score has been a drawback with the MAST-G. Recently, a shorter 10-question version called the *SMAST-G* was developed. Early validation and reliability testing with older adults who had recently had a stroke indicated it was comparable to the MAST-G in efficacy. Additional testing in varied populations of older adults is needed (Blow et al., 1992; Johnson-Greene, McCaul, & Roger, 2009; Reed, 2006).

AUDIT is an acronym for the *Alcohol Use Disorders Identification Test* that is a third screening tool for alcohol misuse. It is an effective 10-item screening tool for use in primary care to identify high-risk alcohol consumption among adults in a variety of populations. The AUDIT is a reliable and valid tool in men, but there has been some concern about it being too specific and not sensitive enough in women. In different studies, the results of the AUDIT in older adults have been conflicting. There have been several modifications that shortened the original tool. Further evaluation is needed with older adults (Bradley et al., 2007; Fiellen, Reid, & O'Connor, 2000; Reinert & Allen, 2007).

Assessment Following Screening

When there are positive results from the screening tool, follow-up assessment is needed by the HCP. At a minimum, follow-up questions should attempt to determine

■ quantity and frequency of alcohol consumption

■ type of alcohol consumed

■ any instances of blackouts (if so, ascertain how frequently have they occurred)

■ any falls or injuries sustained while consuming alcohol

■ the presence of any alcohol-related illness (Widlitz & Martin, 2002)

Interventions

Many of the interventions, which are available to assist older adults who misuse or abuse alcohol, are the same or similar as those who misuse or abuse other substances. The following interventions have been recommended specifically for older adults for whom there is concern about their alcohol consumption. Additional interventions that may also be appropriate for older adults who have problematic behavior with alcohol follow the section on substance abuse.

It is important to ensure that the most appropriate intervention is selected for the older adult based upon culture, needs, and individual preferences (Marlatt & Witkiewitz, 2002).

BRIEF PHYSICIAN OR HCP INTERVENTION

FRAMES is an acronym for an immediate intervention approach suggested by SAMHSA. It includes the following:

- **F**eedback needs to be given to older adults about their screening results and the implications for their health, including risks of impairment as well as actual impairments.
- **R**esponsibility for change is with the older adult who needs to accept that responsibility.
- **A**dvise older adults clearly that it is important to change alcohol behaviors. Educate regarding consequences of abusing alcohol, reasons to reduce or eliminate alcohol, and limits of reasonable alcohol consumption.
- **M**enu of options will increase the chances that older adults will identify a treatment that will be effective (i.e., "Drinking Agreement" or contract, Alcoholics Anonymous [AA]).
- **E**mpathic counseling style will help to engage rather than antagonize older patients.
- **S**elf-efficacy enhancement is important initially and through follow-up interactions (US DHHS, 2001).

This is consistent with research studies that used similar brief physician intervention models used internationally. They reported success when the focus was on assessment and screening, providing feedback on the screening, education, goal setting, and contracting for improved behavior (Fleming et al., 1999, 2002).

EDUCATION

Education is an important component both for the older adult who is assessed as having an abuse issue and those who are at risk for abuse. Older adults and families need to know the following:

■ With aging, there is less water in the body, which results in the amount of alcohol having a more profound effect of intoxication than when younger.

■ There is an increased sensitivity with a decreased tolerance to alcohol

■ With aging, the metabolism is reduced and the serum alcohol level is elevated for a longer time and the liver consequently suffers an increased strain.

■ Appropriate alcohol consumption for people older than 65 years include
  ■ one drink per day (12 ounces beer, 1.5 ounces whiskey or liquor, 5 ounces wine, or 4 ounces sherry, liqueur, or aperitif)
  ■ older women need to limit this "somewhat lower"
  ■ on special occasions, maximum is two drinks

■ Alcohol consumption can trigger or intensify
  ■ cardiac disorders
  ■ stroke risk
  ■ liver disease including cirrhosis
  ■ Gastrointestinal bleeding including esophageal varices
  ■ mental health disorders including depression and anxiety (US DHHS, 2001)

> *Pearls*
>
> Alcohol consumption is part of socialization in many cultures and communities.
> Risky alcohol consumption among older adults is increasing.
> Screening and intervention are important to prevent injuries and morbidity.

SUBSTANCE ABUSE AND MISUSE AMONG OLDER ADULTS

Substance abuse and misuse among older adults is not as well researched as alcohol use and abuse with older adults. The information is scarce. It is expected that the prevalence will dramatically increase as baby boomers age. There are six main reasons:

1. They are a very large cohort.
2. They have benefited from improvements in health care and are expected to live longer than previous generations.
3. They were not exposed to sanctions of prohibition as were previous older adults.
4. Their youth culture was tolerant of substances and in some cases embraced them.
5. Adults older than 65 use more prescription medications than any other age group.
6. Current substance abusers are living to older ages (Patterson & Jeste, 1999; US DHHS, 2001).

CLARIFICATION OF TERMS

When substance abuse is discussed in the literature, one criticism is that there often is not a definition of the terms used (Simoni-Wastila & Yang, 2006). It is not possible to correct that problem in existing literature, or to suggest what the authors may have considered as definitions. American Psychiatric Association Diagnostic and Statistical Manual-IV (APA DSM-IV) (APA, 2000) provides complete diagnostic criteria for substance dependence and substance abuse. The reader is referred to that source for full diagnostic criteria.

In 2001, the American Academy of Pain Medicine (AAPM), America Pain Society (APS) and American Society of Addiction Medicine (ASAM) issued a consensus statement defining terms involved with the use of opioids. The following explanations are based upon information in that statement:

- *Physical dependence* occurs when an opioid has been taken for a period of time (generally 2 weeks or longer) and withdrawal symptoms develop if the dose is significantly reduced, the substance is abruptly stopped, or an antagonist (i.e., naloxone) is administered. This is a response that is considered normal.
- *Tolerance* occurs when an opioid has been taken for a period of time (days or weeks) and there is a reduction in effect (i.e., analgesia or sedation). Increased dosing may be required to attain the previous effect.
- *Addiction* is a chronic neurobiological disease involving genetic, psychosocial, and environmental features. It involves impaired control over using the substance and/or compulsive use of the substance, and/or continuing use despite harm, and/or craving the substance (AAPM, APS, & ASAM, 2001).

The following explanations of terms are also offered:

■ *Pseudoaddiction* is a phenomenon that occurs when pain is undertreated, resulting in the person exhibiting behaviors similar to those seen in addictive behavior (i.e., repeated requests for the substance, "clock watching"). Pseudoaddiction is differentiated from true addiction because once the pain is treated, the behaviors resolve in the former (APS, 2003).

■ *Problem use or abuse* is a pattern of use (alcohol or other substance) that incurs or places the older adult at risk of incurring unfavorable physical, psychological, or social effects or outcomes. The extent of impairment is the critical element regardless of the frequency or quantity used (Oslin & Mavandadi, 2009).

Prescription medication misuse and abuse occurs more frequently than abuse of illegal substances among older adults. This is a challenging situation because the older adult is generally prescribed prescription medications (i.e., opioids, muscle relaxants) because of chronic pain. The HCP often must assess the difference between tolerance and misuse or abuse.

Misuse of psychoactive analgesic and adjuvant medications, including muscle relaxants, anxiolytics and opioids, can take several forms. Older adults may

■ unwittingly consume alcohol while using psychoactive medications
■ not understand instructions for appropriate and safe use (Culberson & Ziskar, 2008; US DHHS, 2001)

Illegal substance use is not common among older adults but HCPs need to know that it does occur. In April 2011, two women aged 62 and 73 were arrested, and in May 2011, a third woman aged 72 was arrested in Brunswick County, North Carolina, who were charged with counts of "opium or heroin trafficking." The undercover detective involved in the case said that such arrests with seniors are increasing, and that sale of narcotics and pain medicines crosses all ages (Etheridge, 2011).

A recent study assessed misusing medications and substances to manage pain among 343 veterans whose ages ranged from 23 to 89 with a mean age of 61 years. The group was predominantly Caucasian (50%) and male (95%). Of the participants, 64% reported chronic pain. Histories of substance abuse, alcohol abuse, depression, and anxiety were common. Among the veterans, 11.7% admitted to buying illegal substances to manage their pain and 16.3% reported sharing prescription medications (Goebel et al., 2011).

SCREENING TOOLS TO IDENTIFY SUBSTANCE ABUSE IN OLDER ADULTS

Unfortunately no tools for screening substance abuse or misuse in older adults have been validated.

Some states have *surveillance programs* that record all opioid prescriptions filled at all pharmacies. Some programs include a list of the providers who wrote the prescription. When an older adult "doctor shops" (obtaining multiple prescriptions for the same or similar medication from different HCPs) that information will appear on the record. Participating HCPs can review these records and discuss the information with the older adult.

Urine or serum testing can be done on a routine or periodic basis to determine the presence of the prescribed mediation as well as other substances not prescribed. There are limitations in accuracy of medication and concentration (Culberson & Ziskar, 2008; Simoni-Wastila & Yang, 2006; Trescot et al., 2006).

Signs and symptoms of substance abuse in older adults are similar to indicators of alcohol misuse or abuse. They can easily be attributed to other age-related illnesses (i.e., dementia). Indicators include
- disturbed sleep
- cognitive problems (confusion, slurred speech)
- changes in mood or disposition, including irritability, depression, anxiety, restlessness, agitation
- poor hygiene
- falling and injuries
- persistent concern about pain medications
- problems in relationships (Culberson & Ziskar, 2008; Goldberg, 2008; US DHHS, 2001)

Managing pain in older adults with comorbid substance misuse or abuse can be challenging. It is imperative to remember that pain and substance abuse are not mutually exclusive. Older adults who have pain can also have substance abuse. Older adults who have histories of substance abuse can have pain or chronic pain. Opioids can be prescribed for older adults who have comorbid substance abuse issues or who are recovered from the disease of addiction. It is important for the HCP, older adult, and family to understand that pain is being treated and the goal is to improve quality of life. Gourlay and colleagues wrote that for people with chronic pain, opioids are the solution; for people with substance abuse issues, opioids are the problem; and for those

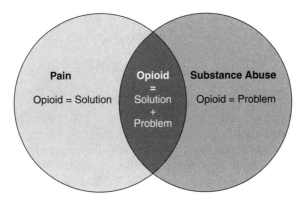

Figure 23.1 ■ Pain and substance abuse. *Source:* Figure developed from information in Gourlay, Heot, and Almahrezi (2005).

who have comorbid pain and substance abuse issues, opioids have a mixed role (see Figure 23.1) (Gourlay et al., 2005).

Cancer Pain Management Comorbid with Substance Abuse in Older Adults

Appropriate management of cancer pain in patients with a history of substance abuse is based upon concepts of palliative care that were discussed in Chapter 13. Although oral analgesia is the route of choice whenever possible, significant doses may be required to manage pain. If the oral route is not possible, subcutaneous administration of opioids may be needed. The following points are important:

■ A single physician should be responsible for analgesic management.
■ Confusion may be a result of the disease process.
■ Requests for dose escalation of opioid may be related to increasing pain but may also be related to disease-related stress or anxiety (Hanks, Cherny, & Fallon, 2005; Passik and Theobald (2000).

Intervention for Withdrawal

Intervention for withdrawal is important to prevent complications that are potentially life threatening and at a minimum can complicate comorbid conditions. Older adults who routinely use alcohol, benzodiazepines, opioids, or other substances are at risk for withdrawal if the substance is abruptly stopped. Clinicians need to be aware

- that older adults may be at risk for withdrawal from legal or illegal substances
- of the signs of acute withdrawal
- of the difference between withdrawal and delirium (see Chapter 22)
- of the need to identify the substance used
- what time frames are involved in the withdrawal process
- what is the most appropriate intervention for the substance from which withdrawal is occurring (Oslin & Mavandadi, 2009)

Withdrawal from opioids results when neurotransmitter release increases. It is characterized by particular symptoms that include

- hyperalgesia (increased sensitivity to pain)
- shivering
- diarrhea
- mydriasis
- rhinitis
- severe anxiety (Bie, Peng, Zhang, & Zhizhong, 2005; Culberson & Ziskar, 2008; Trescot et al., 2006)

TREATMENT OPTIONS FOR OLDER ADULTS WITH ALCOHOL AND SUBSTANCE ABUSE OR MISUSE

Information available indicates that treatment is at least as effective among older adults who misuse or abuse substances as it is among their younger counterparts.

Brief interventions for alcohol or substance misuse and abuse are based upon concepts of motivational interviewing to encourage the older adult to change behavior. The FRAMES intervention described previously in discussion of alcohol misuse is an example of a brief intervention (Blow et al., 2004; Oslin & Mavandadi, 2009; US DHHS, 2001).

Psychosocial treatments generally consist of cognitive behavioral techniques used either individually or in groups. One study with older veterans had promising results for abstaining over time (Oslin & Mavandadi, 2009).

Twelve-step programs are readily available in most communities. Depending upon the substance, Alcoholics Anonymousbe

(AA) and Narcotics Anonymous are designed to help the participants achieve and maintain sobriety as they work through the 12 steps intrinsic in the program design. Reports of 12-step program success with older adults, are conflicting. It is not known what percentage of older attendees have aged as members compared with older adults joining as senior citizens.

Some older adults are reluctant to join because they

■ perceive a stigma with the groups
■ are reluctant to disclose personal information that is part of the programs
■ consider the group focus geared to younger participants
■ have logistic challenges, including schedule of meetings and transportation (AA, 2004; Oslin, Slaymaker, Blow, Owen, & Colleran, 2005; Satre, Mertens, Arean, & Weisner, 2004).

Outpatient treatment centers may involve case management, psychiatric evaluation and therapy, and self-help programs. These programs may be appropriate for older adults who have transportation to an available center (Gunter & Arndt, 2004).

In-patient medical management and treatment is appropriate for older adults with substance abuse issues who

■ require detoxification
■ are frail
■ have physical comorbidities
■ have comorbid psychiatric diagnosis
■ need close observation/supervision (Gunter & Arndt, 2004).

GUIDELINES AND RESOURCES

National Aging Information Center. http://www.aoa.gov/naic 202-619-7501.

National Center on Addiction and Substance Abuse at Columbia University. www.casacolumbia.org 212-841-5200.

National Council on the Aging. www.ncoa.org 202-479-1200.

National Institute on Aging. http://www.nih.gov/nia/ 800-222-2225 800-222-4225 (TTY).

Substance Abuse and Mental Health Services Administration. (2001). http://samhsa.gov 800-729-6686 800-487-4889 (TTY).

Substance Abuse among Older Adults Physician's Guide (no cost for the guide). http://store.samhsa.gov/product/Substance-Abuse-Among-Older-Adults-Physician-s-Guide/SMA10-3394

Case Study

Paul Nash is an 82-year-old musician who was diagnosed 4 months ago with head and neck cancer. He was treated with radiation and was fairly comfortable for the last 3 months. Pain management has been challenging. Paul's girlfriend confided that he still smokes some marijuana and last week tried to buy some heroin. He used heroin for many years but stopped about 15 years ago. Today, when he arrives, you smell alcohol on his breath.

He says that the long-acting morphine (60 mg every 8 hours) is not working. He says that he has to take 20 of the short-acting morphine (30 mg) for breakthrough pain. He tells you that you have to do something about this pain or he is going to end it himself.

Questions

1. What is the first thing that you assess in Paul?
2. What else do you need to assess?
3. What do you think may be happening with Paul?
4. What interventions are appropriate for him?
5. What education do you provide to him and his girlfriend?
6. What changes in analgesia may be appropriate?

REFERENCES

Alcoholics Anonymous. (2004). *Alcoholic Anonymous services: Twelve steps and twelve traditions*. New York, NY: Alcoholics Anonymous.

American Academy of Pain Medicine (AAPM), American Pain Society (APS), & American Society of Addiction Medicine (ASAM). (2001). *Definitions related to the use of opioids for the treatment of pain*. Glenview, IL: American Academy of Pain Medicine.

American Pain Society (APS). (2003). *Principles of analgesic use in the treatment of acute pain and cancer pain* (5th ed.). Glenview, IL: American Pain Society.

American Psychiatric Association (APA). (2000). *Diagnostic and statistical manual of mental disorders* (4th text revised ed.). Washington, DC: American Psychiatric Association.

Barefoot, J. C., Grobaek, M., Feaganes, J. R., McPherson, S., Williams, R. B., & Siegler, I. (2002). Alcoholic beverage preference, diet, and health habits in the

UNC Alumni Heart Study. *The American Journal of Clinical Nutrition, 76,* 466–472.

Barry, K. L., & Blow, F. C. (1999). Screening and assessment of alcohol problems in older adults. In P. A. Lichtenberg (Ed.), *Handbook of assessment in clinical gerontology* (pp. 243–269). Danvers, MA: John Wiley & Sons Inc.

Berks, J., & McCormick, R. (2008). Screening for alcohol misuse in elderly primary care patients: A systematic literature review. *International Psychogeriatrics, 20,* 1090–1103.

Bie, B., Peng, Y., Zhang, Y., & Zhizhong, Z. P. (2005). CAMP-mediated mechanisms for pain sensitization during opioid withdrawal. *The Journal of Neuroscience, 25,* 3824–3832.

Blow, F. C., Brockmann, L. M., & Barry, K. L. (2004). Role of alcohol in late-life suicide. *Alcohol: Clinical and Experimental Research, 28,* 48S–56S.

Blow, F. C., Brower, K. J., Schulenberg, J. E., Demo-Danaberg, J. E., Young, J. P., & Beresford, T. P. (1992). The Michigan Alcoholism Screening Test-Geriatric Version (MAST-G): A new elderly-specific screening instrument. *Alcoholism: Clinical and Experimental Research, 19,* 372.

Bradley, K. A., Debenedetti, A. F., Vok, R. J., Williams, E. C., Frank, D., & Kivlahan, D. R. (2007). AUDIT-C as a brief screen for alcohol misuse in primary care. *Alcoholism: Clinical and Experimental Research, 31,* 1208–1217.

Brennan, P. L., Schulte, K. K., & Moos, R. H. (2005). Pain and use of alcohol to manage pain: Prevalence and 3 year outcomes among older problem and non-problem drinkers. *Addiction, 100,* 777–786.

Brody, J. E. (2002). Hidden plague of alcohol abuse in the elderly. *The New York Times.* Retrieved from http://www.nytimes.com

Culberson, J. W., & Zaskar, M. (2008). Prescription drug misuse/abuse in the elderly. *Geriatrics, 63*(9), 22–31.

Eliopoulos, C. (2001). *Gerontological nursing* (5th ed.). Philadelphia, PA: Lippincott.

Etheridge, K. (2011). More senior citizens being charged with drug trafficking. *WECT News.* http://www.wect.com/story/14620436/more-senior-citizens-being-charged-with-drug-trafficking

Fiellen, D. A., Reid, M. C., & O'Connor, P. G. (2000). Screening for alcohol problems in primary care: A systematic review. *Archives of Internal Medicine, 160,* 1977–1989.

Fleming, M. F., Manwell, L. B., Barry, K. L., Adams, W., & Stauffacher, E. A. (1999). Brief physician advice for alcohol problems in older adults: A randomized community-based trial. *The Journal of Family Practice, 48,* 378–384.

Fleming, M. F., Mundit, M. P., French, M. T., Manwell, B., Stauffacher, E. A., & Barry, K. L. (2002). Brief physician advice for problem drinkers: Long-term efficacy and benefit-cost analysis. *Alcoholism: Clinical & Experimental Research, 26,* 36–43.

Goebel, J. R., Compton, P., Zubkoff, L., Lanto, A., Asch, S. M., Sherbourne, C. D., & Lorenz, K. A. (2011). Prescription sharing, alcohol use, and street drug use to manage pain among veterans. *Journal of Pain and Symptom Management, 41,* 848–858.

Goldberg, R. J. (Ed.). (2008). Substance abuse and the aging brain: Screening diagnosis and treatment. *The Brown University Geriatric Pharmacology UP-DATE, 12*(4), 1, 4–6.

Gourlay, D. L., Heot, H. A., & Almahrezi, A. (2005). Universal precautions in pain medicine: A rational approach to the treatment of chronic pain. *Pain Medicine, 6,* 107–112.

Gunter, T. D., & Arndt, S. (2004). Maximizing treatment of substance abuse in the elderly. *Behavioral Health Management, March/April,* 38–43. Retrieved from www.behavioral.net

Han, B., Gfroerer, J. C., Colliver, J. D., & Penne, M. A. (2009). Substance use disorder among older adults in the United States in 2020. *Addiction, 104,* 88–96.

Hanks, G., Cherny, N. I., & Fallon, M. (2005). Opioid analgesic therapy. In D. Doyle, G. Hanks, N. Cherny, & K. Calman (Eds.), *Oxford textbook of palliative care* (3rd ed., pp. 316–341). New York, NY: Oxford University Press.

Johnson-Greene, D., McCaul, M. E., & Roger, P. (2009). Screening for hazardous drinking using the Michigan Alcohol Screening Test-Geriatric Version (MAST-G) in elderly persons with acute cerebrovascular accidents. *Alcoholism: Clinical and Experimental Research, 33,* 1555–1561.

Klein, W. C., & Jess, C. (2002). One last pleasure? Alcohol use among elderly people in nursing homes. *Health & Social Work, 27,* 193–203.

Marlatt, G. A., & Witkiewitz, K. (2002). Harm reduction approaches to alcohol use: Health promotion, prevention, and treatment. *Addictive Behaviors, 27,* 867–886.

Mayfield, D., McLeod, G., & Hall, P. (1974). The CAGE questionnaire: Validation of a new alcoholism screening instrument. *American Journal of Psychiatry, 131,* 1121–1123.

Moore, A. A., Giuli, L., Gould, R., Hu, P., Zhou, K., Reuben, D., . . . Karlamangla, A. (2006). Alcohol use, comorbidity, and mortality. *Journal of the American Geriatrics Society, 54,* 757–762.

Moore, A. A., Whiteman, E. J., & Ward, K. T. (2007). Risks of combined alcohol/medication use in older adults. *The American Journal of Geriatric Pharmacology, 5,* 64–74.

O'Keefe, J. H., Bybee, K. A., & Lavie, C. J. (2007). Alcohol and cardiovascular health. *Journal of the American College of Cardiology, 50,* 1009–1014.

Oslin, D. W., & Mavandadi, S. (2009). Alcohol and drug problems. In D. G. Blazer & D. C. Steffens (Eds.), *The American Psychiatric Publishing textbook of geriatric psychiatry* (4th ed., pp. 409–428). Washington, DC: The American Psychiatric Publishing Inc.

Oslin, D. W., Slaymaker, V. J., Blow, F. C., Owen, P., & Colleran, C. (2005). Treatment outcomes for alcohol dependence among middle-aged and older adults. *Addictive Behaviors, 30,* 1431–1436.

Passik, S. D., & Theobald, D. E. (2000). Managing addiction in advanced cancer patients. Why bother? *Journal of Pain and Symptom Management, 19,* 229–234.

Patterson, T. L., & Jeste, D. V. (1999). *The potential impact of the baby-boom generation on substance abuse among elderly persons. Psychiatric Services, 50,* 1184–1188.

Ray, L., Lipton, R. B., Zimmerman, M. E., Katz, M. J., & Derby, C. A. (2011). Mechanism s of association between obesity and chronic pain in the elderly. *Pain, 152,* 53–59.

Reed, M. J. (2006). Substance abuse. In S. E. Meiner & A. G. Lueckenotte (Eds.), *Gerontologic nursing* (3rd ed., pp. 365–381). St. Louis, MO: Mosby Elsevier.

Reinert, D. F., & Allen, J. P. (2007). The Alcohol Use Disorders Identification Test: An update of research findings. *Alcoholism: Clinical and Experimental Research, 31,* 185–199.

Satre, D. D., Mertens, J. R., Arean, P. A., & Weisner, C. (2004). Five-year alcohol and drug treatment outcomes of older adults versus middle-aged and younger adults in a managed care program. *Addiction, 99,* 1286–1297.

Simoni-Wastila, L., & Yang, H. K. (2006). Psychoactive drug abuse in older adults. *The American Journal of Geriatric Pharmacotherapy, 4,* 380–394.

Trescot, A. M., Bosewell, M. V., Atluri, S. L., Hansen, H. C., Deer, T. R., Abdi, S., Manchikanti, L. (2006). Opioid guidelines in the management of chronic non-cancer pain. *Pain Physician, 9,* 1–40.

U.S. Department of Health and Human Services (US DHHS). (2001). *Quick guide for clinicians: Based on TIP 26 substance abuse among older adults.* Retrieved June 25, 2011, from http://kap.samhsa.gov/products/tools/cl-guides/pdfs/QGC_26.pdf

U.S. Department of Health and Human Services (US DHHS). (2005). *Older adults in substance abuse treatment: Update.* Retrieved June 24, 2011, from http://www.oas.samhsa.gov/2k5/olderAdultsTX/olderAdultsTX.pdf

U.S. Department of Health and Human Services (US DHHS). (2009). *Illicit drug use among older adults.* Retrieved June 24, 2011, from http://www.oas.samhsa.gov/2k9/168/168OlderAdultsHTML.pdf

Widlitz, M., & Martin, D. (2002). Substance abuse in older adults: An overview. *Geriatrics, 37,* 29–34.

Wollin, S. D., & Jones, P. J. (2001). Alcohol, red wine and cardiovascular disease. *Journal of Nutrition, 131,* 1401–1404.

Zautcke, J. L., Cocker, S. B., Morris, R. W., & Stein-Spencer, L. (2002). Geriatric trauma in the state of Illinois: Substance use and injury patterns. *American Journal of Emergency Medicine, 20,* 14–17.

Index

AAPM. *See* American Academy of Pain Medicine (AAPM)

Abdominal pain, with suicide ideation (SI), 19

Abuse. *See* Alcohol and substance abuse, by older adults

2-Acetaminophen, 93

Acetaminophen, 39, 92, 94, 96, 232, 264, 287
  aspirin versus, 338
  hydrocodone with, 102, 104
  tramadol with, 101, 102, 104, 265

Active therapies, 217

Activities of daily living (ADLs), 9, 40–41, 48, 84

Acupuncture, 176–177, 199, 270, 286, 321

Acute flares, 271

Acute pain, 2, 4, 42

Acyclovir, 306

AD. *See* Alzheimer's disease (AD)

Addiction, 412. *See also* Alcohol and substance abuse, by older adults; Pseudoaddiction

Adequate assessment, of older people, 231

Adjunct medications. *See* Coanalgesia

ADLs. *See* Activities of daily living (ADLs)

Aerobic endurance exercise, 366–367

Aerobic exercise, 217, 366

AGS. *See* American Geriatric Society (AGS)

ALA. *See* Alpha ipoic acid (ALA)

Alcohol and substance abuse, by older adults, 405–406
  barriers to recognizing, 404–405
  cancer pain management comorbid with, 415
  with chronic pain, 406–407
  clarification of terms, 412–413
  diagnosis of, 407–408
  education, 411
  epidemiology of, 403–404
  HCP interventions for, 410
  intervention for withdrawal, 415–416
  and misuse, 411–412
  screening tools
    for alcohol behavior, 408–409
    assessment for, 409
    to identify substance abuse, 414–415
  treatment options for, 416–417

Alcohol Use Disorders Identification Test (AUDIT), 409

Allodynia, 300, 302, 318–319

Alpha ipoic acid (ALA), 312

Alternative medicine, 183
Alzheimer's disease (AD), 47
America Pain Society (APS), 412–413
American Academy of Pain Medicine
(AAPM), 412–413
American Geriatric Society (AGS),
50, 120, 145, 184
American Geriatric Society Panel
on Persistent Pain in Older
Persons, 5
American Pain Society
Monograph, 35
American Pain Society/American
College of Physicians Clinical
Practice Guideline, 176
American Psychiatric Association
Diagnostic and Statistical
Manual-IV (APA
DSM-IV), 388
American Society of Addiction
Medicine (ASAM), 412–413
American Society of
Anesthesiologists Task
Force on Acute Pain
Management, 119
Amitryptiline (Elavil), 112, 124,
125, 126, 128–129
Analgesia, PRN administration of,
151–152
Analgesic medications
avoiding with older adults, 112
in older adults, 93
principles for, 232–235
Analgesic trial, 51
Analgesics and adjuvants
medication, 152–153
elimination, 149
metabolism, 148
side effects, 154–155
confusion, 157–158
dizziness, 158–159
Anger, 19–20

Animal assisted therapy, 191
Annuloplasty. *See* Intradiscal
electrothermal
therapy (IDET)
Anti-spasmotic medication, for
coanalgesia, 135–136
Anticholinergic effects
of orthostatic hypotension, 308
of tricyclic antidepressants,
127, 308
"Anticipatory grief," 236
Anticonvulsants, 319
for coanalgesia
carbamazepine (tegretol), 123
gabapentin (neurontin),
119–120, 121, 122
pregabalin (lyrica), 120,
121, 122
Antidepressants
for coanalgesia
amitryptiline (elavil), 125,
126, 128–129
desipramine (norpramine),
124–127
nortriplyline (pamelor,
aventyl), 125, 126,
127–128
tricyclic antidepressants
(TCAs), 123–124
SSRIs, 393
Antiepileptic medications. *See*
Anticonvulsants
Antiviral therapy, 306
Anxiety, 20
assessment, in older adults
signs and symptoms of, 391
tools, 392
epidemiology, among older
adults, 388–389
multimodal management, in
older adults, 392
and pain, 389

and depression, 390–391
  physiology, 390
pharmacological management
  antidepressants, 393
  benzodiazepines, 393
  buspirone, 392–393
  risperidone, 393
  symptoms, 394–395
  therapeutic interventions, 393, 396
  types, 388
APP. *See* Assuming pain is
  present (APP)
APS. *See* America Pain Society (APS)
Aquatic therapy, 218
Aromatherapy, 199, 342
Arthritic pain, 21
Arthritis, epidemiology of, 257.
  See also Osteoarthritis (OA)
Arthritis Foundation Exercise
  Program, 261–262
ASAM. *See* American Society
  of Addiction
  Medicine (ASAM)
Aspercreme, 267
Aspirin, 92, 112, 232
  versus acetaminophen, 338
"Assess the Patient's Understanding of
  His or Her Prognosis," 251
Assistive devices, physical therapy
  (PT) and, 218, 220
Assuming pain is present (APP), 70
ASUs. *See* Avocado soybean
  unsaponifiables (ASUs)
Asymptomatic tissue deposition, 271
Ataxia, 157
Avocado soybean unsaponifiables
  (ASUs), 268–269

Baclofen, 135, 173, 320, 330
Balanced Budget Act, 237
Balloon compression, 331

Balloon vertebroplasty/kyphoplasty,
  175–176
Balneotherapy, 217–218
Behaviors, pain-related, 49–50.
  See also Cognitive
  behavioral therapy (CBT)
BenGay, 267
Benzodiazepines, 393
Bereavement care, for family
  members, 252
Bergamot, 199
Biofeedback, 199–200
Black box warning, 137
Botulinum toxin (Botox)
  injections, 168
BPI. *See* Brief pain inventory (BPI)
Breathing techniques, 189–190
Brief pain inventory (BPI), 64–65
Buspirone, 392–393
Butorphanol (Stadol), 112, 113

CAGE, screening tool for risky
  alcohol consumption in
  older adults, 408–409
Cancer pain management, with
  substance abuse in older
  adults, 415
Canes, assistive devices, 264
CAPC. *See* Center to Advance
  Palliative Care (CAPC)
Capsaicin (Zostrix, Qutenza),
  138–139, 267, 307
Carbamazepine (Tegretol), 121,
  122, 123, 329–330
CBT. *See* Cognitive behavioral
  therapy (CBT)
Ceiling effect, for NSAID, 98
Celecoxib, 93, 94, 339
Celiac plexus blockade, 235
Center to Advance Palliative Care
  (CAPC), 227, 228

Centering prayer, 197
Central nervous system (CNS), 3,
   97, 355, 356
   side effects, 157
Central poststroke pain (CPSP)
      syndrome
   complementary interventions,
      321–322
   definition of, 317
   diagnosis, 318–319
   epidemiology, 317–318
   interventional efforts, 320–321
   nonpharmacological
      interventions, 321–322
   pharmacological interventions,
      319–320
Central sensitization, 356
Cerebral vascular accident (CVA), 48
Certified registered nurse
      anesthetist (CRNA), 110
Checklist for nonverbal pain
      indicators (CNPI), 66–68
Chemoreceptors, 3
Chiropractic treatment, 177, 200
Chlamydia pneumonia, 325
Choline magnesium (Tricosal,
      Trilisate), 93, 95
Chondroitin, 268
Chronic gout, 271
Chronic low back pain (CLBP),
   16, 113, 169, 171, 176.
   See also Low back
   pain (LBP)
Chronic nonarthritic pain
   with suicide attempts (SA), 19
Chronic nonspecific low back pain
   (CNLBP), 196
Chronic pain, 2, 42
   alcohol uses among older adults
      with, 406–407
   caffeine and alcohol uses, 16
   and depression

conundrum, 377–378
   low back pain, 378
   suicidality in, 387
with fatigue, 21
obesity, 20–21
related to spine, 169
sleep disturbances and falling
   risk, 22
suicide ideation (SI), 19
Chronic renal disease, 149
CLBP. *See* Chronic low back
   pain (CLBP)
Clonazepam, 330
Clonidine, 173
CNLBP. *See* Chronic nonspecific
   low back pain (CNLBP)
CNPI. *See* Checklist for nonverbal
   pain indicators (CNPI)
CNS. *See* Central nervous
   system (CNS)
Coanalgesia
   additional medications for,
      138–140
   anti-spasmotic medication for,
      135–136
   anticonvulsant/antiepileptic
      medications for, 119–123
   antidepressants for, 123–129
   local anesthetics as, 136–138
   muscle relaxants for, 134–135
   serotonin–norepinephrine-
      reuptake inhibitor (SNRI),
      129–132
   steroids for, 132–134
Coblation, 172–173
Cockroft–Gault serum creatinine
   clearance formula, 149
Cognition, 16–17, 381
Cognitive behavioral (CB)
   interventions, 263, 322
Cognitive behavioral techniques,
   186, 212, 416

Cognitive behavioral therapy
(CBT), 213, 385
for fibromyalgia (FMS)
symptom management,
366–367
for generalized anxiety disorder
(GAD) treatment, 393, 396
low back pain (LBP), 285
for pain management, 341–342
Cognitive domain, in pain
assessment, 42
Cognitive impairment. *See also*
Nonverbal/cognitive
impairments
anticholinergic side effects, 127
checklist for nonverbal pain
indicators (CNPI),
66–68
Colchicine, as second-line
therapy, 273
Cold, application of. *See*
Cryotherapy
Combined thermometer scale, 65
Communication, in pain
assessment, 43–44
Communication skills, patient
barrier, 35
Community setting, 237
Comorbidities, 6–7, 8
Complementary care, 183
Complementary interventions
chronic low back pain (CLBP),
285–287
for pain management, in
older adults
additional complementary
modalities, 199–201
American Geriatrics Society
(AGS), 184
breathing techniques,
189–190
devices, 198–199

energy-based interventions,
193–195
environment, modification of,
185–186
healing arts, 190–191
improve comfort of older
adult, 185
National Center for
Complementary and
Alternative Medicine
(NCCAM), 183
pet visitation and animals
assisted therapy, 191
physical interventions,
192–193
Complex regional pain syndrome
(CRPS), 120, 200
Confusion, 157–158
Constipation, 161
Continuous peripheral nerve
blocks. *See* Continuous
regional analgesia
Continuous regional analgesia,
110–111
Conventional medicine, 183
Coping skills training, 263–264
Corticosteroids, 132, 273, 340
Corticotrophin-releasing
factor (CRF)
in depression and pain, 380
Couples therapy, 342
COX-2 inhibitor, 339
COX-2-selective inhibitor NSAID
(celecoxib), 265
COX-2 selective NSAIDs, 98, 100
CPSP syndrome. *See* Central
poststroke pain (CPSP)
syndrome
Cranial arteritis. *See* Temporal
arteritis (TA)
CRF. *See* Corticotrophin-releasing
factor (CRF)

CRNA. *See* Certified registered
    nurse anesthetist (CRNA)
CRPS. *See* Complex regional pain
    syndrome (CRPS)
Cryotherapy, 192, 214, 331
Cultural factors, in pain
    assessment, 33
CVA. *See* Cerebral vascular
    accident (CVA)

Dame Cicely Saunders, 245
DBS. *See* Deep brain stimulation
    (DBS)
Decognition, 358
Deep brain stimulation (DBS),
    320–321
"Define the Patient's Goals for
    Care," 251
Dehydration, 90
Dejerine–Roussy syndrome. *See*
    Central poststroke pain
    (CPSP) syndrome
Delirium, 158
  versus depression and
    dementia, 381
Dementia, 48
  versus depression and
    delirium, 381
  pain assessment in advanced
    dementia (PAINAD), 68–70
Depression, 18
  assessment, in older adults
    signs and symptoms, 382
  and chronic pain relationship,
    among older adults
    conundrum, 377–378
    low back pain, 378
    suicidality in, 387
  versus dementia and
    delirium, 381
  differential diagnosis, 382–383

epidemiological information, 377
geriatric depression scale (GDS),
    71–72
multimodal management, in
    older adults, 383–384
and pain
  physiology of, 379–380
  psychosocial mechanisms,
    380–381
pharmacological management,
    384–385
therapeutic interventions
  CBT, 385
  electroconvulsive therapy
    (ECT), 386
  interpersonal psychotherapy,
    385–386
  problem-solving therapy
    (PST), 386
World Health Organization
    (WHO), description of, 376
Desipramine (Norpramine),
    124–127, 129
Desire, in pain assessment, 33
Devil's claw. *See* Harpagophytum
    procumbens
Dexamethasone (Decadron®), 132
Dextromethorphan
  side effects, 140
Diabetic neuropathy (DN)
  diabetic peripheral neuropathy
    (DPN), 309–312
  National Health and Nutrition
    Examination Survey, 309
  nonpharmacological
    treatments, 312
Diabetic peripheral neuropathy
    (DPN), 309–312
Diaphragmatic breathing, 189
Diclofenac, 94, 266–267
Diclofenac sodium (oral), 99
Diclofenac sodium (topical), 99

Diffuse noxious inhibitory control (DNIC), 356
Distraction activities and techniques, 187
Dizziness, 158–159
DN. *See* Diabetic neuropathy (DN)
DNIC. *See* Diffuse noxious inhibitory control (DNIC)
Doctor shops, 414
Dog rose. *See* Rosa canina
Doleur neuropathique en 4 questions (DN4) tool, 303
DPN. *See* Diabetic peripheral neuropathy (DPN)
Dronabinol
  side effects, 140
Duloxetine (Cymbalta), 129, 130, 131, 310, 384
Duloxetine hydrochloride (cymbalta), 363
Dysesthesia, 123, 302, 318–319

Education
  health care providers in pain assessment, 34–35
  for low back pain, 284
  multimodal management of osteoarthritis (OA), 260–261
  for older adults with gouts, 272
  pain management component, 186–187
  to patients, 82–83
Eicosapentaenoic acid (EPA), for gout persons, 273
Electric shock-like pains, 328
Electroconvulsive therapy (ECT), 386
Electrotherapy, 215–216
Elimination
  analgesic medications and adjuvants, 149
  metabolism and, 90–96

Emergency departments, 347
  alcohol and substance abuse, by older adults, 406
Energy-based interventions, 193–195
Environment, modification of, 185–186
  cognitive behavioral techniques, 186
  distraction activities and techniques, 187
  education, 186–187
  guided imagery, 188–189
  hypnosis, 187–188
  imagery, 188
  interpersonal interactions, 186
  lighting, 185
  position, 186
  relaxation techniques, 188
  rest and sleep, 186
  sounds, 185
  temperature, 185
Epidural corticosteroid injection, 169–170
Equianalgesic dosing in opioids, 109
"Establish the Medical Facts," 251
Etodolac, 339
European Federation of Neurological Societies (EFNS) Task Force, 304
European Male Ageing Study, 17
Exercise, 195–196
  aerobic, 217
  high-intensity weight bearing, 217
  for low back pain, 284–285
  multimodal management of OA, 260–261
  for older adults with gouts, 272
  progressive resistance, 217
  strength training, 217
  stretching, 217
  in water versus land, 217–218

Faces pain scale-revised (FPS-R), 59–60
Facet joint injection, 170–171
Facial expressions, 50
Facial pain
   associated with temporal arteritis/trigeminal neuralgia, 325–331
Famiclovir, 306
Fatigue, 21, 213, 361, 363, 382, 393
FDA. *See* Federal Drug Administration (FDA)
Fear, in pain assessment, 33
Federal Drug Administration (FDA), 92
Fentanyl, 103, 106, 108
Fibro-fog, 358
Fibromyalgia (FMS)
   clinical manifestations of, 357–361
   conditions frequently comorbid with, 355
   demographic and social factors associated with, 354
   diagnosis of, 357–361
   duloxetine hydrochloride (cymbalta), 363
   epidemiology of, 353–354
   etiology and factors associated with, 354–355
   exercise, 366–367
   genetic factors associated with, 354
   medication management of, 361
   milnacipran hydrochloride (savella), 363–364
   multimodal treatment approach, 361
   other medications used in, 364–365
   pathophysiology aspects of, 355–357
   patient and family education, 365
   patient global impression of change (PGIC) scale, 361, 362
   psychological factors associated with, 354
   referrals and consultations, 367–368
   US FDA-approved medications to, 362–364
Fibromyalgia Impact Questionnaire (FIQ), 358–360
Finances, in pain assessment, 34
FIQ. *See* Fibromyalgia Impact Questionnaire (FIQ)
Flavocoxid (Limbrel), 268
FMS. *See* Fibromyalgia (FMS)
Folic acid, for gout persons, 273
FRAMES intervention, 410, 416

Gabapentin (Neurontin), 119–120, 121, 122, 307, 310, 319, 330
GAD. *See* Generalized anxiety disorder (GAD)
Gait, 213–214
   disturbance, 157, 219
Gastrointestinal (GI)
   absorption, 146
   bleeding, 160
   tract side effects, 160–161
Gate control theory of pain, 375, 376
GDS. *See* Geriatric depression scale (GDS)
Gel phenomenon, 260
Gender differences, in musculoskeletal pain, 259
Generalized anxiety disorder (GAD), 388, 390, 392, 393, 396

Genitourinary system side effects, 162
Geriatric anxiety scale, 394–395
Geriatric assessment scale, 392
Geriatric depression scale (GDS), 71–72, 383
Geriatric syndromes, 7
Giant cell arteritis (GCA). *See* Temporal arteritis (TA)
Glucocorticosteroids, 326
Glucosamine sulfate, 268
Goal setting, 264
  for physical therapy (PT), 212–213
Gout
  diagnostic criteria, 272
  epidemiology and prevalence, 271–272
  four phases of, 271
  multimodal management, 272–273
Guided imagery, 188–189, 341, 367

Hand massage, 193
Harpagophytum procumbens, 269
HCPs. *See* Health care providers (HCPs)
Head pain, 19
Healing arts, 190–191
Health care providers (HCPs), 9, 17–18, 44
  barriers to pain
    communication skills, 35
    cultural factors, 34
    education, 34–35
    system barriers, 35
  barriers to timely hospice referral, 249
Heat modalities, 214–215
Herbal preparations, 201, 287

Herbal remedies, for osteoarthritis (OA), 269
High-intensity weight bearing exercises, 217
Home palliative care, 237
Hospice care
  bereavement care, 252
  as best option, 248–249
  communication to facilitate, 250–252
  concept of, 245
  evolution of, 245
  HCP barriers to, 249
  and palliative care, 227–238
  profile of, 245–248
Hospital anxiety and depression scale, 392
Hospital-based palliative care programs, 237–238
Hot packs, 214
Hydrocodone (Vicodin, Lortab, and Narco), 101, 233
  with acetaminophen, 102, 104
Hydromorphone, 103, 106, 108
Hydrotherapy, 217–218
Hyperalgesia, 300, 302
Hyperpathia, 300
Hypnosis, 187–188, 367
Hypoalbuminemia, 90

IASP. *See* International Association for the Study of Pain (IASP)
IBT. *See* Inflatable bone tamp (IBT)
Ibuprophen (Motrin), 94, 99
Ice packs, 341
Icy hot, 267
ID-Pain tool, 303
"Identify Needs for Care," 252
IDET. *See* Intradiscal electrothermal therapy (IDET)

IFC. *See* Interferential
currents (IFC)
IIT pumps. *See* Implanted intrathecal
pumps (IIT) pumps
Imagery techniques, 188
Impaired descending inhibition of
pain, 356
Implanted intrathecal pumps (IIT)
pumps, 173–174
In-patient medical management
and treatment, for older
adults, 417
Incident pain, 151
Indomethacin, 112
Inflatable bone tamp (IBT), 175
Integumentary system side
effects, 162
Intercritical segments, 271
Interferential currents (IFC),
215–216
International Association for the
Study of Pain (IASP), 123,
299, 304
Interpersonal psychotherapy, 385–386
Interview, pain assessment, 36–38
Intra-articular corticosteroid (IAC)
injections, 269–270
Intra-articular hyaluronic acid
(IAHA) injections, 270
Intra-articular injections, 269–270
Intradiscal electrothermal therapy
(IDET), 171
Intrathecal (IT) injections, 173
Intravenous lidocaine, 320
"Introduce Hospice," 252
Ionotophoresis, 216
Iowa pain thermometer (IPT),
60–61, 65
IPT. *See* Iowa pain
thermometer (IPT)
Itching. *See* Pruritus
Iyengar yoga, 286

Ketamine
side effects, 140
Ketaprophen (Actron, Orudis), 94, 99
Ketorolac (Torodol), 94, 99
Kyphoplasty, 175–176

Lamotrigine, 320, 330
LANSS tool. *See* Leeds assessment
of neuropathic symptoms
and signs (LANSS) tool
Lavender oil, 199
LBP. *See* Low back pain (LBP)
Leeds assessment of neuropathic
symptoms and signs
(LANSS) tool, 61–62, 303
Levetiracetam, 330
Lidocaine, 267, 307
Lidocaine transdermal patch,
136–137
Lidoderm patches, 308
Liver/renal dysfunction, 39
LKM. *See* Loving kindness
meditation (LKM)
LLLT. *See* Low-level laser
therapy (LLLT)
Local anesthetics
as coanalgesia
lidocaine transdermal patch,
136–137
mexiletine (Mexitil), 137–138
injection, 167–168
Long-term care facilities, 238
Longitudinal Aging Study
Amsterdam, 390
Loving kindness meditation
(LKM), 198
Low back pain (LBP), 378
cognitive behavioral therapy
(CBT), 285
complementary modalities,
285–287

diagnostic criteria, 284
epidemiology and prevalence,
283–284
medication management, 287
multimodal management,
284–285
surgical intervention, 288
Low-dose aspirin, 327
Low-level laser therapy (LLLT), 215

Magnets, 198–199
Manipulation and mobilization
techniques, 216
Manual therapies, 216–217
Marijuana, 404
Massage, 216, 367
hand, 193
therapeutic, 192–193
MCS. *See* Motor cortex
stimulation (MCS)
Mechanoreceptors, 3
Medicare
alcohol and substance abuse,
by older adults,
405–406
hospice care, 250–251
Medication, for pain complaint,
87–88. *See also* Coanalgesia
administration limitations,
87–88
aging, physiologic changes, 88
analgesic selection process, 93
absorption, 89
anti-inflammatory
medications, 94–95
distribution, effect of, 89–90
availability for patients, 88
comorbid illnesses, 88
cultural influences and beliefs, 88
current medications
interactions, 88

discontinuation of opioid
medications, 111
epidural and regional infusions,
110–111
financial assistance to
pharmaceutical
companies, 88
health literacy, 88
mechanism of action
lortab/vicodin and ultracet, 101
opioids, 102–109
oxycodone 5mg, 101
tapentadol, 101
tramadol, 101
metabolism and elimination
acetaminophen, 92, 96
general pharmacokinetics, 90
World Health Organization
(WHO) pain relief ladder,
91–92
NSAIDs. *See* Nonsteroidal
anti-inflammatory drugs
(NSAIDs)
older adults monitoring and
reassessment
analgesic medications to avoid
with, 112–114
pain assessment, 38–39
pain etiology and severity, 87
patient beliefs, 87
safety, 88
concerns with opioids, 111
issues, 87
Medications management, specific
recommendations
age-related physiological
changes
absorption via integumentary
system, 147
distribution, 147–148
elimination, 149
GI absorption, 146

Medications management, specific
  recommendations (*cont.*)
    metabolism, 148
    transmucosal absorption, 147
  analgesia, needed or PRN
    administration, 151–152
  analgesic and adjuvant
    medications, 152–153
  benefits and risks of, 145–146
  clock scheduled administration,
    150–151
  routes of administration,
    analgesic medication
    oral route, 150
    parenteral routes, 150
    transdermal, topical, oral
      transmucosal, and rectal
      routes, 150
  side effects management, 154
    analgesic and adjuvant-
      related, 154–155
    ataxia/gait disturbance, 157
    central nervous system
      (CNS), 157
    confusion, 157–158
    constipation, 161
    genitourinary system
      side effects, urinary
      retention, 162
    GI tract side effects, 160–161
    integumentary system side
      effects, pruritus, 162
    myoclonus, 159
    respiratory effects, 155–157
  specialists coordination,
    153–154
Meloxicam (Mobic), 99
Meperidine (Demerol), 112, 113
Metabolism
  analgesic medications and
    adjuvants, 148
  and elimination, 90–96

Methadone (Dolophin and
    Methadose), 103, 106,
    112–113
Methylprednisolone (Medrol®), 132
Mexiletine (Mexitil), 137–138
Michigan Alcohol Screening
    Test-Geriatric
    (MAST-G), 409
Microvascular decompression
    (MVD), 330
Migraine headaches
  with anxiety disorders, 20
  with suicide ideation (SI), 19
Milnacipran hydrochloride
    (Savella), 363–364
Minacipran (Savella), 130,
    131, 132
Mindfulness meditation, 198
Mini mental status exam
    (MMSE), 49
Mirror therapy, 200–201
Misconceptions, in pain
    assessment, 32
MMSE. *See* Mini mental status
    exam (MMSE)
Morphine, 102, 105, 107–108, 232
Motor cortex stimulation
    (MCS), 321
Movement therapies, 195–197
MPS. *See* Myofascial pain
    syndromes (MPS)
Mu-agonist opioids, 107
Mu opioids, 265–266
Multidimensional pain scales
  short-form McGill pain
    questionnaire (SF-MPQ),
    62–64
  short-form McGill pain
    questionnaire revised
    (SF-MPQ-2), 64
Multimodal analgesia
    management, 319

Muscle relaxation therapy, 396
Musculoskeletal system, changes in, 147
Music therapy, 190–191, 263
Myoclonus, 159
Myofascial pain syndromes (MPS), 167–168

Nabumetone (Relafen), 99
Naloxone (Narcan®), 157
Naproxen (Aleve Anaprox), 94, 99
National Center for Complementary and Alternative Medicine (NCCAM), 183
National Consensus Project For Quality Palliative Care (NCPQPC), 228
National Hospice and Palliative Care Organization (NHPCO), 227
National Pharmaceutical Council & American Pain Society (NPC APS), 119
Nausea and vomiting, 160–161
NCCAM. *See* National Center for Complementary and Alternative Medicine (NCCAM)
NE. *See* Norepinephrine (NE)
Necrotizing arteritis, 326
Neuroleptic malignant syndrome, symptoms of, 364
Neuromatrix theory of pain, 375
Neuropathic pain (NP), 1–2, 42–43
    characteristics of, 300
    clinical assessment of, 301–304
    economic impact of, 301
    Leeds assessment of neuropathic symptoms and signs (LANSS), 61–62

multimodal management of, 304–305
on quality of life (QOL), 300–304
screening of, 301–302
Neuropathic Pain Questionnaire (NPQ) tool, 303
Neuropathic Pain Special Interest Group (NeuPSIG), 301
Neurotransmitter roles, in depression and pain, 379–380
NHPCO. *See* National Hospice and Palliative Care Organization (NHPCO)
Nightingale, Florence, 191
NMDA receptor blockers, 140
Nociceptive pain process
    modulation, 3
    nociceptors, 3
    occurrence, 2
    perception, 3
    transduction, 2–3
    transmission, 3
Nonacetylated NSAID, 265
Nonpharmacological interventions, 40, 235–236
Nonsteroidal anti-inflammatory drugs (NSAIDs), 264–265
    colchicine, as second-line therapy, 273
    COX-2 selective NSAIDs
        mechanism of action, 98
        safety concerns, 98, 100
    mechanism of action, 96–97
    nonselective NSAID medications, 93, 94, 99
    rheumatoid arthritis (RA) management, 338–339
    safety concerns with, 97–98
    salicylates, 100–101
    side effects

Nonsteroidal anti-inflammatory
drugs (NSAIDs) (*cont.*)
GI bleeding, 160
nausea and vomiting,
160–161
Nonverbal/cognitive impairments
Alzheimer's disease (AD), 47
analgesic trial with medications, 51
assessment of pain in older
adults, 47–52
assessment tools, 49
barriers, 48–49
common painful conditions, 50
dementia, 48
family members or caregivers, 49
mild or moderate cognitive
impairment, 47–48
pain-related behaviors, 49–50
traditional assessment, 47
Norepinephrine (NE)
in depression and pain, 379, 380
Nortriplyline (Pamelor, Aventyl), 125,
126, 127–128, 129, 384
NP. *See* Neuropathic pain (NP)
NPQ tool. *See* Neuropathic Pain
Questionnaire (NPQ) tool
NRS. *See* Numeric rating
scale (NRS)
Nucleoplasty. *See* Coblation
Numeric rating scale (NRS), 32,
57–58
Nursing
diagnosis, 78
hospice care, 251
Nutrition preparation, 201

OA. *See* Osteoarthritis (OA)
Obesity, 20–21, 147
Ofirmev, 92
OLD CARTS, 43
One-dimensional pain scales

numeric rating scale, 57–58
verbal descriptor scale/verbal
rating scale, 58–59
visual analog scale, 56–57
Ophthalmologist, 347
Opioid(s), 112, 304, 307, 311,
312, 340, 412
administration, 109
discontinuation of, 111
dosing, 108–109
IIT pumps, 173
medications, 102–103, 107–108
and opioid-like medications,
104–106
safety concerns with, 111
side effects
constipation, 161
pruritus, 162
respiratory depression,
155–157
urinary retention, 162
use of, 107
Oral analgesia, 233
Oral route, 150
Oral transmucosal route, 150
Osteoarthritis (OA)
assistive devices for, 264
diagnostic criteria for, 260
herbal remedies, 269
interventional options, 269–270
medication management,
264–266
multimodal management of,
260–264
prevalence of, 257–258
gender differences, 259
racial and ethnic differences,
258–259
risk factors associated with,
259–260
supplements and food products,
268–269

surgical interventions, 270–271
topical analgesic preparations,
    266–267
Osteoporosis
    balloon vertebroplasty/
        kyphoplasty, 175–176
    with resulting fractures
        diagnostic criteria, 289–290
        epidemiology and
            prevalence, 289
        multimodal management of,
            290–293
Outpatient treatment centers, 417
Oxcarbazepine, 329
Oxycodone, 102, 105, 108, 232
Oxycontine, 102, 105

Pacemakers, 215
Pain assessment in advanced
        dementia (PAINAD),
        68–70
Pain assessment, in older adult
        patient. *See also* Nonverbal/
        cognitive impairments;
        Medication, for pain
        complaint
    activities of daily living, 40–41
    alcohol and substance use,
        39–40
    assessment guides, 43
    barriers
        health care provider, 34–35
        patient, 32–34
    cognitive domain function, 42
    communication, 43–44
    experience, 38
    finance, 39
    follow up and ongoing
        assessment, 44
    goal, pain-related, 38
    interview of pain

        aggravates, 37
        character, 37
        duration, 37
        location identification, 36–37
        relieves, 37
        severity, 38
        timing aspects, 37
    medication use, 38–39
    nonpharmacological
        interventions, 40
    objectives, 31
    pain screening, 35
    pain types
        acute pain, 42
        chronic pain, 42
        neuropathic pain, 42–43
    patient history, 36
    physical and emotional
        assessment, 31
    physical domain function, 41
    physical examination, 36
    physical, psychosocial, and
        cognitive function, 40
    psychosocial domain function, 41
    strengths and assets, 42
    tools, 55–72. *See also specific tools*
Pain behavior checklist (PBC), 66
Pain intensity, 232
Pain locus of control, 17–18
Pain-related behaviors, 49–50
Pain significance, in older adults
    and aging body, 7
    barriers, pain management, 9
    categories, 4
    communication and
        terminology, 4
    diagnosis, 5–6
    experience
        comorbidities, 6–7
        older healthy adult versus
            younger healthy adults, 6
    locations/site of, 5

Pain significance, in older
  adults (*cont.*)
  management challenges, 7–8
    analgesic medications,
      absorption and excretion, 8
    comorbidities, 8
    financial concerns, 8–9
  prevalence of, 5
  residence, 5
  in United States, 4
PainDETECT tool, 303
Painful physical symptoms (PPS), 390
Palliative care
  caregiver issues with older
    adults, 236
  components of
    adequate assessment, 231
    patient- and family-centered
      care, 230
  definition and concepts, 227–229
  need for
    community setting, 237
    home setting, 237
    hospitals, 237–238
    long-term care facilities, 238
  among older adults, importance
    of, 229–230
  pharmacological management of
    symptoms, 231–235
    nonpharmacological
      interventions, 235–236
    surgical interventions for, 235
Palliative medicine, definition of, 228
Paraffin treatments, 214
Parenteral routes, 150
Paresthesia, 300
Paroxysms, 300
Pasero Opioid-Induced Sedation
  on Scale (POSS), 156
Passive range of motion, 216
Patient- and family-centered care,
  230, 245

Patient and family education, 111
  fibromyalgia, 365
  for polymyalgia rheumatic
    (PMR), 345
  for rheumatoid arthritis, 341
Patient barriers, to pain assessment
  beliefs, 32, 34
  cultural factors, 33
  desire, 33
  fear, 33
  finances, 34
  misconceptions, 32
  sensory impairments, 33
Patient controlled analgesia (PCA),
  109, 151
Patient controlled epidural
  analgesia (PCEA), 110
Patient's global impression of
  change (PGIC), 361, 362
PBC. *See* Pain behavior
  checklist (PBC)
PCA. *See* Patient controlled
  analgesia (PCA)
PCEA. *See* Patient controlled
  epidural analgesia (PCEA)
PENS. *See* Percutaneous electrical
  nerve stimulation (PENS)
Pentazocine (Talwin), 112, 113
Percutaneous-controlled
  radiofrequency trigeminal
  rhizotomy (RF-TR), 330
Percutaneous disc decompression,
  172–173
Percutaneous electrical nerve
  stimulation (PENS), 216
Percutaneous intradiscal
  radiofrequency
  thermocoagulation
  (PIRFT), 171–172
Perineural analgesia. *See*
  Continuous peripheral
  nerve blocks

Peripheral sensitization, 355–356
Persistent pain, 2
Pet ownership, 191
Pet therapy. *See* Animal
    assisted therapy
Pet visitation, 191
PGIC. *See* Patient's
    global impression of
    change (PGIC)
Phantom limb pain (PLP)
  mirror therapy, 200
Pharmacokinetic considerations,
    older adults
  anticonvulsant/antiepileptic
    medications, 121
  antidepressants for
    coanalgesia, 130
Pharmacokinetics, of
    medications, 233
Pharmacological management of
    symptoms, 231–235
Phenytoin, 330
PHN pain. *See* Postherpetic
    neuralgia (PHN) pain
Physical domain in pain
    assessment, 41
Physical therapy (PT)
  and assistive devices, 218
  and education, 218
  interventions for, 214–218
  living environments, evaluation
    of, 220
  in older adults' chronic pain and
    reconditioning, 212–214
  with older adults in falls
    prevention, 219–220
  referral, 285
  rehabilitation role, 212
Physiological factors and pain
    processing, in older adult
  acute pain, 2
  chronic/persistent pain, 2

neuropathic pain (NP), 1–2
nociceptive pain. *See* Nociceptive
    pain process
pain significance. *See* Pain
    significance
somatic pain, 1
unrelieved pain
    complications, 10
visceral pain, 1
Placebo effect, 194
Plan, for pain management
  assessment, 77–78
  diagnosis, 78–79
  implementation of plan, 83
  multidisciplinary team member
    identification, 79–80
  outcomes and goals, 79
  patient education, 81–83
  progress reassessment and
    evaluation towards
    goals, 84
  review of plan, 83
  specific plan development, 80–81
PLP. *See* Phantom limb pain (PLP)
Polymyalgia rheumatica
    (PMR), 343
  clinical manifestations, 344–345
  complementary interventions
    for, 347
  diagnosis, 344–345
  epidemiology of, 343–344
  etiology of, 344
  nonpharmacological
    intervention for, 346
  pain management, 345
  patient and family education
    for, 345
  pharmacological
    management, 345
  referrals and consultations,
    346, 347
  risk factors of, 344

Postherpetic neuralgia (PHN) pain
    complementary therapies
        for, 309
    herpes zoster (HZ) rash, 305
    nonpharmacological
        interventions for, 308
    pharmacological management of,
        306–308
    risk factors for, 305–306
Postoperative nausea and vomiting
        (PONV), 161
Posture training, 213–214
PPS. *See* Painful physical
        symptoms (PPS)
Pregabalin (Lyrica), 120, 121, 122,
        307, 310, 319–320, 362
Prescription medication misuse and
        abuse, 413
Prialt, 173
PRN analgesic medications, 151–152
Problem-solving therapy
        (PST), 386
Progressive muscle relaxation, 190,
        341, 367, 396
Progressive resistance exercises, 217
Pruritus, 162
Pseudoaddiction, 412–413
PST. *See* Problem-solving
        therapy (PST)
Psychosocial domain in pain
        assessment, 41
Psychosocial impact of pain, 15
    anger, 19–20
    anxiety, 20
    caffeine and alcohol use, chronic
        pain, 16
    cognition, 16–17
    daily living activities,
        interference with, 21
    depression, 18
    interpersonal relationships,
        22–23

mobility, 21–22
obesity, 20–21
pain locus of control, 17–18
social environment
    chronic pain, 23–24
    cultural considerations, pain
        management, 24–25
    factors, 24
and social influences, 16
social withdrawal, 23
suicide, 18–19
Psychosocial treatments, 416
PT. *See* Physical therapy (PT)

Quality of life (QOL), 145
    neuropathic pain (NP) on,
        300–304

RA. *See* Rheumatoid arthritis (RA)
Racial and ethnic differences,
        258–259
"Recommend Hospice and
        Refer," 252
Reconditioning exercises, for older
        adults, 213
Rectal route, 150
Red wine, 405
Reflexology, 195
Reiki, 194–195
Relaxation
    breathing, 189
    techniques, 188
Renal function with ageing, 149
Renal/liver dysfunction, 39
Respiratory depression
    monitoring, 155
    naloxone (Narcan®), 157
    occurrence, 155
    Pasero opioid-induced sedation
        scale (POSS), 156

"Respond to Emotions Elicited and Provide Closure," 252
Restless sleep, 21
Revised Fibromyalgia Impact Questionnaire (FIQR), 358, 360
Rheumatoid arthritis (RA)
 aspirin versus acetaminophen, 338
 clinical manifestations, 337
 complementary interventions for, 341–343
 corticosteroids, 340
 COX-2 inhibitor, 339
 diagnosis of, 336–337
 epidemiology of, 335–336
 etiology of, 336
 nonpharmacological intervention for, 341–342
 pain assessment in, 337
 patient and family education for, 341
 pharmacological management in, 337–340
 referrals and consultations, 342–343, 346
 risk factor of, 336
Rheumatological conditions
 polymyalgia rheumatica (PMR). *See* Polymyalgia rheumatica (PMR)
 rheumatoid arthritis (RA). *See* Rheumatoid arthritis (RA)
Rheumatologist, 347
Risperidone, 393
Ropinirole (Requip), 139–140
Rosa canina, 269
Rose hip powder. *See* Rosa canina
Routes of administration, analgesic medication, 150

S-adenosyl L-methionine (SAMe), 269
SA. *See* Suicide attempts (SA)
Sacroiliac joint injection, 170
Salicylates
 categories, 100
 mechanism of action, 100
 medications, 101
 opioids, 100
Saline, 167–168
Salsalates (Disalcid, Salflex, Mono-Gesic), 93, 95
SAMHSA. *See* Substance Abuse and Mental Health Services Administration (SAMHSA)
SC. *See* Suicide completions (SC)
SCS. *See* Spinal cord stimulation (SCS)
Sedation, 159–160
Self-management strategies, 263
Self-report of pain, 49, 51
Sensory impairments, in pain assessment, 33
Serotonin
 in depression and pain, 379, 380
 syndrome, symptoms of, 364
Serotonin-specific reuptake inhibitor (SSRI), 384
Serotonin–norepinephrine reuptake inhibitor (SNRI)
 antidepressant medications, 393
 duloxetine (Cymbalta), 129, 130, 131
 minacipran (Savella), 130, 131, 132
 venlafaxine (Effexor), 129–132
Serum testing, 414
"Set the Stage," 251
Sham acupuncture, 176

Short-form McGill pain questionnaire (SF-MPQ), 62–64

Short-form McGill pain questionnaire revised (SF-MPQ-2), 64

Short-wave diathermy, 214–215

SI. *See* Suicide ideation (SI)

Side effect management of medication, 154

Sleep disturbances, 21, 355

S.M.A.R.T., 262

Snoring, 155

Sodium oxybate, 365

Soft belly breathing. *See* Diaphragmatic breathing

Somatic pain, 1

Spinal cord stimulation (SCS), 174–175, 321

Spinal manipulation, 177

Spirituality
    fibromyalgia (FMS), 367
    and prayer, 197–198
    for rheumatoid arthritis, 341

Spontaneous pain, 151

Square breathing technique, 189–190

SS scale. *See* Symptom severity (SS) scale

SSRI. *See* Serotonin-specific reuptake inhibitor (SSRI)

"Start low and go slow" axiom, 91

Stereotactic cingulotomy, 235

Steroid(s)
    therapy, 345
    for coanalgesia, 132–134
        corticosteroids, 132
        indications, 132–133
        pharmacokinetic considerations, 133–134

Stool softeners, 161

Strength training exercises, 217

Stress management, for central poststroke pain syndrome, 321–322

Stretching exercise, 217

Substance abuse. *See* Alcohol and substance abuse, by older adults

Substance Abuse and Mental Health Services Administration (SAMHSA), 407

Substance P, in depression and pain, 379–380

Suicide, 18–19, 387

Suicide attempts (SA), 18

Suicide completions (SC), 18

Suicide ideation (SI), 18

Superficial heat, 192

Supplement preparation, 201

Surgical interventions
    for osteoarthritis (OA), 270–271
    for palliative pain management, 235

Symptom Impact Questionnaire, 361

Symptom severity (SS) scale, 357

System barriers in pain assessment, 35

TA. *See* Temporal arteritis (TA)

Tai chi, 196–197, 218, 262, 291

Tapentadol (Nucynta), 101, 102, 105

Tapering, 326

TCM. *See* Traditional Chinese Medicine (TCM)

Temporal arteritis (TA), 325–327

Tendonitis, 216

TENS. *See* Transcutaneous electrical nerve stimulations (TENS)

Terminal illness, 248

Therapeutic ergonomics, 213–214
Therapeutic exercise, 219
Therapeutic massage, 192–193
Therapeutic touch (TT), 193–194, 341, 367
Thermal therapies, 214–215
Thermoreceptors, 3
Thoracoscopic splanchnicectomy, 235
Tic douloureux. *See* Trigeminal neuralgia
Tiger balm, 267
Topical analgesic preparations, 266–267
Topical NSAIDs, 266–267
Topical route, 150
Traditional Chinese Medicine (TCM), 176
Tramadol (Ultram), 101, 102, 104, 152, 160, 232, 304, 311, 312
with acetaminophen, 101, 102, 104, 265
Transcutaneous electrical nerve stimulations (TENS), 198, 215, 321
Transdermal route, 150
Transmucosal absorption, 147
Tricyclic antidepressants (TCAs), 307, 310, 312, 319, 384
anticholinergic side effects, 127, 308
for coanalgesia, 123–126
Trigeminal neuralgia (TGN)
classical, 329
diagnosis of, 329–330
epidemiology, 328
surgical interventions, 330–331
symptomatic, 329
treatment options, 329–330
Trigger point injections, 167–168
TT. *See* Therapeutic touch (TT)
Twelve-step programs, 416–417

Types of pain
acute pain, 2, 4, 42
chronic pain. *See* Chronic pain
neuropathic pain. *See* Neuropathic pain (NP)

Ultrasonography, for temporal arteritis, 326
Ultrasound diathermy, 214–215
Unidimensional pain scale. *See* One-dimensional pain scales
United States
alcohol and substance abuse, by older adults, 403–404
aromatherapy, 199
hospice in 2011, profile of, 245–248
low back pain in, 283
palliative care among older adults, 229–230
Unrelieved pain complications, 10
Urinary retention, 162
Urine testing, 414

Valaciclovir, 306
Valproate, 330
VAS. *See* Visual analog scale (VAS)
VCF. *See* Vertebral compression fractures (VCF)
VCS. *See* Vestibular caloric stimulation (VCS)
VDS. *See* Verbal descriptor scale (VDS)
Venlafaxine (Effexor), 129–132, 311
Verbal descriptor scale (VDS), 58–59
Verbal rating scale. *See* Verbal descriptor scale (VDS)

Vertebral compression fractures (VCF), 175–176
Vertebroplasty
  facet joint injection, 170–171
  myofascial pain syndromes, interventions for, 167–168
  nerve blocks, 168–170
  percutaneous disc decompression using coblation, 172–173
  percutaneous thermocoagulation intradiscal techniques, 171–172
  sacroiliac joint injection, 170
  spine-related interventions and surgery, 173–177
Vestibular caloric stimulation (VCS), 320
Viniyoga style yoga, 286
Visceral pain, 1
Visual analog scale (VAS), 56–57
Vitamin E, for gout persons, 273
Vocalizations, 50

Voltaren, 99
Vomiting, nausea and, 160–161

Water versus land, exercise in, 217–218
Weight management, 262–263, 285
WHO. *See* World Health Organization (WHO)
Widespread pain index (WPI), 357
World Health Organization (WHO), 376
  pain relief ladder, 91–92, 100, 107, 232
WPI. *See* Widespread pain index (WPI)

Yoga, 197

Zygapophysial joints, 170